HEALTH CARE OF WOMEN AND CHILDREN IN DEVELOPING COUNTRIES

HEALTH CARE
OF WOMEN AND CHILDREN
IN DEVELOPING COUNTRIES

HELEN M. WALLACE, M.D., M.P.H.
Professor of Maternal and Child Health
Graduate School of Public Health
San Diego State University
San Diego, California, U.S.A.

KANTI GIRI, M.B.B.S., DG.O., F.I.C.S., F.R.C.O.G.
Regional Advisor in Family Health
World Health Organization
New Delhi, India

THIRD PARTY PUBLISHING COMPANY
Oakland, California

HEALTH CARE OF WOMEN AND CHILDREN
IN DEVELOPING COUNTRIES
International Standard Book Number 0-89914-031-9
Library of Congress Number 89-051547

Printed in the United States of America
First Impression 1990
Third Party Publishing Company
A Division of Third Party Associates, Inc.
P.O. Box 13306, Montclair Station E
Oakland, California 94661-0306, U.S.A.

Managing Editor and Designer, Paul R. Mico
Electronic Page Composition and Graphics, Patrick Kammermeyer

Cover art. Kollwitz, "Boy With Arms Around Mother's Neck."
Etching, 1931

DEDICATION

This book "Health Care of Women and Children in Developing Countries" is dedicated to the service providers of the developing countries in maternal and child health/family planning at all levels for their consistent and sincere efforts to improve the health of mothers and children and thereby make a happier and healthier family.

ACKNOWLEDGEMENTS

The editors of this book wish to acknowledge the important role played by many organizations and people in making this publication possible. For example, three Universities (the University of Minnesota, the University of California at Berkeley, and San Diego State University) have been generous in granting time to the senior editor to work at the international level. The World Health Organization provided opportunity to work within it and with developing countries greatly enriching the background knowledge of the editors. Colleagues in the Division of Maternal and Child Health in WHO and in developing countries around the world who have knowledge and vast experience about the needs of women, children and families and how best to meet these needs. Lastly, the vital role played by Paul Mico, our publisher, has been far beyond the mechanical tasks in this book. He has been most helpful in developing the outline and contents as well.

Helen M. Wallace

Kanti Giri

CONTENTS

SECTION I INTRODUCTION

CONTRIBUTORS

Anna Alisjabana, M.D. Professor, Department of Child Health, Padjadjaran University Medical School, Bandung, West Java, Indonesia.

James Allman, Ph.D. Consultant, Center for Population and Family Health, Columbia University School of Public Health, New York, New York, U.S.A.

Kenneth J. Bart, M.D., M.P.H. Director of Health, U.S. Agency for International Development, Washington, D.C., U.S.A.

Mark A. Belsey, M.D. Director of Maternal and Child Health, World Health Organization, Geneva, Switzerland.

Vilai Benchakan, M.D. Emeritus Professor of Obstetrics and Gynecology, Ramathibodi Medical School, Bangkok, Thailand.

F. John Bennett, M.B., CH.B., D.P.H., F.F.C.M. Director, Health Learning Materials Department, African Medical and Research Foundation, Nairobi, Kenya.

Ruth A. Brandwein, Ph.D, M.S.W. Dean, School of Social Work, State University of New York at Stony Brook; Commissioner, Suffolk County Department of Social Services, Hauppauge, New York, U.S.A.

John H. Bryant, M.D. Professor and Chairman, Department of Community Health Sciences, The Aga Khan University, Faculty of Health Sciences, Karachi, Pakistan.

Birgitta Bucht, Fil. Kand (M.A.) Chief, Population Trends and Structure Section, Population Division, United Nations, New York, New York, U.S.A.

Nimrod O. Bwibo, M.D., M.P.H. Principal, College of Allied Health Sciences, University of Nairobi, Nairobi, Kenya.

Carole Chan Technical Officer, Expanded Programme on Immunization, World Health Organization, Geneva, Switzerland.

K. Chaturachinda, M.B., CH.B., F.R.C.O.G. Professor of Obstetrics and Gynecology, Ramathibodi Hospital and Medical School, Bangkok, Thailand.

M.M.A. Faridi, M.D., D.C.H. Department of Pediatrics, University College of Medical Sciences and Guru Teg Bahadur Hospital, New Delhi, India.

M.F. Fathalla, M.D., Ph.D., F.A.C.O.G. Director of WHO Special Programme of Research, Development and Research Training, World Health Organization, Geneva, Switzerland.

B. Jane Ferguson Adolescent Unit, World Health Organization, Geneva, Switzerland.

Herbert L. Friedman, M.D. Director of Adolescent Unit, World Health Organization, Geneva, Switzerland.

O.P. Ghai, M.D. Professor and Head, Department of Pediatrics, University College of Medical Sciences, Guru Teg Bahadur Hospital, New Delhi, India.

Shanti Ghosh, M.D., F.A.M.S. New Delhi, India; formerly, Professor and Head of Department of Pediatrics, Safdarjung Hospital, New Delhi, India.

Duff G. Gillespie, Ph.D. Director For Population, U.S. Agency For International Development, Washington, D.C., U.S.A.

Kanti Giri, M.B.B.S., DG.O., F.I.C.S., F.R.C.O.G. Regional Advisor in Family Health, World Health Organization, New Delhi, India.

Trinidad A. Gomez, M.D., M.P.H. Director, Institute of Community and Family Health, Quezon City, Philippines.

C. Gopalan, M.D., Ph.D., D.Sc., F.R.C.P. President, Nutrition Foundation of India, New Delhi, India.

James P. Grant, Director, U.N.I.C.E.F. United Nations Children's Fund, New York, New York, U.S.A.

Jerome Grossman, Ph.D. Professor of Public Health, University of Hawaii School of Public Health, Honolulu, Hawaii, U.S.A.

Richard J. Guidotti, M.D. Scientist, Maternal and Child Health, World Health Organization, Geneva, Switzerland.

Gregory F. Hayden, M.D. Associate Professor, Department of Pediatrics, University of Virginia Medical School, Charlottesville, Virginia, U.S.A.

Ralph H. Henderson, M.D. Director, Expanded Programme on Immunization, World Health Organization, Geneva, Switzerland.

Jodi L. Jacobson Senior Researcher, World Watch Institute, Washington, D.C., U.S.A.

Pamela R. Johnson, Ph.D. Applied Research Division, Office of Health, U.S. Agency for International Development, Washington, D.C., U.S.A.

Kauser S. Khan, M.D. Department of Community Health Sciences, The Aga Khan University, Faculty of Health Sciences, Karachi, Pakistan.

U Ko Ko, M.B.B.S., D.P.H., D.T.M. & H., F.R.C.O.P. Regional Director, World Health Organization, South East Asia Regional Office, New Delhi, India.

Suporn Koetsawang, M.D. Director, Family Planning Research Center, and Chair, Department of Obstetrics and Gynecology, Siraras Hospital and Medical School, Bangkok, Thailand.

Ajit Kumar, M.D. Professor of Pediatrics, Osmania Medical College, Hyderabad, India.

Lata Kumar, M.D. Additional Professor, Department of Pediatrics, Postgraduate Institute of Medical Education and Research, Chandigarh, India.

Amelia Mangay-Maglacas, R.N., Dr.P.H. Formerly, Chief Scientist for Nursing, Health Manpower Development Unit, World Health Organization, Geneva, Switzerland.

Deborah Maine, M.P.H. Associate Research Scientist, Center for Population and Family Health, Columbia University School of Public Health, New York, New York, U.S.A.

Jonathan Mann, M.D. Director, AIDS Program, World Health Organization, Geneva, Switzerland.

Y.C. Mathur, M.D. Professor of Social Pediatrics, Institute of Child Health, Niloufer Hospital, Hyderabad, India; President, Indian Academy of Pediatrics.

David Morley, M.D. Professor, Institute of Child Health, Emeritus, University of London, England.

Janet Nassim, M.A. Consultant, Population, Health and Nutrition Division, World Bank, Washington, D.C., U.S.A.

S. Olu Oduntan, M.D., M.P.H. Professor of Public Health, University of Ibadan Medical School, Ibadan, Nigeria.

Winit Phuapradit, M.D., M.P.H. Department of Obstetrics and Gynecology, Ramathibodi Hospital and Medical School, Bangkok, Thailand.

Phyllis T. Piotrow, Ph.D. Director, Center for Communication Programs, Johns Hopkins School of Hygiene and Public Health, Baltimore, Maryland, U.S.A.

S. Pongthai, M.D. Department of Obstetrics and Gynecology, Ramathibodi Hospital and Medical School, Bangkok, Thailand.

Anna-Marie Masse-Raimbault, M.D. International Children's Centre, Paris, France.

Bhasker Rao, M.D. Emeritus Professor of Obstetrics and Gynecology, Madras Medical College, Madras, India.

S.S. Ratnam, M.D. Professor of Obstetrics and Gynecology, National University of Singapore, Singapore.

Jack Reynolds, Ph.D. Senior Scientist, University Research Corporation, Department of Social Services, East-West Population Institute, Honolulu, Hawaii, U.S.A.

Milton I. Roemer, M.D., M.A., M.P.H. Professor of Public Health, University of California School of Public Health, Los Angeles, California, U.S.A.

Erica Royston Division of Maternal and Child Health, World Health Organization, Geneva, Switzerland.

Nafis Sadik, M.D. Director, United Nations Population Fund, New York, New York, U.S.A.

Fred T. Sai, M.D. Senior Advisor, Health and Population, World Bank, Washington, D.C., U.S.A.

Stephen A. Sapirie, Dr.P.H. Division of Family Health, World Health Organization, Geneva, Switzerland.

Helmut Sell, M.D. Regional Advisor in Mental Health, World Health Organization, New Delhi, India.

Judith R. Seltzer, Ph.D. Chief, Policy Development Division, Office of Population, U.S. Agency For International Development, Washington, D.C., U.S.A.

Pramilla Senanayake, M.B.B.S., D.T.P.H., Ph.D. Assistant Secretary General, International Planned Parenthood Federation, London, England.

Carlos V. Serrano, M.D., Ph.D. Regional Advisor in Maternal and Child Health, Pan American Health Organization, Washington, D.C., U.S.A.

Jacqueline D. Sherris, Ph.D. Center for Communication Program, Johns Hopkins School of Hygiene and Public Health, Baltimore, Maryland, U.S.A.

Kuldip Singh, M.B.B.S., M.R.C.O.G. Senior Lecturer, Department of Obstetrics and Gynecology, National University of Singapore, National University Hospital, Singapore.

Surjit Singh, M.D. Assistant Professor of Pediatrics, Postgraduate Institute of Medical Education and Research, Chandigarh, India.

S. Sudhutoravut, M.D. Department of Obstetrics and Gynecology, Ramathibodi Hospital and Medical School, Bangkok, Thailand.

N.B. Thapa, M.D. Director, Integrated National Injury Prevention Program, Kanti Childrens Hospital, Kathmandu, Nepal.

Inayat Thaver, M.D. Department of Community Health Sciences, The Aga Khan University, Faculty of Health Sciences, Karachi, Pakistan.

Somsak Varakamin, M.D., M.P.H. Permanent Secretary, Ministry of Health, Bangkok, Thailand.

B.N.S. Walia, M.D., D.C.H., F.A.M.S. Professor and Head, Department of Pediatrics, Postgraduate Institute of Medical Education and Research, Chandigarh, India.

Helen M. Wallace, M.D., M.P.H. Professor of Maternal and Child Health, Graduate School of Public Health, San Diego State University, San Diego, California, U.S.A.

Beverly Winikoff, M.D., M.P.H. Senior Medical Associate, Population Council, New York, New York, U.S.A.

PREFACE

Women and children comprise almost three-fourths of the people of the "developing" world. Furthermore, they are the most vulnerable people of all populations in all parts of the world. Indicators of the outcome of their health care dramatically provide a picture of the vulnerability and sensitivity to exposure to unfavorable influences in their environment – whether it is poor nutrition, toxic substances, infection, poor sanitation, crowding, inadequate health care, or lack of education.

With this picture of vulnerability one would expect that the health care of women and children in all countries would be given the highest priority. Yet this is not so, and especially in developing countries. The need for increased effort to expand and improve the health status and care of women and children is overdue.

Primary responsibility for the improvement of health status and care of women and children rests with health workers at all levels, with government officials and with the people themselves. All of these groups and individuals must be able to recognize the problems and needs, and be able to achieve improved solutions together.

In recent years the concern on children's health has been emphasized, resulting in UNICEF's Child Survival and Development program. The Declaration of Talloires, supported by UNICEF, WHO, UNDP, World Bank, and the Rockefeller Foundation, has further reiterated the global targets for immunization and eradication of polio by the year 2000. The Joint UNICEF/WHO Statement of 1989 of Health of Mothers and Children further stresses the need to accelerate the programme. The International Conference on Safe Motherhood Initiative, February 1987, highlighted the appalling high maternal mortality rates in the developing countries and drew the attention of the policy makers to plan programmes for the reduction.

The follow-up conference of the 1978 Alma-Ata Conference held in Riga,* in March 1988, included in its recommendations for action the following:

1. Maintaining health for all as a permanent goal of all nations up to and beyond the year 2000;
2. reviewing and strengthening strategies for health for all;
3. intensifying social and political action for health;
4. developing and mobilizing leadership for health for all;
5. empowering people;
6. making inter-sectoral collaboration a force for health for all.

The Riga 1988 statement reported that solutions must be found to problems such as very high maternal and under-five mortality rates; under-development, population growth and environment. The Riga statement further reported that special and urgent priority be given to support the poorest countries particularly those with highest infant, under-fives and maternal mortality rates. More extensive resources and stronger commitment are urgently needed.

The purpose of this book is to inform those in leadership positions in the health field, in government, and in community activities at national, provincial, state, district, and local levels of the prevailing situation in order to further expand and improve health care of women, infants, children, and youth throughout the developing world.

Helen M. Wallace, M.D., M.P.H.
Kanti Giri, M.B.B.S., DG.O.,F.I.C.S., F.R.C.O.G.

---

* World Health Organization. Alma-Ata Reaffirmed at Riga. A Statement of Renewed and Strengthened Commitment To Health For All By the Year 2000 and Beyond. March 1988.

FOREWORD

Women are firmly at the centre of local and national life and of prospects for development. Their health and wellbeing are not only desirable in themselves, but essential for the future. This is not yet reflected in the priorities assigned by the development plans of governments or international institutions; it should be the task of everyone concerned with development to ensure that this situation changes.

In a world which likes to see results, and to see them quickly, it is not easy to argue the case that better health care for women and children should take precedence. The benefits are slow to appear, and largely invisible when they do. Healthier mothers and children do not obviously contribute to economic growth, to the protection of the environment, or to slower population growth. Yet we know that it is so. Women who have the choice will usually opt for later and fewer pregnancies than their mothers had. It is a crucially important part of health care to give them the choice, for two reasons: First, because spacing pregnancy is itself a contribution to better health among mothers and children; and second, because improved maternal and child health in one generation is usually translated into smaller families in the next.

There is a third reason. Choice in the matter of family size implies choice in other areas as well. Once women take the step of spacing their pregnancies by their own decision, they are one step further towards decision-making in other areas of their lives. Power over decision-making is a crucial mark of status; and a higher status for women will ensure that their contribution to development is valued at its true worth. This book will be a valuable contribution to all these ends.

Nafis Sadik, M.D.
United Nations Population Fund

DECLARATION OF TALLOIRES
12 March, 1988

Remarkable progress in health has been achieved during the past decade. Global recognition that healthy children and healthy families are essential for human and national development is steadily increasing. Consensus has been reached on the strategy for providing primary health care programmes. The international community has become engaged in partnership with national governments in the creation of successful global programmes, ensuring the availability of financial support and appropriate technologies. These include:

1. *immunization programmes* which now protect over 50% of infants in developing countries with polio or DPT vaccines, preventing some 200,000 children from becoming paralyzed with poliomyelitis and over a million children each year from dying of measles, whooping cough, or neonatal tetanus;

2. *diarrhoeal diseases control programmes* which now make available for 60% of the developing world population life-saving fluids (particularly oral rehydration salts), the use of which may be preventing as many as a million deaths annually from diarrhoea;

3. *initiatives to control respiratory infections* which hold promise in the years ahead of averting many of the 3 million childhood deaths from acute respiratory infections occurring each year in developing countries and that are not prevented currently by immunization;

4. *safe motherhood and family planning programmes* which are so important in protecting the well-being of families.

Progress, to date, demonstrates that resources can be mobilized and that rapid and effective action can be taken to combat dangerous threats to the health of children and mothers, particularly in developing countries.

This progress is the result of:

- enthusiastic world-wide agreement on the development of health strategies based on primary health care;
- the commitment of national governments, multi- and bilateral development agencies, non-governmental organizations, private and voluntary groups, and people in all walks of life to give priority to these programmes;
- coordinated action by the sponsors of The Task Force for Child Survival: WHO, UNICEF, The World Bank, UNDP, and The Rockefeller Foundation.

We, The Task Force for Child Survival, conveners of the meeting "Protecting the World's Children — An Agenda for the 1990s" in Talloires, France, 10-12 March, 1988:

1. EXPRESS appreciation and admiration for the efforts made by the developing countries to reduce infant and child deaths through primary health care and child survival actions;

2. COMMIT OURSELVES to pursue and expand these initiatives in the 1990s;

3. URGE national governments, multi- and bilateral development agencies, United Nations agencies, non-governmental organizations, and private and voluntary groups to commit themselves to:

   - increase national resources from both developing and industrialized countries devoted to health in the context of overall development and self-reliance;
   - improve women's health and education, recognizing the importance for women themselves, recognizing women's contributions to national development, and recognizing that mothers are by far the most important primary health care workers;
   - accelerate progress to achieve universal childhood immunization by 1990 and to sustain it thereafter;
   - accelerate progress to eliminate or markedly reduce as public health problems the other main preventable causes of child and maternal mortality and morbidity, striving to reach sustained universal coverage of children and mothers by the year 2000;
   - assure the development of new vaccines and technologies and their application, particularly in developing countries, as they become appropriate for public health use;
   - promote expanded coverage of water supply and sanitation;
   - pursue research and development, including technology transfer, in support of the above actions;

4. SUGGEST that the following be considered by national and international bodies as targets to be achieved by the year 2000:

- the global eradication of poliomyelitis;
- the virtual elimination of neonatal tetanus deaths;
- a 90% reduction in measles cases and a 95% reduction in measles deaths compared with pre-immunization levels;
- a 25% reduction in case/fatality rates associated with acute respiratory infection in children under 5 years;
- reduction of infant and under-5 child mortality rates in all countries by at least half (1980-2000), or to 50 and 70 per 1,000 live births respectively, whichever achieves the greater reduction;
- reduction of current maternal mortality rates in all countries by at least half.

Achievement of these strategies would result in the avoidance of tens of millions of child deaths and disabilities by the year 2000, as well as a balanced population growth as parents become more confident their children will survive and develop. The eradication of poliomyelitis would, with the eradication of smallpox, represent a fitting gift from the 20th to the 21st century.

5. DRAW world attention to the potential for enlarging upon the successes outlined above to encompass low-cost, effective initiatives to:

- improve the quality and coverage of educational services so as to obtain universal primary education and 80% female literacy, and
- reduce to less than 1% severe malnutrition in children under 5 while also significantly reducing moderate and mild malnutrition in each country.

6. WELCOME the progress being made in drafting the Convention on the Rights of the Child and join the United Nations General Assembly in urging completion of the Convention in 1989, the 10th anniversary of the International Year of the Child.

We are convinced that vigorous pursuit of these initiatives aimed at protecting the world's children will ensure that children and mothers – indeed whole families – will benefit from the best of available health technologies, making an essential contribution to human and national development and to the attainment of Health For All By The Year 2000.

—Talloires, France

Section I
INTRODUCTION

1

HEALTH CARE OF CHILDREN IN DEVELOPING COUNTRIES

Helen M. Wallace, M.D., M.P.H.

INTRODUCTION

From a global perspective, the most vulnerable parts of our society are mothers and children. This is true both in "developing" and "developed" countries. Many of the health problems and health needs faced by mothers and children in "developing" countries today are similar to those faced by mothers and children in previous decades in "developed" countries. Infant mortality (the rate of babies dying before their first birthday per 1,000 live births) is one of the most valuable indicators of the status of development of a society or a country. As an indicator, it is closely related to the overall level of well-being in a country or region. It distinguishes clearly between a society of some sufficiency and a society of stark deprivation. It reflects not only food, clean water, medical and health care, but also the actual availability of such basic resources to all segments of a population. High infant mortality is associated with certain societal problems – environmental contamination, lack of education of mothers, poor health care, the disadvantaged position of women, etc. In searching out the explanation of infant deaths, two levels of analysis are needed: One to identify the immediate causes of death, and another to examine the social, economic, or environmental conditions that make infants vulnerable to these immediate causes.[1]

The immediate cause of a baby's death may be lack of food, a disease, a severe birth defect, extreme low birth weight, or an injury. But underneath most infant deaths is likely to be a mosaic of low family income, lack of sanitation, crowding, high fertility, or exposure to toxic substances. Many of these direct and indirect causes interact, so that it may be difficult to pinpoint one single factor alone which causes the death of an infant. Because infant mortality is so closely tied to broad social and economic conditions, the most

3

decisive gains to be made in reduction of infant mortality involve improvements in sanitation, water supply, nutrition, access to medical and health care, fertility control, and education.

Factors Influencing Infant Mortality

1. Education of the mother (Figure 1)
2. Provision of clean water (Figure 2, page 5)
3. Interval between births (Figure 3, page 5)
4. Birth order (Figure 4, page 5)
5. The type of feeding of the infant (Figure 5, page 6)
6. Birth weight of the baby (Table 3, page 10)
7. Maternal health care (Figure 6, page 6)

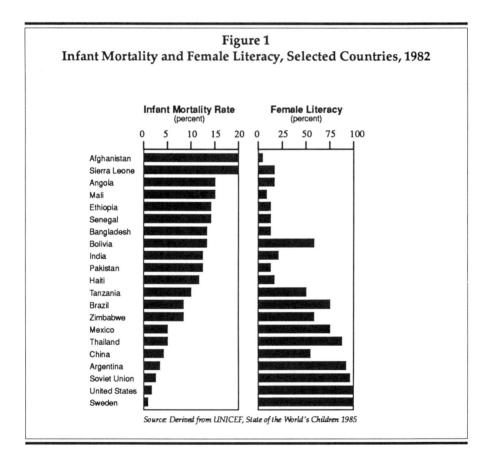

Figure 1
Infant Mortality and Female Literacy, Selected Countries, 1982

Source: Derived from UNICEF, State of the World's Children 1985

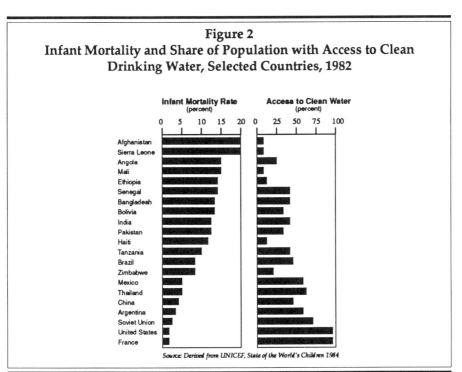

Figure 2
Infant Mortality and Share of Population with Access to Clean Drinking Water, Selected Countries, 1982

Source: Derived from UNICEF, State of the World's Children 1984

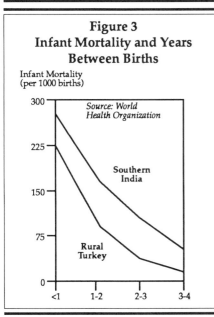

Figure 3
Infant Mortality and Years Between Births

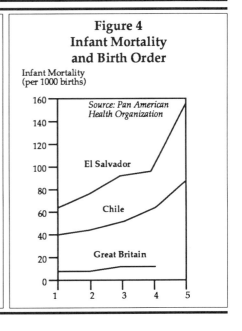

Figure 4
Infant Mortality and Birth Order

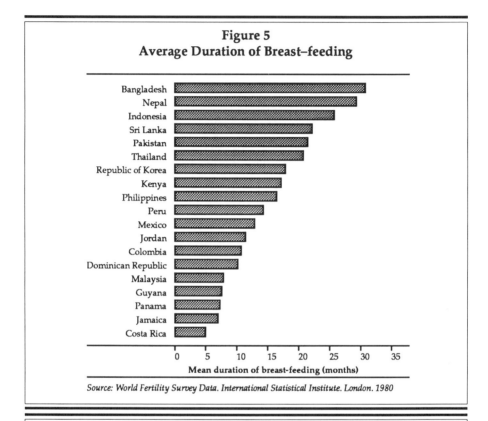

Figure 5
Average Duration of Breast–feeding

Source: World Fertility Survey Data. International Statistical Institute. London. 1980

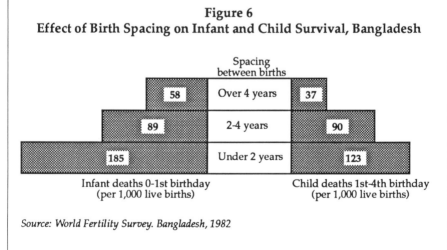

Figure 6
Effect of Birth Spacing on Infant and Child Survival, Bangladesh

Source: World Fertility Survey. Bangladesh, 1982

THE EXTENT OF THE PROBLEM OF MORTALITY IN CHILDREN TODAY

Approximately 17 million children in the world die each year from the combined effects of poor nutrition, diarrhea, malaria, pneumonia, measles, whooping cough, and tetanus (Table 1). Virtually all these deaths could be prevented with relatively simple measures already available to us. Six diseases (measles, whooping cough, tetanus, tuberculosis, polio, and diphtheria) kill 5 million children a year in the developing world, and account for approximately one-third of all childrens' deaths; we have effective immunizing agents against all six of these diseases.

Each day, more than 40,000 young children in the world die from a combination of malnutrition and infection. For every child who dies, six now live in hunger and ill-health, which may have a long term damaging effect on their lives. It is estimated that the use of specific measures (ORT, immunization, the growth chart, and breast feeding) could reduce these 40,000 deaths of children a day down to 20,000 a day.

It is estimated that one out of every 20 children born in the developing world dies before reaching the age of 5 years.

Table 1
Estimates Of Major Causes Of Death In Children

Cause	Estimated Number of Children Dying Per Year
Dehydration due to Diarrhea	5 million
Pneumonia	3 million
Measles	2 million
Whooping Cough	1-1/2 million
Tetanus of Newborn	1 million
Poliomyelitis	50,000
Diphtheria	5,000

Source: World Health Organization

RECENT LEVELS OF INFANT AND
EARLY CHILDHOOD MORTALITY

Study of levels and trends in infant and early childhood (0-4 years) mortality reported to the UN/WHO shows a wide range. The highest reported U5MRs* are in general from Africa south of the Sahara, followed by Asia, Latin America, Europe and Oceania in that order (Table 2, next page).

In all countries studied, mortality has declined over time. On the average, there were 43 fewer deaths under the age of five years per 1,000 births than 15-19 years earlier, a 28% reduction in mortality. The number of deaths prevented per 1,000 births is about evenly divided between infants (20 deaths) and other ages (10 toddlers and 13 pre-schooler deaths averted).

Countries with the greatest reported declines are Malaysia, Panama, Jordan, and Jamaica. The region with the greatest decline was Western Asia. Countries in Africa had the least decline.

INCIDENCE OF LOW BIRTH WEIGHT (LBW)

At least 10-15% of babies are born with low birth weight (under 5-1/2 pounds at birth); they account for 30-40% of all infant deaths in the developing world.[2] One of the specific factors known to have an effect on birth weight is maternal nutrition.

A review at the end of 1983 of data from 90 countries shows that there has been a slight decrease in the incidence of low birth weight. Of the 127 million infants born in 1982, some 20 million (16.0%) had low birth weight, a decrease from 16.8% in 1979. For developing countries the percentage decreased from 18.4 to 17.6 (Table 3, page 10).

The incidence of LBW by region varies from 13.1% in Middle South Asia and 19.7% in Asia as a whole, to 14.0% in Africa, 10.1% in Latin America, 6.8% in North America, and 6.5% in Europe.[3]

In Africa, the percentage for 1982 (at 14.0%) is 1% lower than for 1979. This fall is due largely to changes in Northern and Southern Africa.

The overall percentage of LBW infants born in Asia declined slightly, but in Middle South Asia there is no change. Rates in the region remain between 20% and 50%.

---

* U5MR = Under-five mortality rate.

Table 2
Under Five Mortality Rate (1987)

Low (30 & Under)	Middle (31-94)	High (95 - 170)	Very High (over 170)
USSR - 30	Iran - 94	Pakistan-169	Afghanistan-304
Mauritius - 30	Vietnam - 91	Zaire - 164	Mali - 296
Romania - 28	Ecuador - 89	Laos - 163	Mozambique - 295
Yugoslavia - 28	Brazil - 87	Togo - 156	Angola - 288
Chile - 26	El Salvador - 87	Camaroon - 156	Sierra Leone-270
Trinidad/Tobago-24	Tunisia - 86	India - 152	Malawi - 267
Kuwait - 23	Papua N.G.-85	Liberia - 150	Ethiopia - 261
Jamaica - 23	Domin.Rep. - 84	Ghana - 149	Guinea - 252
Costa Rica - 23	Philippines -76	Ivory Coast - 145	Burkina Faso-237
Bulgaria - 20	Mexico - 70	Lesotho - 139	Niger - 232
Poland - 19	Colombia - 69	Zambia - 130	Chad - 227
Cuba - 19	Syria - 67	Egypt - 129	Guinea Bissau-227
Hungary - 19	Paraguay - 63	Peru - 126	Central Afr. Rep- 226
Portugal - 19	Mongolia - 61	Libya - 123	Somali - 225
Greece - 17	Jordan - 60	Morocco - 123	Mauritania - 223
Czecho - 17	Lebanon - 53	Indonesia - 120	Senegal - 220
Belgium - 13	Thailand - 51	Congo - 117	Rwanda-209
USA- 13	Albania - 48	Kenya - 116	Kampuchea-208
N.Zealand - 13	China - 45	Zimbabwe - 116	Yemen Dem-202
Israel - 13	Sri Lanka - 45	Algeria - 111	Bhutan-200
Austria - 12	Venezuela- 45	Honduras - 111	Nepal - 200
Singapore - 12	Guyana - 39	Guatemala - 103	Yemen - 195
Italy - 12	Argentina - 38	Saudi Arabia-102	Burundi - 192
Ger.Dem.Rep-12	Panama - 35	Nicaragua - 99	Bangladesh-191
U.K. - 11	Korea-Dem.Rep-34	Burma - 98	Benin - 188
Ireland - 11	Korea-Rep - 34	S. Africa - 98	Madagascar-187
Ger.Fed.Rep.-11	Malaysia - 33	Turkey - 97	Sudan - 184
Denmark - 11	U.Arab Em - 33	Iraq - 96	Tanzania-179
Spain - 11	Uruguay - 32	Botswana - 95	Nigeria - 177
Australia - 10			Bolivia-176
France - 10			Haiti - 176
Hong Kong - 10			Gabon - 172
Canada - 9			Uganda - 172
Netherlands - 9			
Norway - 8			
Switzerland - 8			
Japan - 8			
Finland - 7			
Sweden - 7			

Source: The State of The Worlds Children 1989. New York, NY.1989 116 pages

In Latin America, there is evidence of improvement in many countries. Data from Cuba, Panama, Uruguay, and Venezuela all show a downward trend.

MALNUTRITION

Rates of malnutrition are a good indicator of overall child health. A crude estimate of global trends in malnutrition in children under 5 years of age indicates no change in relative terms, but a growing malnutrition problem in absolute numbers. (Malnutrition here is defined as below 70% body weight for age, using U.S. norms.) The number of children malnourished in the Sixties and early Seventies totaled about 125 million, compared to 145 million in the Seventies and Eighties (Table 4, next page). Africa experienced an

Table 3
Estimated Low-weight Births, by World Regions and by Subregions of the Americas, in 1979 and 1982

Regions and subregions	Live births,1982 (in thousands)	low-weight births, 1982(in thousands)	% infants with low birth-weight 1979	1982
Africa	23,148	3,233	15.0	14.0
Asia	74,855	14,750	20.3	19.7
Europe	6,857	445	7.7	6.5
Oceania	507	59	12.2	11.6
Union of Soviet Socialist Republics	5,111	409	8.0	8.0
Northern America	4,402	299	7.3	6.8
Latin America and the Caribbean	12,490	1,259	10.2	10.1
Middle America	3,669	448	12.0*	12.0
The Caribbean	867	102	13.0	12.0
Tropical South America	7,033	647	9.0	9.0
Temperate South America	921	62	8.0	7.0
The World	127,400	20,450	16.8	16.0
Developed countries	18,200	1,250	7.4	6.9
Developing countries	109,200	19,200	18.4	17.6

* Previous estimate for Middle America corrected
Source: PAHO Bulletin 18:404, 1984

increase of 2 million malnourished children, and Asian malnourished children increased from 95 to 115 million. Altogether, an estimated 25% of the world's children under age 5 years can be described as malnourished.

Malnutrition in infants and young children commonly consists of protein-energy malnutrition, marasmus, vitamin A deficiency including severe xerophthalmia in South East Asia, and severe iodine deficiency in countries like Nepal and Bhutan.

Malnutrition is the result of a variety of causes and circumstances – food shortage, due to inadequate food production; inadequate food storage; inadequate food distribution; failure to establish food priorities for the more vulnerable groups of any society (pregnant and lactating women, and infants and children); and lack of information about the proper and safe use of available foods.[4] Unquestionably, one of the serious causes of malnutrition in each generation with equally serious implications for the next generation is the practice in some countries of having the mother of the family eat last, after everyone else in the family has eaten.

Malnutrition caused by poor child feeding practices usually claims over 10 times as many children as actual famine. Coupled with dehydration due to diarrhea, malnutrition is the leading killer in the world, killing 5-8 million

Table 4
Estimates of Annual Cases of Malnutrition in Children Ages 0-4, by Region[1]

Region	1963-73		1973-83	
	(millions)	(percent)	(millions)	(percent)
Africa	19.9	31.1	21.9	25.6
Asia	94.8	50.6	114.6	54.0
Latin America	10.8	25.9	8.6	17.7
Total	125.5	26.0	145.1	26.0

[1]The figures are decade averages extrapolated for the regions from country specific surveys. They are approximate and should be used with caution. Asia excludes the Soviet Union, China, and Japan, but includes India, Pakistan, Bangladesh, Burma, Indonesia, Malaysia, Nepal, and other smaller nations.

Source: "Global Trends in Protein-Energy Malnutrition," *Bulletin of the Pan American Health Organization*, Vol. 18, No. 4, 1984.

children a year, at least 10% of all deaths. It is caused by a combination of poor sanitation, infectious diseases such as measles, failure to breast feed, poor weaning practices, especially the failure to safely and adequately supplement breast milk after 5 or 6 months of age. The most effective defense against diarrhea, malnutrition, and infections includes nutrition education, breast feeding, safe and careful food supplementation, safe and careful weaning, oral rehydration therapy, immunization, and safe basic sanitation (water supply and sewage disposal).

GLOBAL TRENDS IN PROTEIN – ENERGY MALNUTRITION

Data collected by the U.S. National Center for Health Statistics for 1963-73 and for 1973-83 used weight-for-age as the malnutrition indicator for children under five years of age. The data show improvement in the Americas and in Africa. No improvement was found in Asia, where in 1973-83 the estimate of children malnourished was 114.6 million. (Table 4).

BREAST FEEDING

When a baby is breast fed, its exposure to contaminated water, food, and utensils is usually limited. One of the major protections to babies in developing countries is the breast feeding that most of them have during the first several months of life or longer. Furthermore, mother's milk contains antibodies that increase the baby's resistance to infection. In the first 5-6 months of life, breast milk contains the nutrients essential for early growth.

In studies done in a number of countries around the world, among the young children of poor parents, bottle-fed babies were between 3-4 times more likely to be malnourished. Bottle-fed babies for the first 3 months of life were 3-4 times more likely to die than babies who are exclusively breast fed. Bottle-fed babies are more likely to have three times as many episodes of diarrhea.

Within the past decade, great concern has been expressed about the decrease in breast feeding in developing countries. In 1981, the WHO Health Assembly adopted a new international code on marketing breast milk substitutes. A joint WHO/UNICEF Statement on "Practicing, Promoting and Supporting Breast Feeding - The Special Role of Maternity Services" is available.

THE EXPANDED PROGRAM OF IMMUNIZATION

The WHO Expanded Programme on Immunization (EPI) began in 1974. The aim is to immunize all children by 1990. Also termed "Universal Child Immunization" (UCI-1990) WHO/UNICEF have set the target to eradicate poliomyelitis by the year 2000.

The toll of childrens' deaths in developing countries from the five communicable diseases of childhood is enormous (Table 5). It is estimated that five million such deaths occur each year, as follows:

Table 5

Estimated Annual Number of Deaths From Neonatal Tetanus, Measles and Pertussis and Annual Number of Cases of Poliomyelitis in Developing Countries Excluding China

(October, 1988)

	Neonatal tetanus(1)	Measles(2)	Pertussis(3)	Total deaths	Cumulative % of total deaths	Polio-myelitis cases (4)	Cumulative % of cases
		(thousands)			%	(thousands)	%
25 largest developing countries	592	1,263	403	2,257	79	159	76
Other developing countries	166	325	117	608	21	50	24
Total, developing countries	757	1,587	520	2,865	100	209	100

(1) Neonatal tetanus: based on survey data or, in the absence of survey, extrapolated from countries with similar socioeconomic conditions.

(2) Measles: it is assumed that the vaccine efficacy is 95% and that all unimmunized children will acquire measles. Coverage is assumed to be zero in countries from which data are not available.

(3) Pertussis: it is assumed that the vaccine efficacy is 80% and that 80% of unimmunized children will get pertussis. Coverage is assumed to be zero in countries from which data are not available.

(4) Poliomyelitis: in view of the narrow limits of variation of results of poliomyelitis surveys, and in the absence of an immunization programme, a fixed incidence rate of 5 cases per thousand newborns is used. A vaccine efficacy of 95% is assumed. Coverage is assumed to be zero in countries from which data are not available.

Source: Reference 6

Disease	Annual No. of Deaths
Measles	2.2 million
Pertussis	1.6 million
Neonatal Tetanus	1.2 million
Poliomyelitis	50,000
Diphtheria	5,000

Every six seconds, a child dies and another is disabled from a disease for which there is an effective immunizing agent.

The common communicable diseases of childhood are also causes of malnutrition in children, especially measles and whooping cough. All of the immunizable communicable diseases are driving forces in the cycle of malnutrition and infection, which retard the growth of millions of children who survive the infections themselves. In one study in Africa, measles was found to be the precipitating cause in half of the cases of hospitalization for malnutrition. Immunization against the six communicable diseases is also a preventive measure against malnutrition.

During the past 15 years the expanded immunization services in the developing countries have been accelerated and now administer a dose of measles vaccine to half the children of the world (generally by early 2nd year), and a third dose of polio + DPT to 60% of children before reaching their first birthday and BCG to over 60% (Table 6, page 16-17; and Figure 7).

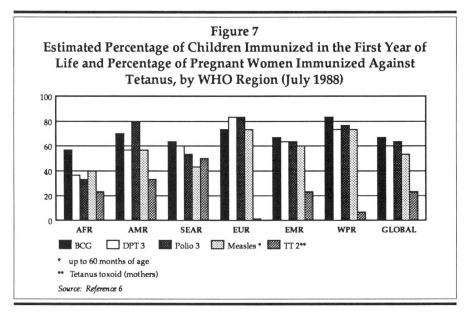

Figure 7
Estimated Percentage of Children Immunized in the First Year of Life and Percentage of Pregnant Women Immunized Against Tetanus, by WHO Region (July 1988)

Legend: BCG · DPT 3 · Polio 3 · Measles * · TT 2 **

* up to 60 months of age
** Tetanus toxoid (mothers)

Source: Reference 6

A major problem with immunization campaigns is the drop-out rate for the second and third injections in the usual series of immunizations. The reasons for the drop-out are: (1) The need for re-visits by mothers bringing their children to clinic; (2) transport; (3) the fact that populations are scattered in rural areas; (4) illiteracy of parents; (5) absence of electricity and shortage of fuel to protect the potency of the vaccines; (6) scarcity of trained manpower; (7) limited outreach of health services; and (8) reluctance of parents to bring their children back for second and third injections if they have fever, aches, restlessness from the first injection.

The breakdown in the cold chain frequently interferes with immunization efforts. There is needed a method of refrigeration storage, and transport of vaccines. The sensitivity to heat of several vaccines has contributed one of the main constraints to the expansion of immunization programs. Work is under way to develop more stable and more effective vaccines.

There have been recent technological breakthroughs, consisting of new vaccines which retain their potency for longer periods and at higher temperatures; solar-powered refrigerators; low-cost sterilization techniques; and improvement in cold chain technology.

The cost of immunizing a child against the six communicable diseases of childhood is $5 per child. To immunize each one of the 100 million children born each year in the developing world would cost $500 million per year. Most of the $5 is for the delivery system; the vaccines themselves cost $0.05.

At present $72 million is spent in immunizing children, according to present estimates. Of this, 80% is provided by the developing countries themselves, with the remainder from the international agencies.

Present needs in the EPI Program are more effective efforts at parent education, community involvement, funds, improved management, organization, and training of staff. A permanent system is needed, capable of delivering vaccines to every infant each year and capable of educating the new generation of parents each year. There is also need to provide immunizations at times and places more convenient for mothers and babies.

DIARRHEA AND ORAL REHYDRATION THERAPY (ORT)

It is estimated that 500 million children have attacks of diarrhea 3-4 times a year. Each year, four million young children in developing countries die due to diarrhea. The majority of these diarrhea deaths are due to dehydration, which could be prevented by oral rehydration (ORT). If applied correctly, it can prevent an estimated 90% of the current 4 million diarrhea deaths in

Table 6
Estimated Immunization Coverage With BCG, DPT, Poliomyelitis, Measles, and Tetanus Vaccines
(October 1988)

Developing Countries	Newborn Surviving to 1 year of age (millions)	Cumulative percentage of infants %	Immunization coverage (%)				Pregnant women
			Children less than 1 year of age				
			BCG %	DPT III %	Polio III %	Measles* %	Tetanus II %
1. India (S)	22.56	25	72	73	64	44	58
2. Indonesia (S)	5.15	31	74	61	62	55	29
3. Nigeria (6&7)	4.59	36	37	21	21	24	17
4. Bangladesh (7)	4.15	40	14	9	8	8	7
5. Brazil (7)	4.07	45	68	57	90	55	62
6. Pakistan (7)	4.03	49	72	62	62	53	27
7. Mexico (7)	2.68	52	71	62	97	54	42
8. Ethiopia (6&7)	1.99	55	27	16	6	13	7
9. Iran (7)	1.98	57	56	74	74	76	12
10. Philippines (6&7)	1.83	59	92	73	73	68	49
11. Viet Nam (7)	1.78	61	68	61	75	60	—
12. Egypt (7)	1.78	63	72	81	81	86	1
13. Thailand (7)	1.44	64	61	48	47	34	38
14. Turkey (7)	1.41	66	34	71	70	50	—
15. Zaire (6&7)	1.29	67	52	32	36	41	28
16. South Africa	1.28	69	—	—	—	—	—

17. Burma (7)	1.17	70	45	23	13	14	24
18. Kenya (7S)	1.13	71	86	75	75	60	37
19. United Rep. Tanzania(5&7)	1.07	72	94	81	65	88	54
20. Republic of Korea (7)	0.95	74	95	85	93	95	—
21. Sudan (7)	0.94	75	46	29	29	22	12
22. Algeria (7S)	0.90	76	95	66	66	59	—
23. Colombia (7)	0.88	77	80	58	82	59	6
24. Morocco (7)	0.85	77	87	78	78	76	33
25. Argentina (7)	0.75	78	91	75	85	81	—
Total (above countries)	70.63	78	63	57	58	46	35
Other developing countries	19.56	22	63	50	51	47	24
Sub-total developing countries (excluding China)	90.19	100	63	56	56	46	32
China (7S)	19.94		85	75	77	77	—
Total developing countries (including China)	110.13		68	60	61	53	27
Total industrialized countries	18.11			59	66	68	76
Global total	128.24		66	60	61	55	23

¹Ranked by number of surviving infants. Figures in brackets denote the following:
(4) 1984 coverage data.   (5) 1985 coverage data.
(6) 1986 coverage data.   (7) 1987 coverage data.
(S) Survey data.   - no information available.
*Up to 60 months of age.

Source: Reference 6

children under 5 years in the developing countries. But less than 15% of the world's families are using this low cost treatment for preventing and treating diarrheal dehydration which is the biggest single killer of children in the world today (Figure 8).

During the process of weaning from breast feeding, great care is needed in the safe introduction of supplementary foods. In the developing countries the risk of introducing infections is great, causing diarrhea and dehydration in the infants. The hazards are due to unsafe water, contaminated foodstuffs, unhygienic sanitation, infrequent washing of hands, and poor domestic and personal hygiene. The average child in a poor community of the developing world will have 6-16 bouts of diarrheal infection each year and often the mother's response is to withhold food and fluid. The result is that the child is malnourished by both the illness and the treatment. Each episode of infection can increase malnutrition and each increase in malnutrition increases the risk

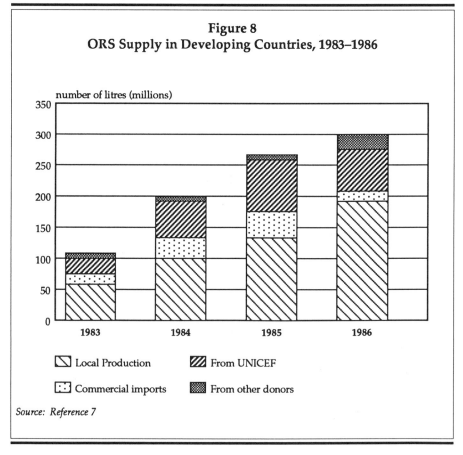

Figure 8
ORS Supply in Developing Countries, 1983–1986

Source: *Reference 7*

of another infection. Most children recover but many fall into sudden and severe dehydration. In only 2-3 days, 15% of the body weight can be lost, and at that point, death is imminent.

With the discovery of ORT, treatment can be given by the mother at home, using the right mix of sugar, salt, and water. ORT consists of a simple sugar and salt solution to correct the biochemical imbalance in the body that results from loss of fluid due to diarrhea. The use of ORT prevents death in 90% of diarrheal dehydration cases. In countries that have adopted ORT, hospital admission rates and mortality from diarrheal dehydration have been cut in half.[5]

The use of ORT in treating and preventing diarrhea is based on the knowledge that glucose stimulates the absorption of salt and water in the small intestine. The first step was the development by WHO and UNICEF of a formula for ORT.

An important recent development was the introduction by WHO of a more stable formula containing tri-sodium citrate in place of sodium bicarbonate. Research is still going on to develop mixtures that will replace the glucose in ORT with cereals such as rice powder which are readily available in some areas. This increases the absorption of sodium and water by the intestine and thus reduces the volume and duration of diarrhea.

Home therapy is based on the use of either fluids or foods already available in the home, such as rice water, carrot soup, or a drink made up from sugar, salt, and drinking water – to prevent dehydration from diarrhea. But almost all home remedies lack the sodium bicarbonate or citrate and potassium chloride contained in oral rehydration salts (ORS), and therefore are not as effective in treatment of diarrhea.

Only about 10% of the children who are at serious risk of diarrheal dehydration ever receive ORT. UNICEF points out that even this low rate of coverage has already saved 1/2 million children's lives each year. Ninety-six countries are now implementing plans for diarrheal control programs, within which ORT is one component. UNICEF is playing a leading role in production of ORS (oral rehydration salts) and in the crucial area of information activities relating to ORT.

Over 96 countries have begun ORT programs so far. UNICEF and WHO have assisted 46 countries to begin local manufacture. (Figure 8).

One of the major needs is the training of health staff at all levels – national, regional, district and local – before an ORT program is introduced.

Health staff need to be trained in the details of the technique of introducing the use of ORT. Village health workers and their supervisors especially need detailed meticulous training if they are to be able to teach the mothers the safe use of ORT.

MONITORING OF GROWTH

This consists of the large-scale use of simple cardboard child growth charts kept by the mothers in their own homes as a stimulus and a guide to the proper feeding of the infant and preschool child. Regular monthly weighing and the entering of the results by the mother herself can make early malnutrition visible to the one person who cares most and can do the most about improving the child's diet.

Usually growth charts have been kept in clinics rather than in homes, and the weighing, monitoring, and evaluating have been the responsibility of health personnel rather than of the mothers. The potential value of the growth chart will be when the weighing and chart use involve the mother and help the mother to improve her child's nutrition.

Regular monthly weight gain is the most important single indicator of a child's normal healthy growth.

About 1% of the world's children are visibly and obviously malnourished. But more than 24% of the developing world's children suffer from invisible malnutrition. The very invisibility is one of the main barriers to prevention or cure; making the problem visible to the mother is an important step toward protecting and promoting the normal healthy growth of many millions of infants and children in those vulnerable early years.

Problems in the use of this approach include the need for accurate weighing of the child and the need for monthly contact with a trained person to assist in plotting the child's growth and giving advice. There are severe limitations in the outreach of the growth monitoring idea. Needs include the training of more community health workers in growth monitoring and advice to mothers; and the need for a cheap, light and accurate means of weighing children, and involvement of the community itself such as organization, mothers group, etc.

FAMILY PLANNING

Each year in the poorer countries of the world, between 10 and 20% of children never live to see their first birthday – a total of 10 million infant deaths in the developing world. Most of these deaths are preventable. High levels of neonatal, infant and childhood mortality, as well as maternal mortality, are associated with or result from the poor health and nutritional status of women, complications of pregnancy and childbirth, low birth weight and conditions of the perinatal period, such as malnutrition and infection. Regulated fertility can prevent both maternal and infant mortality.

Children born of very young mothers are more likely to die than those born to women aged 20 to 30. They tend to have lower birth weight, which itself decreases the chances of survival and healthy development. Children born to mothers over 35 run the risk of having birth defects. In addition, fetal and neonatal mortality rates increase with high maternal age.

One of the greatest threats to infant and child health is close spacing of births. Both the child born before and the child born after a short birth interval run the increased risk of illness and death. For the older child, new pregnancy may mean early or abrupt weaning from the mother's breast. The early introduction of breast milk substitutes and weaning foods carries with it the risk of contamination, diarrhea, and malnutrition. Recent data show that mortality rates for children aged 1-2 years are up to four times higher if their birth were followed by another within 18 months. (Figure 6).

The younger child born after a short birth interval also suffers. Studies show that there is a higher perinatal and infant mortality rate in babies born less than 2 years after a previous birth.

Infant and childhood mortality is also closely related to birth order. Children of birth order 7 or more have mortality rates one-third higher than those of birth order 2 or 3. Children of high birth orders are likely to be born of mothers who are older and physically exhausted. They have to compete for food, attention, perinatal care, and love with older brothers and sisters. Children from large families often have more frequent illnesses and grow more slowly.

The recent developments in making family planning education and services available to women and couples make it possible to change this picture. By preventing births to teenagers as well as to women of high parity and by lengthening the birth interval, many unnecessary deaths and much ill-health among women and children can be prevented. Few preventive health measures can have so great an effect as providing easy access to effective methods of family planning.

Family planning acceptance and utilization are closely related to the socio-economic status, education, and employment of women, as well as to age at marriage. They are closely related to the provision of easily accessible services and supplies. They are especially related to the issues of women's status in society, and to the development of women's roles.

TRADITIONAL BIRTH ATTENDANTS

It is estimated that 45% of the women of the world are delivered at home by an untrained birth attendant. Thus, we may say that the one person most likely to be used to provide primary care to women of the child bearing age around the world is the untrained traditional birth attendant. It is for this reason that the TBA is now looked upon by the World Health Organization and by many Ministries of Health around the world as one of the major resources to provide primary care in the network of organized MCH services in developing countries.

In India, an estimated 600,000 dyahs attend 80% of all births. In Thailand, 17,000 Moh tam yae attend 80% of all births; in Nicaragua the parteras deliver 68% of all babies. In total, 60-80% of all mothers in the developing world turn to traditional midwives for help with the process of bearing and caring for children. (Figure 9, next page).

Unlike modern health practitioners, TBAs are concentrated among the poor and in rural areas.

The TBAs are the MCH services for the vast majority of the poor. In many poor communities, they are therefore one of the greatest of all potential re-sources for providing mothers with knowledge and practical on-the-spot help in the task of protecting their children's lives and health.

Experience has shown that most TBAs welcome training in techniques new to them, when it is offered in a helpful, constructive way – i.e., hand washing, cord care, nutrition. Training has reduced both perinatal and infant mortality caused by neonatal tetanus and sepsis. TBAs can be persuaded to refer their patients for prenatal care. They can be persuaded to refer their patients with complications for special care, if such special care is available. Many Ministries of Health now have an organized program to train TBAs as part of their MCH Program.

PROGRESS MADE IN THE HEALTH CARE OF CHILDREN AND MOTHERS IN DEVELOPING COUNTRIES

Within the past 25 years, there is evidence of considerable progress hav-ing been made in the health care of children and mothers in developing countries around the world. Some of the examples of this progress include the following:

1. The introduction of family planning education and services, and its successful adoption by some countries.
2. The gradual decrease in the infant mortality rate in some countries.
3. The increased number of well trained health professionals in some Ministries of Health.
4. Specific steps taken by WHO and UNICEF to assist Ministries of Health to focus on specific problems such as immunization; prevention of death due to dehydration resulting from diarrhea; increased promotion of breast feeding and discouragement of

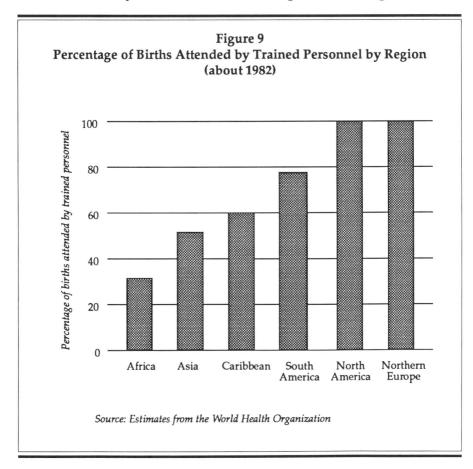

Figure 9
**Percentage of Births Attended by Trained Personnel by Region
(about 1982)**

Source: Estimates from the World Health Organization

bottle feeding; efforts at monitoring growth to identify earlier young children with malnutrition.

5. Efforts to improve maternity care through training of traditional birth attendants and to include them in the health system.

6. Efforts to study and quantify such major problems as perinatal and infant mortality, the incidence of low birth weight, the incidence of malnutrition; collaborative studies of causes and prevention of infant and perinatal mortality.

GENERAL REFERENCES

1. UNICEF. United Nations Children's Fund:

    A. The State of The World's Children 1982-83. 11 pages.
    B. The State of The World's Children 1984. 78 pages.
    C. The State of The World's Children 1989. 116 pages.

2. United Nations Fund For Population Activities:

    A. The State of World Population 1983. 8 pages.
    B. The State of World Population 1985. 11 pages.

3. United Nations. The State of The World's Women 1985. 19 pages.

SPECIFIC REFERENCES

1. Puffer, R.R. and C.V. Serrano. Patterns of Mortality In Childhood. Washington, D.C. Pan American Health Organization, 1975. 470 pages.

2. Division of Family Health, World Health Organization. The incidence of low birth weight: a critical review of available information. World Health Statistics Quarterly 33:197-224, 1980.

3. Bulletin of Pan American Health Organization. 18:404-406, 1984.

4. Royston, E. The prevalence of nutritional anemia in developing countries: a critical review of available information. World Health Statistics Quarterly, no. 2: page 52-91, 1982.

5. Ayres, D. Oral rehydration therapy. World Health, June 1985: pp. 9–11.

6. World Health Organization. Progress report on the expanded programme of immunization. Geneva, Switzerland: WHO, Jan. 23-25, 1989. 41 pages.

7. UNICEF/WHO Joint Committee on Health Policy. Progress report on diarrhoeal diseases control programme. Geneva, Switzerland: WHO, Jan. 23-25, 1989. 13 pages.

2

THE DEMOGRAPHY OF MATERNAL AND CHILD HEALTH IN DEVELOPING COUNTRIES

DEBORAH MAINE, M.P.H. AND JAMES ALLMAN, PH.D.

INTRODUCTION

The demography of maternal and child health is a study in dramatic contrasts between developed and developing countries. In broad terms, most of the women and children in the world live in developing countries, where fertility and mortality are high, and health services are inadequate. Furthermore, high fertility means that the actual number of women and children to be served by health programs is growing rapidly. For this reason, a great deal of effort in the international health field is being devoted to finding ways to target services efficiently. After review of statistics on population distribution, fertility and mortality, we will return to the subject of services.

POPULATION

The world's population is said to have reached five billion people on July 11th, 1987. As Figure 1 (next page) shows, about six out of every 10 people in the world live in Asia.[1] Another two in 10 live in Africa or Latin America. Thus, more than four out of five people in the world live in the developing world.

Of the world's population, 23 percent are women of reproductive age, and 12 percent children under 5 years old.[1,2] In other words, the target population of MCH programs makes up more than one-third of the total population. Due to regional variations in birth rates, however, this understates the situation in developing countries. The proportion of the population that is less than five years old is only 7-8 percent in Europe and North America, compared to 12 percent in Asia, 14 percent in Latin America and 18 percent in Africa.[1]

FERTILITY

The difference in the proportion of the population made up of young children (noted above) is due to regional variations in fertility rates. One measure of fertility is the Total Fertility Rate (TFR). This is a synthetic rate, representing the number of children an average woman would have during her lifetime if she conformed to the age-specific rates current at the time of the survey.

According to the United Nations, during 1975-80, the TFR for the more developed countries of the world was 2.0, compared to 4.5 for the less developed nations.[2] During the period 1980-85, the TFR for the more developed countries was unchanged at 2.0, while the TFR for the less developed coun-

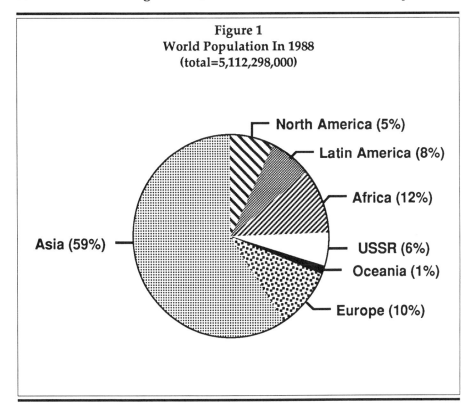

Figure 1
World Population In 1988
(total=5,112,298,000)

North America (5%)
Latin America (8%)
Africa (12%)
Asia (59%)
USSR (6%)
Oceania (1%)
Europe (10%)

tries declined by about 10 percent, to 4.1. A sizable proportion of this decline took place in Asia, specifically China, which is famous for its vigorous family planning program. By 1985, the TFRs were as follows in various regions: Asia, 3.6; Latin America, 4.1; Africa, 6.3. Kenya has the highest TFR in the world – 8.1.

Figure 2 shows the impact of fertility on the future population of the world.[1] From the point of view of MCH programs in Africa, for example, these data remind us that over the next few decades the number of people to be served by health programs will more than double.

INFANT AND CHILD MORTALITY

An infant born in a developing country today is, on average, more than five times as likely to die during the first year of life as one born in a developed country.[1] Figure 3 (next page) shows the proportion of all births and infant deaths that take place in various regions of the world.[1] The region with largest discrepancy between births and infant deaths is Africa, which has 20

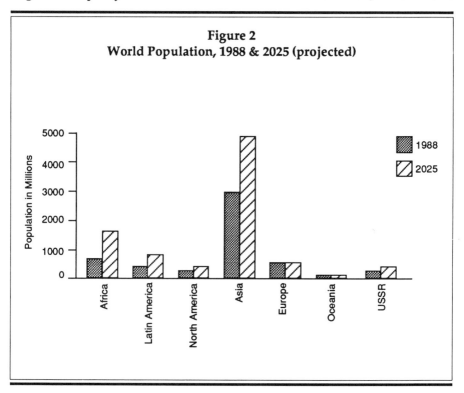

Figure 2
World Population, 1988 & 2025 (projected)

percent of births and 29 percent of deaths. Looking at such large regions, however, conceals substantial differences within them. For example, the infant mortality rate in mainland China is less than one-third the rate for Southern Asia, which includes India, Bangladesh and Pakistan (32 deaths per 1,000 live births in China, compared to 102 in South Asia).

Between 1950 and 1980 infant death rates fell by 44 percent in developing countries.[3] While economic development, increases in food production and availability, and sociocultural advances (such as increases in female literacy) contributed to this decline, changes in health care policy and provision have probably also played an important role.

A broad range of demographic and epidemiological studies shows that the major causes of illness and death among young children in developing countries are malnutrition, diarrheal and other infectious diseases (such as measles and pneumonia).[4]

MATERNAL MORTALITY

The World Health Organization estimates that 500,000 women die every year from complications of pregnancy, including abortion. Figure 4 (next page) shows that virtually all of these deaths take place in developing countries (99 percent).[2,5] By comparing the data used to develop Figures 3 and 4, it

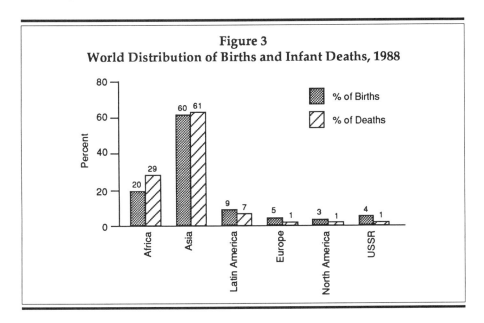

Figure 3
World Distribution of Births and Infant Deaths, 1988

can be shown that the discrepancy between the population at risk and the proportion of deaths taking place in developing countries is even greater for maternal than for infant deaths. Fifteen percent of all births and three percent of all infant deaths take place in developed countries. By comparison, 25 percent of the women in the world live in developed countries, and only one percent of maternal deaths occur in these countries.

The frequency of maternal death in a country depends not only on the risk of an average pregnancy, but on the fertility rate as well. Unlike the risk of infant mortality (to which each person is exposed only once), the risk of maternal death accumulates with each successive pregnancy.

The risk of an average pregnancy is indicated by the maternal mortality ratio (often incorrectly called the "maternal mortality rate") which is the number of maternal deaths per 100,000 live births. Ratios of 500-800 maternal deaths per 100,000 births are common in developing countries, compared to ratios of less than 30 in developed countries.[6]

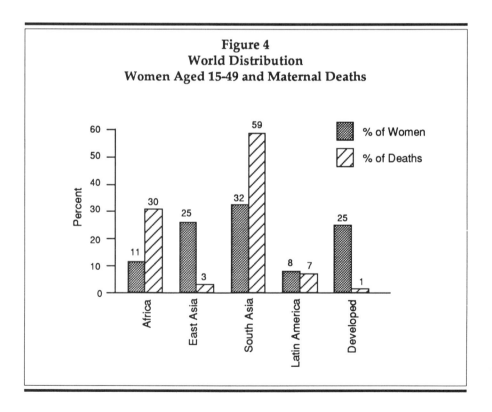

Figure 4
World Distribution
Women Aged 15-49 and Maternal Deaths

Not only do women in developing countries have higher risks of death with each pregnancy, they become pregnant more often. Consequently, an average woman's lifetime risk of dying a maternal death ranges from 1 in 21 in Africa, to one in 9,850 in Northern Europe.[5]

The major causes of maternal death in developing countries today are the same as they were in industrialized countries 40 years ago – hemorrhage, infection, toxemia, obstructed labor and complications of illicit abortion.[5]

FAMILY PLANNING AND HEALTH

Family planning deserves its own section in a chapter such as this because it has unique attributes. First of all, it can help reduce both mortality and population growth. This is unusual because most initiatives that reduce mortality (particularly infant mortality) increase population growth, which can, in the long run, aggravate problems of health care delivery.

Secondly, family planning is one of the few initiatives that has the potential to substantially reduce both maternal and infant deaths.[7]

Family planning can reduce maternal mortality in a number of ways. Firstly, when women do not get pregnant they are not at risk of complications of pregnancy or childbirth. Secondly, if women are able to avoid unwanted pregnancies, they will not have to choose between induced abortion or an unwanted birth. In most developing countries, induced abortion is illegal. Even where it is legal (as in India) it is not accessible to most women. Consequently, deaths from illicit abortion are responsible for an estimated one-fifth of all maternal deaths in the Third World.[8]

Finally, women who have many children, or who give birth at either extreme of their reproductive years, are more likely to die of obstetric complications than are other women.[9] Births to such high-risk women are common in the developing countries. In many countries in Africa, for example, more than 30 percent of all births are to women aged 35 or older.[10]

Although some people still believe that women in developing countries want very large families and are not interested in fertility control, data from the World Fertility Survey show that there are significant numbers of women who do not want another child. In countries such as Bangladesh, Colombia, Egypt, Jamaica, Mexico, Pakistan, Philippines and Venezuela, more than two out every five married women say that they do not want any more children.[11] Even in sub-Saharan Africa, where the proportion of women saying that they do not want any more children is smaller than elsewhere, that proportion is as high as 17 percent in such countries as Kenya and Sudan. Furthermore, the proportions of women who want no more children increases among older women and women with at least three children – a fortunate fact, since these women are also at high risk of poor pregnancy outcomes.[9]

Unfortunately, many women who want no more children are not using effective contraceptives. This proportion ranges from about 50 percent in Egypt and Indonesia to more than 75 percent in Pakistan and Lesotho.[8] If all women who want to limit their families could do so, maternal mortality would be reduced substantially, by from 15 percent in sub-Saharan Africa to 40 percent or more in Sri Lanka and Pakistan.[8]

Through somewhat different mechanisms, family planning can help reduce infant as well as maternal mortality. Pregnancy and birth among women at either end of their reproductive years and women who have already had at least four births carry a higher risk of death for the infant as well as for the mother.[9] Even more important for infant and child health, however, is the effect of the spacing of births within the family.[12] Data from World Fertility Studies in two dozen countries in Africa, Asia and Latin America show that infants born less than two years after the birth of their next older sibling are twice as likely to die as are infants born after a longer birth interval.[12]

Promoting and providing family planning services to allow women to space births and stop childbearing when this is desired should be a high priority in MCH programs throughout the developing world.

THE NEED FOR HEALTH SERVICES

During the past 15 years, considerable attention has been paid to adapting medical systems in developing countries to their needs and resources rather than simply patterning services on Western models. During the colonial period, health systems in most developing countries concentrated on providing the small, urban elite with curative treatment by highly trained personnel using modern technology. Since most people in these countries are poor and/or live in rural areas, few were being served. Independence, economic development and modernization generally did not greatly improve (and in many ways exacerbated) this situation.

A major expression of reorientation was the primary health care (PHC) strategy which was adopted at the World Health Organization's Alma Ata conference in 1978.[13] This initiative has received support worldwide. Although the implementation of PHC is still in progress and the results controversial, the move away from Western models and toward PHC is a major improvement.

REDUCING CHILD MORTALITY

To reduce mortality among infants and young children, and bring about a "Child Survival Revolution" as called for by UNICEF and other international and national agencies, several relatively simple, low cost preventive measures are being actively promoted. These include oral rehydration for diarrheal diseases, immunization, growth monitoring, breastfeeding, family planning, and food supplementation in cases of malnutrition.[14]

Progress in these areas has been substantial. The immunization coverage of children in developing countries (not including China) against diphtheria, whooping cough, tetanus, tuberculosis, and polio has reached 50 percent; 40 percent for measles.[15] Oral rehydration of children with diarrhea (which was almost unknown outside specialist circles until 1980) is now being used by an estimated 18 percent of cases.[15]

In some countries, however, child survival interventions are not gaining ground or are actually losing momentum. Part of the problem seems to be that health institutions are not in place at the grassroots level. Often the poorest developing countries do not have the basic physical facilities to provide PHC services. In some areas the physical structure exists, but it lacks trained and motivated staff, essential drugs, and community support. Conversely, in developing countries where good health care at low cost has been provided, a great deal of attention has been paid to basic services at the grassroots level. China, Sri Lanka, and Costa Rica are examples studied in a recent report.[16] Certainly, political will is an essential element in such success stories.

REDUCING MATERNAL MORTALITY

Complications of pregnancy and childbirth are the leading cause of death among women of reproductive age in developing countries, yet little attention has been paid to this topic until recently.[5] Part of the problem may be that it is commonly assumed that whatever is good for the child is good for the mother. However, not only are the causes of maternal deaths quite different from those of child death, but so also are the potential remedies. For example, a well-nourished child with measles is much less likely to die than is a malnourished child with the same disease. However, a woman with obstructed labor who cannot get appropriate medical care (e.g., a cesarean section) will probably die whether she is malnourished or not. And serious obstetric problems are quite common even among healthy women with no complications during pregnancy.[17]

The means to prevent deaths from obstetric complications have existed for decades: Antibiotics for infection, cesarean section for obstructed labor, blood transfusions and oxytocic drugs for hemorrhage, sedatives and other drugs for eclampsia. Unfortunately, such treatment is not accessible to most women in poor countries.

REFERENCES

1. Population Division Department of International Economic and Social Affairs. World Population Chart 1988. New York, NY: United Nations.

2. Population Division Department of International Economic and Social Affairs. Chart: 1987 World Contraceptive Use. New York, NY: United Nations.

3. Prosterman, R.L. The decline in hunger-related deaths. The Hunger Project Paper 1. California, 1984.

4. Rhode, J.E. Why the other half dies: The science and politics of child mortality in the third world. Assignment Children 61/62. Geneva: UNICEF, 35-36, 1983.

5. Starrs, A. Preventing the tragedy of maternal deaths. A Report on the International Safe Motherhood Conference. Nairobi, Kenya, 1987, pp. 4-55.

6. Royston, E., and A.D. Lopez. On the assessment of maternal mortality. Wld Hlth Statis Quart 40:214-224, 1987.

7. Rosenfield, A., and D. Maine. Maternal mortality: A neglected tragedy. Where is the M in MCH? The Lancet 2 (8446) 83-85, 1985.

8. Maine, D., A. Rosenfield, and M. Wallace, et al. Prevention of maternal mortality in developing countries: Program options and practical considerations. Official background paper for the International Safe Motherhood Conference. Nairobi, Kenya, 1987.

9. Maine, D. Family Planning: Its Impact on the Health of Women and Children. New York: Columbia University, 1981, p. 8.

10. Maine, D., R. McNamara, and J. Wray, et al. Effects of fertility change on maternal and child health: Prospects for sub-Saharan Africa. PHN Technical Notes 85:15. Washington, D.C: The World Bank, 1985.

11. Gille, H. World Fertility Survey. Major Findings and Implications. London: Alden Press, 1984, pp. 1-61.

12. Maine, D., and R. McNamara. Birth Spacing and Child Survival. Center for Population and Family Planning, New York: Columbia University, 1985.

13. WHO/UNICEF. Primary Health Care. International Conference on Primary Health Care. Alma Ata, USSR, 6-12 September 1978. Geneva: WHO, 1978.

14. Grant, J.P. The State of the World's Children 1984. UNICEF. London: Oxford University Press, 1983.

15. Grant, J.P. The State of the World's Children 1988. London: Oxford University Press, 1988.

16. Halstead, S.B., J.A. Walsh, and K. Warren (ed). Good Health at Low Cost. New York: Rockefeller Foundation, 1985.

17. Rosenberg, S.N., P.P. Albertson, and E.E. Jones, et al. Complications of labor and delivery following uncomplicated pregnancy. Medical Care XIX:1, 68-79, 1981.

3

PATTERNS OF DELIVERY OF HEALTH CARE FOR WOMEN AND CHILDREN

MILTON I. ROEMER, M.D., M.A., M.P.H.

In almost all countries of the world, small children and expectant mothers have special priority in the organized aspects of the nation's health system. The expression of this priority takes different forms.

TYPES OF NATIONAL HEALTH SYSTEMS

The approximately 160 sovereign countries in the world may be classified in different ways. The commonest method of classification has been along an economic dimension – grouping countries according to their wealth, as measured by gross national product (GNP) per capita per year. By this approach, agencies such as the World Bank classify countries as "high income and industrialized," "middle income," and "low income," with a special place for "rich oil-exporting countries" that are not generally industrialized.[1]

In this perspective the countries of the world in 1985 were distributed approximately as follows:

Economic Level	GNP per capita	Countries
High income and industrialized	$5000 and over	25
Middle income	$500 to $5000	90
Very Low income	Under $500	40
Oil-rich countries	$8000 and higher	5
All levels		160

Provisions for the health care of women and children vary greatly, of course, among countries of these several economic levels. Countries of greater affluence typically have many more health personnel and facilities, they can render higher volumes of health services, and their people enjoy higher standards of living.

There is, however, another approach to analyzing and understanding countries and their health systems, including the patterns of delivering care to mothers and children. This is along a political dimension. At any economic level, countries may organize their health systems according to varying concepts of social policy. Viewed historically, dominant policies in a health system have reflected different degrees of social intervention in the private market of health services.

Political ideology in some countries may result in a minimal degree of intervention in the health service market. Most health service is purchased as a private transaction between patient and provider. For many historical and political reasons, other countries develop varying degrees of health care market intervention, through deliberate planning and through the organization of services, collectivization of their financing, or both. In its most extreme form, the free market for buying and selling health service has been virtually eliminated, and replaced by a centrally planned and highly organized health system. These gradations can be expressed as follows:

Market intervention	Type of Health System
Minimal	Entrepreneurial
Moderate	Welfare-oriented
Extensive	Comprehensive
Virtually complete	Socialist

Combining these two dimensions for analysis of national health systems, we derive a matrix as illustrated in Figure 1 (next page). The resultant 16 conceptual cells are numbered to facilitate discussion.[2]

Patterns of delivering maternal and child health (MCH) services vary in some degree among all 16 types of health systems. Moreover, within each type of system, there may be substantial variations among different population groups – especially between upper and lower social classes. In all but a few of the conceptual cells there are numerous countries – in some as many as 15 or 20. In the space available, however, we can consider MCH patterns in only one country of each conceptual type. Since the most decisive determinant of delivery patterns in health systems is political, our analytical approach will begin along this dimension.

ENTREPRENEURIAL HEALTH SYSTEMS

Entrepreneurial health systems – that is, with minimal market intervention – in high income and industrialized countries are well illustrated in the United States of America (cell 1).[3] Here, services to mothers and children, whether therapeutic or preventive in purpose, are rendered mainly by private physicians and other private health care providers. While MCH clinics, operated principally by local Departments of Health, serve the poorest section of the population, these persons are only a small portion of the total. Of all U.S. infants born in a year, only some 10 to 15 percent are served by governmental MCH clinics.

Prenatal and postpartum care at public health clinics reach even a small percentage of maternity cases. Although governmentally sponsored, many of these clinics require payment of registration fees.

Entrepreneurial health systems in middle-income countries are illustrated by Thailand (cell 5).[4] More than two-thirds of all health expenditures here are in the private sector – modern or traditional. Yet, insofar as the Ministry of Health provides organized services through health centers or health posts, they are oriented very largely to serving mothers and children. The staffing of MCH clinics is mainly by assistant nurses and assistant midwives. As recently as 1977, of all rural childbirths 64 percent were delivered by traditional birth attendants, and only 30 percent of pregnant women had received any prenatal care.

Figure 1
Types of National Health System, Classified by Economic Level and Health System Policies

Economic Level (GNP per capita)	Health System Policies (Market Intervention)			
	Entrepreneurial	Welfare-oriented	Comprehensive	Socialist
High income	1	2	3	4
Middle income	5	6	7	8
Very low income	9	10	11	12
Oil-rich	13	14	15	16

Among entrepreneurial countries of very low income level, <u>Ghana</u> is an example (cell 9).[5] Despite massive poverty, some 70 percent of health expenditures are in the private sector. Much of this is for the services of untrained traditional healers or the purchase of self-prescribed drugs from pharmacies or itinerant drug-sellers. Ministry of Health facilities for primary health care are staffed almost wholly by briefly trained auxiliary personnel; in the public services, physicians are found only in hospitals. Even the meagerly staffed health posts are accessible to only 45 percent of the rural population, who constitute 68 percent of the total. In 1986 only 37 percent of the children had been immunized against diphtheria, pertussis, and tetanus (DPT); of known infant diarrhea episodes, only 26 percent had been treated with oral rehydration salts (ORS). The infant mortality rate in 1987 was 91 per 1000 live births.

<u>Gabon</u> is a small African country with entrepreneurial health system policies, in spite of high wealth from oil extraction (cell 13). Its sudden wealth from finding oil in the 1970s led mainly to a large private sector in health care, patronized by civil servants and others with high salaries. The great majority of physicians are expatriates, attracted by the opportunity for high private earnings. A health care infrastructure for MCH or other services is extremely weak. Although hospital beds are relatively abundant, health centers for MCH service are relatively few, and staffed mainly by nursing auxiliaries. The infant mortality rate in 1985 was 122 per 1000 live births.

WELFARE-ORIENTED HEALTH SYSTEMS

Welfare-oriented countries of high income are numerous, especially in Western Europe; the <u>Federal</u> <u>Republic</u> <u>of</u> <u>Germany</u> may serve as an example (cell 2).[7] Nearly the entire population is protected with respect to the costs of medical care, through local insurance funds. The services are rendered, however, by private health practitioners, and these obviously include the treatment of children as well as adults. For preventive MCH services, nevertheless, local public health agencies maintain networks of MCH clinics both for expectant women and children under age four. Years ago these preventive services were available only at the public MCH clinics, since the insurance did not pay doctors for preventive work. Since the end of World War II, however, preventive service may also be obtained from private practitioners, remunerated by health insurance fees. Attendance at public MCH clinics, therefore, has declined, except for immunizations or for the families of workers who may not be fully insured. Public health agency services must in all cases be limited to prevention.

Middle-income countries with welfare-oriented health systems are also numerous, especially in Latin America and to some extent in the Middle East (cell 6). An example is <u>Mexico</u>, where the Ministry of Health operates a nationwide network of health centers and health stations open to everyone.[8] MCH services are provided by teams of physicians, nurses, and auxiliary health workers. Around 60 percent of the population, however, are also covered by "social security" programs, which provide health service directly; in contrast to Germany, the insurance organizations do not simply pay private doctors for their services, but they established their own polyclinics where physicians and others work on salary. MCH services are regularly available at these polyclinics, which are typically better staffed than the health centers of the Ministry of Health. In addition to the availability of these two large organized health care programs, affluent families may obtain MCH care from purely private practitioners.

Very low income countries with a welfare-oriented health system may be illustrated by <u>Burma</u> (cell 10).[9] Because of its great poverty, there are relatively few physicians (28 per 100,000 people), and nearly all the customary MCH services must be provided by personnel equivalent to nurse-midwives (lady health visitors), assistant nurses, and assistant midwives. A nationwide network of rural and urban health centers, each of which is expected to serve about 20,000 people, is the principal resource. The Director of each rural health center is typically a Health Assistant, who is always male, but he gives treatment rather than preventive services for women and children. The vast majority of persons attending the health centers are, in fact, women and children – for both preventive services (including checkups and immunizations) and for treatment of symptoms. Adult men usually see private physicians for medical care or sometimes go to special clinics maintained by the Ministry of Cooperatives.

A welfare-oriented country, with vast petroleum resources is illustrated by Libya (cell 14).[10] Because of great alienation outside the Arab world, little is known about Libya's health system, except that national government policy calls for general health service being available to everyone. This is done through an extensive network of health centers, staffed by physicians and nurses. There are 161 physicians and 278 nurses (all levels) per 100,000 – an exceptionally abundant supply. MCH services are an integral part of the program of every health center, but Libya has been handicapped by adult literacy among women of only 50 percent in 1985. This may account for the high infant mortality of 84 per 1000 live births, in spite of a GNP per capita of $7170.

COMPREHENSIVE HEALTH SYSTEMS

These health systems have gone further than the welfare-oriented ones, in establishing comprehensive health service as an entitlement of everyone.

This has usually been done by financing health care mainly through general revenues and by mobilizing nearly all health resources (personnel and facilities) under government. The low income countries with such systems may be handicapped by simple lack of resources, but whatever resources may be available are equally accessible to everyone.

Comprehensive health systems in countries of high income, with substantial industrialization, may be illustrated by that in Sweden (cell 3).[11] In this Scandinavian country all forms of health care are available to every resident, with only small charges for drugs and certain ambulatory services. Preventively oriented MCH services, however, are entirely free, and an active educational campaign encourages all expectant mothers to seek prenatal care early and to bring infants for regular check-ups and immunizations. These services are provided mainly by specially trained nurses in general community health centers or in separate MCH clinics. The physicians in both hospitals and health centers are paid by salaries, derived mainly from general revenues. Only about 10 percent of Swedish physicians remain in private practice, but they do little preventively-oriented MCH work. With an infant mortality rate of only 6.0 per 1000 live births in 1987, Sweden has next to the lowest such national rate (Japan's is slightly lower) of any country.

Among middle-income countries, a comprehensive health system may be illustrated by that in Israel (cell 7). The Ministry of Health in Israel maintains a network of health centers, emphasizing MCH services, accessible to everyone in this small country. Home visits by nurses are an important part of the program. At the same time, there is a large nationwide scheme of health insurance – legally voluntary but covering 85 percent of the population – that operates its own network of health centers and polyclinics, with salaried personnel. The latter resources also provide preventive MCH services, although they are devoted mainly to treatment of the sick. Many political attempts have been made to integrate the government services with the large voluntary health insurance scheme. Although they have not been successful, under the two programs the people of Israel receive high quality health services, especially in the MCH field.

Among very poor countries, a comprehensive health system is illustrated by that in Sri Lanka (cell 11).[13] Although many physicians and pharmacies are private, 65 percent of national health expenditures are governmental, and everyone is entitled to health care. This island of 16 million people is divided into an hierarchical framework of districts, divisions, subdivisions, and villages – virtually all of which are served by quite well-staffed health centers or health stations. Hospitals are staffed by physicians, as are the main district and divisional public health headquarters. The subdivisional health centers,

each serving about 20,000 people, are headed by an Assistant Medical Practitioner, who is invariably male. On his staff, and also in more than 4400 village
health stations, are large numbers of registered nurses, assistant nurses, and
midwives. These female personnel are trained to provide a broad scope of
MCH services. With four echelons of administration below the national level,
the services are well supervised and the standard of care is high. Compared
with other south Asian countries, the level of literacy is very high (83 percent
in women in 1985), and good nutrition is provided by regular food supplements for children. All these factors doubtless contribute to Sri Lanka's low
infant mortality in 1987 of 34 per 1000 live births.

Among the oil-rich countries with comprehensive health systems, Kuwait is illustrative (cell 15).[14] This small but extremely wealthy city-state has
used much of its wealth for the education and health care of its people.
Distance is no problem, and everyone is easily accessible to a health center or
polyclinic. MCH and all other health services are entirely free to everyone,
including the 50 percent of people who are "guest workers" with families, and
not citizens. The commonest type of Kuwaiti health center is for general
medical care, but for most preventive services to prenatal women and small
children, there are designated clinics with specially trained doctors, nurses,
and midwives. Practically all childbirths are delivered in hospitals by well-
trained nurse-midwives. The record of DPT as well as measles and polio
immunizations was 95 percent of the children in 1986-87.

SOCIALIST HEALTH SYSTEMS

High income countries with socialist health systems are best illustrated
by the Soviet Union (cell 4).[15] The entire population of this large country is
entitled to comprehensive care, and this is provided through a vast national
network of health facilities, staffed by governmentally employed health personnel. Major emphasis is given to MCH services, but routine prevention is
not separated from treatment; it is provided by the same doctors in the same
facilities. (Special hours of the week may be set aside for preventive activities,
for the sake of efficiency.) "Feldshers" or medical assistants are extensively
used, especially in rural areas, in spite of a vast supply of doctors (some 400
per 100,000); childbirths are delivered by trained midwives, predominantly in
hospitals. In large cities there are many separate polyclinics exclusively for
children, as well as children's hospitals. About one-third of the nation's doctors are pediatricians, whose basic medical studies have been oriented to
pediatrics after the third year of the 6-year curriculum. In the 1970s, problems
appeared, suggesting that the emphasis on vast quantitative expansion of
health care resources had resulted in a deterioration of quality. In the 1980s,

therefore, extensive reorganization, with increased government funding, was undertaken, in order to improve the quality of MCH and all health services.

Cuba (cell 8) illustrates well a middle-income country with socialist health policies.[16] In many ways, it emulates the Soviet patterns, but its human and physical resources are not so abundant. An extensive network of polyclinics – about 400, each serving 25,000 people – blankets the island. Every 5000 people are served, without charge, by a salaried polyclinic health team, including a pediatrician for the children and an obstetrician-gynecologist for women. These doctors do all the necessary preventive as well as therapeutic health work. Midwives and medical assistants are not used, but there are many nurses to assist the physician. Rationing of basic foodstuffs assures an adequate level of nutrition for all families, and illiteracy has been wiped out. As a result, Cuba has achieved an infant mortality rate of 15.0 per 1000 live births, the lowest such rate of any Latin American country.

A very low-income country with socialist health policies is illustrated by Vietnam (cell 12).[17] After 30 years of war before national liberation, the country suffered millions of deaths and massive destruction, and reconstruction since 1975 has been slow and difficult. Vietnam's 40 provinces are divided into 466 districts, each headed by a medical director (who also does clinical work in the district hospital). At the local level, where MCH and other primary health services are provided to the people, there are some 8600 communes, with about 7000 population each. Here assistant doctors, trained for three years, as well as auxiliary nurses and midwives (trained for one year), provide both preventive and treatment services. Educational and personal preventive services, including MCH examinations and immunizations, are done in the afternoons, while treatment of the sick is done in the mornings. Much of the treatment of both adults and children is based on ancient Vietnamese concepts of traditional healing.

There is no oil-rich country with a socialist health system (cell 16) in the current world. One low-income country in the Middle East region, the People's Democratic Republic of Yemen, has socialist health policies and has recently struck oil. One cannot yet tell if it will acquire the type of wealth that transformed Kuwait or Qatar.

This completes very brief accounts of 15 types of national health systems, and the patterns of delivery of MCH services in them. It is evident that politically-determined policies toward a private market for health services are a major determinant of these patterns. In all countries, even the most entrepreneurial, with very strong private medical markets, there is some degree of market intervention, in order to help poor families that could not purchase the health services they need. There are also non-market services for personal prevention and environmental protection in every country. As countries develop greater market intervention – largely through governmentally controlled financing, delivery of care, or both – the patterns of delivery of MCH services tend to reach greater proportions of the population.[18]

These tendencies are inevitably constrained by the economic level of the country. A wealthy nation, with almost any health system policies, can develop greater human and physical resources for health care than a poor nation. Yet a major lesson from the comparative study of national health systems is that political will to implement certain national priorities, can lead to much greater health resources in even a poor country than would be expected. The supply of physicians, nurses, and polyclinics in Cuba, for example, is much greater than that in many countries of higher economic levels. National wealth may set rough limits, of course, on the capabilities of a health system, but political priorities determine whether those limits will be reached or even exceeded. Within the health system of virtually every country, preventive services for children and mothers fortunately occupy a prominent place. The manner of delivery of those services, however, always depends on the general contours of the national health system.

One may be tempted to consider what is the "best" strategy for providing MCH services to the population of any country. Perhaps, from a purely idealistic perspective, many might favor:

1. availability of MCH services to all persons, rich and poor,
2. a comprehensive scope of such services, both preventive and therapeutic,
3. delivery of services by competent and sensitive health personnel organized in efficient teams,
4. integration of MCH care with general health services for families and individuals, and
5. adequate financing by the most egalitarian possible method – progressive taxation.

Unfortunately, the political realities of countries, not to mention the economic constraints, seldom permit an ideal response to the health needs of mothers and children. The optimal MCH strategy in any country must nearly always be a compromise between the ideal and the socially feasible.

REFERENCES

1. World Bank. World Development Report 1987. Washington, D.C.: Oxford University Press, 1987.

2. Roemer, M.I. Analysis of health service systems – A general approach, reorienting health services: Application of a systems approach. C.O. Pannenborg et al., (ed). New York: Plenum Press, 1984, pp. 47-59.

3. Jonas, S., and contributors. Health Care Delivery in the United States. 3d ed. New York: Springer, 1986.

4. Roemer, M.I. The health care system of Thailand, New Delhi, India. World Health Organization Regional Office for South-East Asia, 1981.

5. Sai, F.T. Ghana: health service prospects: an international survey. I. Douglas-Wilson and G. McLachlen (ed). London: The Lancet and Nuffield Provincial Hospitals Trust, 1973, pp.125-155.

6. Blanc, L., and M. Blanc. The role of utilization studies in the planning of primary health care. World Health Forum 2: 347-349, 1981.

7. Light, D.W., S. Liebfried, and F. Tennestedt. Social medicine and professional dominance: The German experience. Am J Public Health 76: 78-83, 1986.

8. Soberon, G., J. Frenk and J. Supulveda. The health care reform in Mexico: Before and after the 1985 earthquakes. Am J Public Health 76: 673-680, 1986.

9. Roemer, M. I. Primary Health Care in Burma's National Health System. San Francisco CA: Western Consortium for the Health Professions, 1986.

10. Raymond, M.S.U. Health and Policy Making in the Arab Middle East, Washington D.C: Georgetown University, 1978.

11. National Board of Health and Welfare: The Swedish Health Services in the 1990s. Stockholm: Liber Tryck Stockholm, 1985.

12. Tulchinski, T.H. Israel health review. Israel J Med Sciences, 18:345-355, 1982.

13. Perera, P.D.A. Health Care Systems of Sri Lanka, Good Health at Low Cost. Halstead, S.B., J.A. Walsh and K.S. Warren (eds). New York: The Rockefeller Foundation, 1985, pp. 93-110.

14. State of Kuwait, Ministry of Public Health. Health Services in Kuwait. Kuwait: MOPH, 1981.

15. Raffel, N.K. Health services in the Union of Soviet Socialist Republics. Comparative Health Systems: Descriptive Analyses of Fourteen National Health Systems. Raffel, M.W. (ed). University Park, PA: Pennsylvania State University Press, 1984, pp. 488-519.

16. Danielson, R.S. Cuban Medicine. New Brunswick, NJ: Transaction Books, 1979.

17. Ladinsky, J.L., and R.E. Levine. The organization of health services in Vietnam. J Public Health Policy 6: 255-268, 1985.

18. Roemer, M.I. Market failure and health care policy. J Public Health Policy 3: 419-431, 1982.

4

SOCIAL BENEFITS

RUTH A. BRANDWEIN, PH.D., M.S.W.

Social benefits are those public provisions collectively afforded a population, either universally or categorically, by society. The type and level of such social welfare benefits vary from nation to nation, and within each nation at different points of time, depending both on the level of surplus wealth that is available for redistribution and the ideology of the government. As Maimonna Kane of Senegal expressed it,

> "...social welfare cannot be perceived in the same way in Europe, in the Eastern countries, in the United States, as in Africa. The difference of context... and of ethics...reflects also differences of perception..." (Kane).[1]

In general, the industrialized "Welfare State" nations of Western Europe and the socialist states of Eastern Europe have been the most generous in their provisions. The United States and the Union of South Africa, while as wealthy as these other nations, have a lower-level of benefits because of their ideology. For example, they are the only industrialized nations without national health insurance or child care.

The Southern Hemisphere nations are, in general, less industrialized and poorer, and so have a lower level of social benefits. (Note: we will refer to these nations as "Southern Hemisphere," which is a descriptive term and with some exceptions, includes most of the nations usually referred to as "developing." The term "developing nations," as the earlier terms "Third World" or "undeveloped" is considered a derogatory, judgmental and inaccurate term.)

It will not be possible to summarize all the social benefits of every Southern Hemisphere nation. Rather, we will provide an overview, discuss general

47

trends, and provide some illustrations regarding such social provisions as maternity leaves and maternity allowances, children's and family allowances, social security pensions and disability insurance, and child care.

STATUS OF WOMEN

Because this book is concerned with women, children, and families, it is important to provide some background information regarding the status of women in these nations as a context for understanding the need and significance of the various benefits. Whether we consider their legal, social, or economic status, that of women is universally lower than men's.

Only 47 of 139 member nations have ratified the United Nations Convention for the Elimination of All Discrimination Against Women. The American and European nations have the highest rate of ratification (the U.S. has merely signed it, but has not ratified it); Asian and African nations have the lowest rates of signing or ratification. Of the seven conventions on the rights of women (the other six include equal political rights, equal marriage rights, equality in education, equal pay for equal value, maternity protection and equality in employment) sixteen nations have not ratified any. Thirteen, including the U.S., have ratified only one (Sivard).[2] These figures are not surprising when one learns that in these Southern Hemisphere nations women hold only seven percent of the seats in national legislatures, and the figure is depressingly similar in many industrialized nations.

Most of these Southern tier states have large proportions of female-headed households. Worldwide, 30 percent of households are headed by women (Seager and Olson).[3] In these nations 70 percent of the poor live in female headed households or are elderly (most of whom are women). In a Physical Quality of Life Index for women, based on a composite of indicators of average life expectancy, infant mortality and literacy, Egypt and Kenya had ratings of 39 and 37, respectively, out of a possible score of 100 (in contrast the U.S. score was 97) (Huston).[4]

WOMEN AND WORK

Social benefits in most of the world are related to membership in the paid labor force. In much of the world, and especially in primarily agricultural societies, much of the work women do is unpaid, either in the home, in subsistence agriculture or in the informal or "unorganized" sector of the economy (such as street vendors or home work). Throughout the world women produce half the world's food; in Africa that figure is 80 percent. If unpaid household labor were calculated it would add one third – $4 trillion – to the world's annual economic product. In all countries, women work longer hours than do men and earn less. Moreover, women are segregated in job ghettos. Nursing, primary school teaching, service workers and child care providers are universally women's jobs. In Africa women do the trading and agricultural work; in Southeast Asia they are ghettoized in low paying jobs in the textile and electronics industries, and in the Caribbean and Latin America they hold domestic service jobs (Sivard, Seager, and Olson).[5]

The International Labor Organization (ILO) standard for maternity leave is twelve weeks or more at full pay. Comparing national legislative policies we find that most of the states of Latin America and the Caribbean conform to this standard as do India, Pakistan and some nations of western Africa. More than half the African states provide at least 12 weeks of maternity leave but without full pay, as do most of the states in Southeast Asia. China and some of the eastern African nations provide maternity leave of less than 12 weeks but at full pay, and most of the Middle East nations (and the United States) provide some leave and pay provisions but below the ILO standards (Seager and Olson).[6]

Most countries have policies providing some level of maternity leave, most typically six weeks prior to and six weeks after delivery. They also provide some time during the day when mothers, upon return to work, can breast feed their children. In practice however, up to 85 percent of women are not in the formal sector. That is, if they are agricultural workers, domestics, street vendors, doing piece work at home, employed seasonally, part-time, or on contract they are in the informal or unorganized sector and so are not eligible for any of these benefits. While usually illegal, employers may fire pregnant workers or not hire women workers at all (Morgan).[7] To counter this, one author recommends that social security payments required of employers should be determined on the basis of the number of workers and not on the sex of the workers. Employers, whether they hire women or not, and regardless of the number of women they employ should contribute to funds for maternity and other benefits....(thus) reducing the probability of discrimination in (women's) job engagement and stability (Charlton).[8]

FAMILY AND CHILDREN'S ALLOWANCES

Family or children's allowances are fairly common in the social welfare states of western Europe and the socialist states, but are uncommon in the poor nations of the Southern Hemisphere. There are some notable exceptions in Latin America. Brazil provides a "Salario Familial" equal to 5 percent of the minimum wage per child. This has the effect of encouraging large families. However, it is given to the father who has complete autonomy as to how it is spent. Chile has recently begun a program paying certain heads of household $110 per month. Nicaragua also provides subsidies to large families (Morgan).[9] The only other Southern Hemisphere nations reportedly providing some kind of allowance are Indonesia, where only government and military employees receive children's allowances, and Senegal, where family allowances are paid to men as heads of household and to some single women with children (Morgan).[10]

SOCIAL SECURITY PENSIONS AND DISABILITY INSURANCE

Unlike family or children's allowances, which are rare in nations struggling for survival and using national resources for such basics as potable water and basic health care, a large number of these nations have some form of national insurance. Typically these plans, some of which are contributory by employee and employer as well as government, cover women retiring at age 55 and men at age 60. Most of them include in addition to these pension benefits, disability insurance, widow's insurance and occasionally, unemployment benefits. In practice, however, the coverage is often quite limited. In Nicaragua the program favors workers earning less than $3000. More typically, as is the situation with maternity benefits, those working part-time, seasonally, in rural areas or in the informal sector are denied coverage. Senegal seems to be an exception as its policy specifically includes domestic workers. Information, however, is lacking on the actual practice. In China, the government guarantees to meet five basic needs (food, clothing, housing, medical care, and burial) for childless seniors (Morgan).[11]

In many of these countries care of the elderly is still a responsibility of the extended family. As this system begins to break down with migration to urban areas and industrialization, more problems will occur if the government does not provide a social benefits system to replace those supports the family can no longer provide.

CHILD CARE

In general, Southern Hemisphere nations are countries of the young. Part of the explanation for the limited pension system is that in many countries, as in India, there are relatively few elderly. In contrast, the high birth rate, especially in Africa, means that there are many children. In Kenya, for example, the average number of children per mother is seven, and it is the fastest growing nation in the world with a population increase of 4 percent per year. In many parts of Africa, notably Kenya, the Sudan and northwest Africa there are more than 800 preschool aged children for every 1000 women of childbearing age. In the rest of Africa, most of Latin America, the Middle East and some Asian nations (Burma, Laos) there are between 650 and 800 preschoolers for every such 1000 women (Seager and Olson).[12]

In a number of nations factory owners are required to provide creches or child care if they employ more than a specified number of women. But, as with the other social benefits, some employers avoid providing child care facilities by not hiring women, or hiring them on contract or part-time. Some nations have embarked on extensive programs of government-built or -run centers. For example, China currently enrolls 25 percent of all preschool age children in 990,000 nurseries. Cuba operates 782 centers for 86,000 children providing meals, medical and dental care in addition to basic child care. Egypt operates over 2,000 daycare centers but of these only 176 are for girls.

In some nations, the voluntary sector or self-help movement provides child care. In Sri Lanka the Sarvodaza movement has developed mothers' centers, providing cooperative child care in 3,000 villages. The Vanasthali Rural Development Centre in India has the goal of providing nursery schools (balwadis) in every village under the guidance of trained women teachers (Muzumdar).[13] Yet in many parts of India girls are still kept out of school in order to provide such care or self-employed women bring their children with them to the worksite (ranging from 85 percent of handcart peddlers to 38 percent of vegetable vendors) (Morgan, SEWA).[14] In Zimbabwe, 1,000 pre-school centers are run by voluntary and women's organizations and the need is pressing because older children who had assumed child care responsibilities are now in school.

LOOKING TO THE FUTURE

Over the last decade a number of international recommendations have been made pertaining to social benefits. In 1975 the United Nations-sponsored Women's International Conference held in Mexico City produced a document entitled *World Plan of Action*. Its major recommendation was that 1975-1985 be named the International Decade of Women by the United Nations. This was done. A mid-decade conference was held in Copenhagen in 1980 and an end-of-the-decade conference held in Nairobi in 1985 counted over 60 percent of the participants at the open forum from the developing world. Out of that conference the United Nations adopted *Forward Looking Strategies for the Advancement of Women to the Year 2000*. While it is one thing for a government to support a document and quite another to implement its provisions, these documents do carry weight in many of the world's nations. They provide some guidelines and directions for governments and a focus and level of credibility for women's advocates. The major themes of the decade were equality, development and peace, with three sub-themes: education, employment and health. Social benefits were not a major area of concern but among the recommendations in these documents are some pertaining to the issues covered in this chapter.

In the *World Plan of Action* nations are urged to consider the role of women in terms of their contribution to families and the value of roles such as parent, spouse and homemaker. By 1985 the *Forward Looking Strategy* document called more specifically for recognition of women's informal and invisible economic contributions to society and stated that the value of housework should be considered equal to financial contributions to the family (United Nations).[15]

Article 11 of The United Nations Convention on the Elimination of All Forms of Discrimination Against Women calls for equality in employment rights – for equality of remuneration and benefits, social security and maternity leave.

In the 1979 United Nations Declaration of Rights of Disabled Persons and its 1982 World Program of Action *Concerning Disabled Persons* governments are called upon to provide occupational and social rehabilitation measures, support services and assistance with domestic responsibilities as well as opportunities to participate in all aspects of life.

Regarding children's and family allowances the *World Plan of Action* urged that social security programs include children and family allowances in order to strengthen the economic stability of family members.

The *Forward Looking Strategies* calls on governments to provide adequate care for children of working parents and specifically calls for childcare facilities for urban poor children.

CONCLUSION

In Europe and the United States, the rural, pre-industrial society, in which needs were met in the family, gave way with different degrees of reluctance in the industrial era to various forms of the welfare state. In such a society the needs of family members are provided by a centralized, national government. A major difficulty in discussing social benefits in the context of Southern Hemisphere nations is that it is a social welfare state model and may not be appropriate to their development.

It would be ethnocentric to assume that countries which are now in a pre-industrial, agricultural stage, and in which the extended family is beginning to break down in its ability to meet familial needs, will necessarily follow the social welfare state model in their development.

In fact, there are indications that the model is being rejected, based on the problems of provisions through a strong, central bureaucratic government experienced by both the Western capitalist and the socialist nations. In addition to the difficulties of centralized governments in nations without developed transportation and communications infrastructures, social welfare is seen as merely relieving distress. Instead some of these nations are exploring a third model, which may be seen as a more advanced stage in meeting human needs than the welfare state. This is the social development model which emphasizes self-help, empowerment, decentralization and social action as well as providing social benefits.

The Maendeleo ya Wanawake Organization in Kenya, which receives funds from the government, but also from foundations, corporations, the U.N. and other nations, is such an example. With operations in Nairobi and in the rural areas it works with women to develop maternal and child health programs, nutrition information, energy conservation, income generation, clean water and a number of other projects.[16]

Another even more impressive example is the Self-Employed Women's Association (SEWA) in India.[17] Originally part of the labor movement, it is a membership organization of vendors, traders and street hawkers, home-based producers, laborers and service workers. They have developed banking services to provide loans for these women, have provided economic development projects by organizing marketing, providing tools and buying in bulk, and are involved in advocacy on behalf of their members. Ela Bhatt, the founder of SEWA is now a member of the Indian parliament.

In the words of Priscilla Musanya of Zambia,

"Social development is a concept which is more comprehensive and move dynamic than social welfare. Social development puts welfare in the context of active participation by local communities in the planning and delivery of social services." (Musanya).[18]

Social development implies more than mere self reliance at the local level without the redistribution of resources. Social development as a way of providing social benefits through self empowerment can lead to a more equitable society.

REFERENCES

1. Kane, M. Paths to the future, preparing the U.N. interregional consultation on development social welfare policies and programmes: Key social issues. Vienna: International Council of Social Welfare, June 1987, p. 12.

2. Sivard, R.L. Women...A World Survey. New York: Carnegie Corporation,1985, pp 30-31.

3. Seager, J., and A. Olson. Women in the World: An International Atlas. New York: Simon and Schuster/Touchstone, 1986, chart 28.

4. Huston, P. Third World Women Speak Out. New York: Praeger, 1979, pp. 150-151.

5. Sivard, R.L. Women... A World Survey, pp. 5-15. Seager, J., and A. Olson. Women in the World Atlas, charts 13, 15, 18.

6. Seager, J., and A. Olson. Op. cit., chart 20.

7. Morgan, R. (ed). Sisterhood is Global: The International Women's Movement Anthology. Garden City, N.Y.: Anchor Press/Doubleday, 1984.

8. Charlton, S.E.M. Women in Third World Development. Boulder: Westview Press, 1984, p. 144.

9. Morgan, R. Op. cit., pp. 78, 136.

10. Ibid., pp. 315, 590.

11. Ibid., p. 145.

12. Seager, J., and A. Olson. Op. cit., chart 12.

13. Muzumdar, K. Case study on Mrs. Nirmala Purandare, feminist visions for social work education. Workshop organized by Streevani and International Association of Schools of Social Work, Tata Institute of Social Sciences and College of Social Work, Bombay, Oct. 27-Nov. 1, 1987.

14. Morgan, R. Sisterhood is Global, p. 298: Self-Employed Women's Association. Ahmedabad, 1984, p. 9.

15. United Nations: World Plan of Action. United Nations World Conference of the International Women's Year, adopted at Mexico City, July, 1975. United Nations: Forward Looking Strategies to the Year 2000, adopted at Nairobi, Kenya, July, 1985, paragraphs 59, 73.

16. Maendeleo ya Wanawake Organization. Projects: a profile in development. Nairobi, Kenya, July 1985.

17. Self-Employed Women's Association, Ahmedabad, July 1984. Annual Activities Report of SEWA, Ahmedabad, 1986.

18. Musanya, P. Self-reliance in social development. Key Social Issues, p. 19.

5

HEALTH EDUCATION: THE LEADING EDGE OF PRIMARY HEALTH CARE AND MATERNAL AND CHILD HEALTH

JEROME GROSSMAN, PH.D.

No idea has had greater impact on our thinking about public health in the second half of the 20th Century than the realization that ordinary people – acting for themselves, their families, their communities – can do more to promote and maintain personal and public health than scores of health workers can do for them.

How people behave – individually and collectively – is now clearly seen as a key factor in health promotion and disease prevention.

"The health sciences and professions are undergoing a revolution in theory and practice that promises to alter radically traditional notions about the nature of human health and disease. At the core of this revolution is the belief that human behavior and its social determinants are critical variables for understanding the etiology, treatment, and prevention of many disorders."[1]

So significant is acceptance of the concept that it has led to calls for dramatic change in our way of thinking.

In the USA, a "second" public health revolution is underway emphasizing health promotion, prevention and protection with a focus on helping people to learn to adopt behaviors which are central to their wellbeing. Participation in organized action to assure a proper environment for such action is also part of the "new look." Internationally, the milestone declaration of Alma Ata and the vision of Health for All by the Year 2000 are similarly directed.

"Throughout the world, it seems to me," observed Dr. Halfdan Mahler, then Director General of the WHO, "in countries rich and poor alike, those who wish to improve the quality of life will do well to reflect on man's behavior as the basis of much of his health."[2]

The leading edge in anticipating and responding to the challenge of these initiatives has been entrusted to the field of health education. From a traditional concern with "health publicity," health education is now, in its most advanced form, the bridge between the practice of public health and the need to integrate social, behavioral and cultural science in public health concept.

"This is a substantial departure from the traditional approach in which the health education component of policies was defined in connection with highly targeted programmes concerned with disease control or family planning and which were carried out according to professional values and expectations. Targeted disease control programmes are still necessary, but they should fall increasingly within the community's own framework of a comprehensive health and development programme."[3]

In this maturation process, we have learned to ask new questions and to look in new places for the information which we need to function intelligently. We become, each in our own way, students of how people learn, and how individual and social change can be facilitated. We have learned to ask questions such as:

- Why do women not take advantage of prenatal care when it is available and accessible?
- Why do families take advantage of only one immunization for their children in an intended series of three?
- Why do people fail to practice the most basic rules of personal hygiene, when the resources for them to do so are easily available?

SCOPE AND NATURE OF HEALTH EDUCATION

Activities sharing the common description of "health education" display enormous reach and contrast. They may range from the distribution of a single page of directions for infant feeding to complex social organization processes.

Such broad scope is not surprising in view of the myriad needs and countless situations in which it is important for people to learn to behave in ways in the pursuit of health and well being.

What does differentiate one type of "health education" from another is, however, not the scope and nature of the activities themselves but the purpose and values which energize them. Health education in the terms presented here refers to a process which takes place as people learn to know, to value and to act in a manner which helps them achieve and sustain adequate levels of health for themselves and their families.

There are many times in public health practice when a choice must be made about the manner in which behavior is to be influenced. At times, we opt for procedures which force compliance through the use of police power or sanctions against those who do not conform. Or we may offer rewards entirely removed from the purpose for which individuals are encouraged to learn. The values in these cases make the individual's decision-making role secondary to the public health purpose as conceived by the service givers or social policy setters.

A wholly different set of purpose and value emphasizes the central role of the individual in learning to know, to value, to assume primary responsibility for his or her decisions and actions.

The direction of this process is first in developing competence for meaningful problem assessment, resource mobilization and personal action, and secondly in utilizing that competence in social action. Fundamental to this concept is the emphasis on the helper's role of facilitating growth in self direction. It is a value which places the individual at the center of our concern and takes into account the role which social, cultural, environmental, and economic factors play in determining the possibilities of acting.

Health education so conceived is a process of planned change: To practice that art is to commit to a helping relationship; to practice the science is to function with understanding of the learning process.

There is much yet to learn about learning. But there are many things we do know. And the practiced application of that knowledge is what will distinguish professionals from amateurs.

People grow and develop in a social and cultural environment. The learning which is inherent in this process is neither formal nor explicit. Its most important elements are an internalization of values – learning what is important and worthwhile – and compliance with the norms, beliefs and expectations of the reference groups which are central to the experience. This is particularly true in more stable cultural situations such as those non-urban areas of the developing world in which values, norms, expectations may pass from one generation to the next with little or no change for long periods.

Thus concern for the process of helping people learn must be acted upon with an awareness that the behaviors of individuals with whom we work are a function of a long and powerful learning process. One must enter into that process with respect for that which has gone before. There are no "blank tablets."

These highlights of conceptual and value concerns of health education can be further explored in the context of the three broad and interrelated perspectives which follow.

THREE PERSPECTIVES

HEALTH EDUCATION AS MEANS

The most conventional and persistent perception of health education among professional and lay persons is that of a series of activities in which the educational effort is a means, strategy, tactic or other intermediate process aimed at facilitating the achievement of a public health goal or purpose by securing a desired behavior on the part of a "target" group.

It is education which is valued primarily as a means to attain specific health goals. This perception of health education is a "top-down" process in which information and recommended practices are passed from knowledgeable sources (the health establishment) to less informed (the public). The implementation of this model usually involves the dissemination of information to reach those assumed to be in need or those whose failure to act is seen as the root cause of the public health problem.

The technology of information dissemination comes into play and individuals versed in the use of that technology play a prominent part in planning and development of strategies.

Among many health service policy makers, these activities are synonymous with health education and a majority of the resources allocated to health education are devoted to them.

Such programs appear to assume that the achievement of behavioral outcomes results from reaching individuals with information, advice and "motivating" material. There is no greater fallacy which contributes to public health failure and resource wastage than this assumption.

The most troublesome aspect of this perspective, moreover, is its repeated tendency to assume that failure to achieve the desired outcome is a failure of the individual concerned. Such a premise has been labeled "blaming the victim" and has become universally apparent in preventive and health risk reduction efforts.[4]

We "blame the victim" when we ignore the social (including political and economic), cultural and environmental context in which lifestyle choices are made. "Blaming the victim" is to ignore the fact that it does no good to implore mothers to utilize food which is not available to them. Or to fail to recognize the irrelevance of long term prevention in an environment which harbors immediate life threats.

However well intentioned and carefully prepared the storehouse of knowledge available to transmit to people, we will experience consistent failure in efforts to help people learn if we pass this knowledge on with indirect, largely anonymous methods which are not supported by other learning opportunities.

As an example, the UNICEF-produced Facts of Life, a compilation of 55 priority messages, is said to be "the most important information now available to help parents protect their children's lives and growth – knowledge which has the potential to drastically reduce child deaths and child malnutrition,"[5] Yet knowledge is an abstraction (without nutritional value) and its conversion to practice is a function of a complex set of variables, many of which lie outside the control of the person or family. The question to be asked is whether UNICEF's plea to "put the knowledge at the disposal of today's parents" will be accompanied by support for the complex of learning experiences which are required. This point is illustrated by Adik Wibowo's review of case studies in Indonesia. She reports an instance in West Java where 74.7% of expectant mothers knew the why and where of obtaining care – but only 29.3% availed themselves of the opportunity.[6]

Certainly efforts to work directly with people on specific problems – advocating specific changes in diet, in choice of caregiver, in responding to emergency, in recognizing problems at an early stage, in promoting preventive action – will always have a place of utmost importance in a comprehensive approach to maternal and child health. But such interaction is without effect if it does not demonstrate an appropriate understanding of the situation or the educational problem.

Authentic health education processes respond to needs as people with problems see them and try to help in terms meaningful to the individual, family or group. It is not selling, preaching, directing or fooling – it will not be accomplished in isolated minutes at the conclusion of a consultation or a picture show in a crowded hallway.

Interaction which results in learning is not restricted to the opportunities provided by contact with health service persons. Much greater results, in fact, occur when we tap into existing communication and trust networks. Members of the community, peers, concerned kin, recognized leaders, are all the most important "educators" we can identify. Many programs are purposely designed to involve these "significant others" in the change process. The involvement of such resources as volunteers and other community-based supporting workers as partners in health development is one of the most significant breakthroughs taking place in the strengthening of health education as part of the primary health care revolution now in progress.

HEALTH EDUCATION AS HUMAN DEVELOPMENT

If we allow ourselves a larger view of need and opportunity for health education, away from specific, limited concern with specific acts, it is apparent that education must be synonymous with human development. This is a perspective in which the goal is helping individuals develop confidence and competence in a whole range of decision making without dependence on specific interventions by professional workers. This perspective has the added dimension of concern with the skills which enable people to be productive participants in collaborative community-based actions.

Human development goals are an expression of empowerment strategies which are now a legitimate aspect of public health. This concept, as elaborated by the political scientist George Kent, is "something more than local people following instructions or answering questions. To be empowered is to increase your capacity to define, analyze and act on your own problems. . . if you do something differently," (breast feed instead of bottle feed, for example) "you do it not because you were told to do that but because you arrived at an understanding of the situation in which you decided for yourself that changing your behavior would be in your best interest."[7]

The probability that health agencies are not yet well equipped to engage fully in this type of educational endeavor has two implications. The first is that preparation of workers, of volunteers, of influential others in the community to enable them to understand, value and carry on this type of assistance is a necessary priority in all programs. A second implication is the need to reach out to community development groups and non-governmental agencies who have the skill and commitment to share in educational efforts.

Whatever the intended direction of work with mothers or youth, a number of common guidelines can be utilized. The following are adapted from a longer set suggested by Lyra Srinivasan.[8]

1. Relate health education to perceived priorities of everyday life.
2. Recognize that "motivation" needs to come from inner conviction rather than external incentives.
3. Adult education requires an opportunity to clarify values, discern cause-effect relationships, make considered judgments and take responsibility for action.
4. In rural development people are their own major resource, and need to be prepared in a variety of leadership roles in support of educational programs.
5. Learning materials can be developed locally with the involvement of learners.

HEALTH EDUCATION AS SOCIAL ACTION

A third perspective of health education moves away from the focus on influencing individual behavior in some specific way to an involvement of people in the kind of social action which will provide or create conditions which are necessary prerequisites for health and for learning. This approach stems from the unavoidable conclusion that many of the barriers to health are in the social and physical environment and that citizens require skill and confidence to participate in collaborative efforts to change those conditions. Health education thus becomes the mechanism "to ensure that individuals and communities can express their views on health policy and take an active part in the planning and delivery of health programs."[9]

These approaches to health education are a far cry from concepts which look on the individual who does not behave as we would wish as the problem. It is important to recognize, for example, that the health services themselves often are "the problem" when they are inappropriate, poorly delivered, inaccessible or insensitive to the cultural imperatives of time and place.

A particularly insightful analysis of the relationship of such approaches to maternal and child health is that of Peggy Antrobus.[10]

"Though attempts have been made to secure participation in decision making processes . . . all too often it is the men who participate. Women's invisibility leads to failure to take their needs, concerns and perspectives into account. When these strategies do focus on women they tend to treat them as 'passive recipients' or 'target groups' for the benefits rather than as adults with their own strengths, wisdom and capacity to manage their own affairs."

ILLUSTRATIONS FROM ASIA

INDONESIA

Posyandu is the Indonesian term for an integrated service post which functions at the community level to provide needed preventive service for mothers and children. Within the Posyandu, a range of previously separate activities is brought together in a single approach. Educational activities, group and individual are an interwoven part of this total package.

A second, equally important concept underlying the Posyandu movement is the involvement of citizens in active leadership functions in the identification of problems, and planning and implementation of community programs, activities carried out in collaborative efforts with the health service and other development staff. The integrated Posyandu system, primarily the responsibility of the Ministry of Health, and the village development system of the National Family Welfare Movement, operate side by side complementing and supplementing each other's responsibility. The glue which holds the concept and its operation together is a constant commitment to health education.[11]

SRI LANKA

Active efforts to enlist the support of the community in the conduct of development efforts are a hallmark of contemporary public health. They are based on the premise that the trust, concern and long-term helping relationship which can be established within a community by individuals who are part of that community are critical elements of an educational process which the health professional cannot easily provide when working alone.

A broad range of different programs designed to enlist such support is in evidence throughout the world. Sri Lanka was among the first to implement a systematic plan to involve volunteer recruits on a long-term basis. The Sri Lanka initiative was based on the happy fact that the island republic has one of the region's most comprehensive educational systems and highest literacy rates. The fact that many well educated young people and older residents in rural areas had communication skills, time, and interest to participate as community health leaders provided a rich resource to build on. So timely was the idea that a nationwide network of volunteers who assumed responsibility for developing long-term helping relationships with the families of their communities came into being in a relatively short time. These citizens, mostly women, engage in a range of tasks which includes helping with immunization and growth monitoring records, matching needs with available resources, assisting in referral to next level of service and keeping the health service and development staff aware and sensitive to the needs and problems of the area. Above all, they provide the kind of help which is the best guarantee of effective health education.[12]

THAILAND

Bangkok, a magnificent metropolis of over six million inhabitants, is in a period of rapid modernization. Its very growth has left in its wake scores of areas in which people live in congested (slum) conditions. To help deal with the problems citizens of such areas face, the Department of Health Education of the Mahidol University Faculty of Public Health has undertaken a service and study project testing the appropriateness of a community development approach within an urban slum area.

The program, supported from both public and private sources, was oriented in its original concept to maternal and child health needs. Instead of a conventional service program, however, the Department embarked on a broad community development venture in which resident groups were organized to assume responsibility to define and work on problems with technical assistance and seed money from the program.

The work has proceeded over a number of years. The first of the community-desired goals was usually environmental clean-up programs which were entered into with enthusiasm by area residents. With the confidence in staff and the increasing competence of community leadership which emerged, maternal and child health service activities were then initiated with the slum area itself a "delivery point" for preventive and care services. Participation by residents in the management of service and recruitment of eligible clients was an important dimension of action.

The program thus avoided the usual campaign and mass information distribution activities which previous efforts by the established agencies had attempted. Health education was, instead, a part of the way things were done and an outcome of the participatory planning and implementation processes which evolved. When information, advice, and suggestions were passed on, as they increasingly were, it was the leadership of the communities and the influential members of the families involved who were the teachers – and the health workers who were the learners.[13]

FEEDBACK AND ASSESSMENT

As with any other program element, health education requires a continuing and systematic feedback and assessment component if it is to function wisely. It is subject to the same evaluative standards which govern all purposeful action – seeking to secure data which can help in the interpretation of progress toward intended outcomes. There is an important need as well to document what we are learning about the task at hand.

There are several significant cautions, however, which are relevant to evaluation of health education. First, health education has not yet developed the full range of indicators which may be more common in assessment of conditions involving morbidity and mortality. Although progress is being made in efforts to identify dimensions of educational effort – knowledge, value clarification, behavior – which can form a basis of assessment, expectations for precision and specificity of measurement in this field are not likely to be easily realized.

Second, educational evaluation contends with the fact that a variety of essentially similar activities may be carried out with different objectives and, as a result, with differing judgments of the value of outcomes. Competing notions of the desired direction and purpose of education must first be clarified before any meaningful assessment is possible.

A third and underlined caution is the contention that educational initiatives never operate in a vacuum. The kinds of changes sought are rarely attributable to any single "cause." Interpretation of outcome must therefore rest on analysis of a range of factors which may be involved and the nature of the assumptions on which the program was based. "Magic bullets" – single interventions acting alone to produce a desired outcome – are not possible to assume in the educational domain.

Last, there is the reality that the kinds of changes to which education addresses itself tend to be more long term in their achievement than the short-term outcomes which are frequently sought.

Particularly relevant for educational evaluation is the concept that programs develop in stages and that the evaluative questions must be appropriate to the stage in which the effort exists.[14] We cannot expect to secure valid impact data, for example, from efforts which have not yet developed to a point where such outcomes can be expected.

Most discussions of evaluation, this one included, start from the vantage point of the service provider. In keeping with a philosophy reiterated through this chapter, however, it would follow that the most meaningful data belong to the people or groups whose needs are the subject of our efforts. Evaluation, then, must certainly reflect data and insights from these individuals. The "learners" must have a key role in evaluation and an opportunity to participate in analysis of how well they are learning, how useful or important the learning has been and to what extent it has an impact on their health and quality of life.

REFERENCES

1. Marsella, A.J., and A.Dash-Scheuer. Coping, Culture and Healthy Human Development, Health and Cross Cultural Psychology. P.R. Dasen, J.W. Berry and N. Sartorus (ed). Berkeley Hills: Sage, 1988, pp. 162-178.

2. Mahler, H. The health of the family. Presented to the International Health Conference of the National Council for International Health, October 1974.

3. World Health Organization. New Approaches to Health Education in Primary Health Care. Technical Report Series 690. Geneva: WHO, 1983.

4. Labonte, R., and S. Porterfield. Canadian perspectives in health education. Health Education, April 1981.

5. Grant, J.P. Teaching health professionals to teach, address presented to Third International Symposium on Health in the Asia Pacific Region, Jakarta 1988. Bangkok: Asia Pacific Consortium for Public Health, 1989.

6. Wibowo, A. National health care, a review of functional studies in Indonesia. Presented to the Third International Symposium on Health in Asia and the Pacific Region, Jakarta, 1988. Jakarta: Faculty of Public Health, 1988.

7. Kent, G. Empowerment for Child Survival. Honolulu: Department of Political Science, University of Hawaii, 1988.

8. Srinivasan, L. Perspective on Non-Formal Adult Learning. New York: World Education, 1977.

9. World Health Organization, op. cit.

10. Antrobus, P. Feminist issues in development, reports. World Education Association, Fall 1987.

11. From material prepared by Dr. S.L. Leimena, Director General of Community Health, Ministry of Health, Jakarta, December 1988.

12. From material prepared by Dr. Walter Patrick, Professor, University of Hawaii and former director of training, Central Health Education Bureau Government of Sri Lanka.

13. From material prepared by Professor Somjit Supannatas, Chairman, Department of Health Education, Faculty of Public Health, Mahidol University, Bangkok.

14. Blum, H. Planning for Health. New York: Human Sciences Press, 1974.

6

AIDS IN MOTHERS AND CHILDREN IN DEVELOPING COUNTRIES

RICHARD J. GUIDOTTI, M.D. AND JONATHAN MANN, M.D.

INTRODUCTION

The AIDS (acquired immunodeficiency syndrome) pandemic is recognized as a new and in some ways unprecedented threat to health. It is estimated that from the beginning of the HIV pandemic in the mid–1970s until mid–1988, approximately 450,000 cases of AIDS have occurred worldwide. At least five million people throughout the world became infected with HIV (the AIDS virus) and of these, it is estimated that 1.5 million are women. Nearly one million of those HIV-infected women live in Africa, and WHO estimates that approximately 80,000 HIV-infected births occurred between 1980 and 1987. These estimates are based on a fertility rate for an HIV-infected woman of one live birth in every three years and a conservative estimate of a 25% perinatal transmission rate (range 12%-65%).[1]

Projections have recently been made regarding the substantial impact of mother-to-infant transmission of HIV on under-five childhood mortality. For example, in a population where 10% of the women are infected with HIV, and given a 25% perinatal transmission rate, the under-five mortality rate will be increased by 18%. This increase will reach 36% in a population where 20% of women are HIV-infected; thus, if the under-five mortality rate is 100 per 1000 live births without HIV infection, an additional 36 deaths per 1000 will be due to HIV, giving a rate of 136/1000.[1]

The importance of the AIDS pandemic to maternal and child health workers became obvious as more was learned about perinatal transmission. Important questions include: How does a virus which affects immune mechanisms, alter the course of pregnancy (a condition which of itself has an altered immune response)? What effect does HIV have on the fetus and newborn?

68

What recommendations should a health worker give an HIV-infected woman regarding breast-feeding and immunization for her child? Are there any known contraindications to prescribing contraceptives to an HIV-infected woman? What precautions should a health worker take when delivering a woman who is HIV-infected?

This chapter will attempt to answer some of these questions using the best information available, bearing in mind that AIDS is a relatively new disease and much is still to be learned.

GEOGRAPHICAL DISTRIBUTION OF AIDS

THREE PATTERNS OF INFECTION:

Since AIDS was first recognized in 1981, three general patterns of HIV infection and AIDS have emerged, all based on the same fundamental routes of HIV transmission (through sexual intercourse, exposure to blood and from infected mother to fetus or infant).[2] In Pattern I countries like the U.S., Canada, many Western European countries, Australia, New Zealand and parts of Latin America, transmission of HIV occurs mainly among homosexual or bisexual males and urban intravenous (IV) drug users. Heterosexual transmission is responsible for a small percentage of cases, but is increasing. Moreover, the male-to-female sex ratio of reported AIDS cases ranged from 10-15 to 1 and perinatal transmission is not common. An exception to this rule exists in some inner cities of Pattern I countries where the epidemiology of AIDS differs because of greater numbers of IV drug users, leading to more heterosexual spread and consequently more perinatal transmission.

Pattern II countries would include most countries in sub-Saharan Africa and increasingly, certain Latin American countries, particularly those of the Caribbean. For MCH health workers in these countries it is important to note that HIV infection is distributed roughly equally among women and men, that the incidence of infection is relatively high and that as a result, HIV infection in pregnant women and their newborns is of major concern. It is also important to note that peak age-specific HIV seroprevalence rates in Pattern II areas generally occur among young (15-24 year-old) women who also have the highest fertility rates.

Pattern III countries include Eastern Europe, North Africa, the Middle East, Asia and most of the Pacific (excluding Australia and New Zealand). Only about one percent of all AIDS cases reported to WHO have come from Pattern III countries. The few reported cases can be traced to IV drug use, homosexual and heterosexual transmission among small well-defined groups.

Imported blood and blood products have also been responsible for HIV transmission in some of these areas. The sex ratio, with respect to HIV infection in these countries varies greatly and in those areas where IV drug use is a large problem, a preponderance of males is infected.

Although these three distinct patterns can serve as a guide to health workers for their particular geographical area, it must be emphasized that the AIDS pandemic is dynamic and continuing to evolve. Updating of HIV epidemiology and surveillance will be needed in order to provide health workers with current accurate information on its distribution patterns.

MODES OF TRANSMISSION

The human immunodeficiency virus (HIV) is transmitted through sexual intercourse (either homosexual or heterosexual), contamination with HIV-infected blood (e.g., blood transfusions, accidental injury with contaminated needles, sharing of needles by drug users), and perinatally. The relative frequency of transmission in utero/transplacental, connatal (at time of birth), or shortly after birth is not known. There are some suggestive data that a large proportion of mother-to-infant transmission of HIV may be transplacental. These three modes are responsible for the global pandemic, although their relative importance varies geographically and temporally. For example, transmission via blood transfusion has become less common with donor deferral and institution of screening methods for HIV infection, while perinatal transmission may increase due to more heterosexual spread.

Maternal Child Health (MCH) care workers should familiarize themselves with all three modes of HIV transmission.

As providers of antenatal care, MCH workers will likely come into contact with pregnant women who may be HIV infected or may want information on AIDS.

As attendants to birth, MCH workers should be aware of the general HIV seroprevalence rates of the population they serve, and knowledge of precautions to take in the delivery of all women (universal precautions).

As providers of postpartum care and well-baby clinics, MCH workers will be confronted with questions on breast-feeding by HIV-infected women as well as decisions regarding immunization of a child born to an HIV-infected mother.

As providers of family planning services, clinical gynecological procedures and treatment of sexually transmitted diseases, health workers must know the facts about AIDS in order to give correct advice.

SCREENING FOR HIV

The question arises whether women attending antenatal clinics should be screened routinely for HIV. In the past, perinatal screening for certain conditions has offered the possibility of being a major tool for prevention. It is, however, important to remember the general problem that screening may lead to either unnecessary anxiety or a false sense of security by yielding false positive or false negative results, respectively. In addition, the profound personal and social impact of HIV infection has led to a heightened awareness of the ethical and legal aspects of screening, particularly regarding informed consent and confidentiality.

Current recommendations by the U.S. Centers for Disease Control (CDC) are that women who fall into so-called "high-risk" groups should be offered HIV testing routinely. These groups usually include IV drug users, women in liaison with HIV-infected men or with men who themselves have an increased risk of HIV infection (e.g., bisexuals, IV drug users), and prostitutes. (For countries where either epidemiological Pattern I or III currently exists, this recommendation may also apply; however, for countries with a Pattern II where the definition of a high-risk group may include a larger percent of the population, the identification of "high-risk" pregnant women may not be practical.)

The requirements for a worthwhile perinatal screening program were outlined by Cuckle and Wald[3] even before AIDS was recognized. It is interesting to see how these requirements apply to screening pregnant women for HIV. The authors listed eight requirements for a successful perinatal screening program.

1. The disorder should be well defined.
2. The prevalence should be known.
3. The condition should be medically important and there should be an effective remedy.
4. The program should be cost-effective.
5. Procedures following a positive result should be generally agreed and acceptable both to the screening authorities and to the patients.
6. Facilities should be available or easily installed.
7. The test should be simple and safe.
8. Distribution of test values in affected and unaffected individuals should be known.

It appears that a voluntary screening program among pregnant women for HIV infection using the ELISA method, and if positive, followed by a supplemental test (such as Western Blot) would satisfy these conditions in some countries. Of course the issue of what constitutes an "effective remedy" remains of primary concern. AIDS differs from other perinatal conditions. Unlike syphilis, there are no curative therapies for HIV infection and AIDS. The probability that the fetus will be HIV-infected is not precisely known, unlike screening for certain genetic conditions. Current studies on intrauterine transmission of HIV provide estimates from 12-65%, complicating decision-making on early therapeutic abortion. At present the only "effective remedy" for a pregnant woman who is HIV-infected consists of providing her with the best information available regarding the risks to herself and her infant. This information must be accompanied by compassionate counseling aimed toward helping her make decisions on her present as well as future pregnancies.

The question of cost-effectiveness always arises when considering screening programs, especially in countries with extremely limited health resources and budgets. In estimating the cost-effectiveness of a screening program, one must consider the prevalence of the condition screened for, the accuracy of the test (number of false positive, as well as false negative results) under "local" conditions, and the cost of individuals tests. At present the false positive rate for the ELISA test is under 1 in 5000, or 0.22% under ideal (reference laboratory) situations; under less than ideal conditions, it has been shown to be 0.6% or higher.

An example would be the testing of 100,000 pregnant women for HIV infection in whom the prevalence of infection is 1 per 10,000 (0.01%). Assuming the test is carried out under ideal conditions and has a false positive rate of 0.02%, then twenty women would be expected to test falsely positive. Therefore, of thirty positive results (10 true positives and 20 false positives) the positive predictive value of the test in identifying an infected person was only 33%. At current prices an ELISA test costs US$0.75, the above disappointing results cost, for the laboratory test alone, a total of US$75,000.[4]

If the prevalence of HIV is assumed to be 8 per 1000 (0.8%), then 800 women would be correctly identified and only 20 would be false positives, which is a more acceptable positive predictive value of over 97%. On the other hand, if the more realistic false positive rate of 0.6% is used we are left with an unacceptable 600 women who test falsely positive and a positive predictive value in this situation of about 57%.[4]

False negative results (women who have the condition and test negative) can occur in two ways. First, the test result is wrong (when the person has antibodies to the HIV, but is interpreted as not having antibodies). Second, when the person has no antibodies, but has nevertheless been infected with

HIV (the so-called "window effect"). It is thought that this time period may vary from between two months to much longer periods (up to a year or two), although most people appear to develop antibodies within three months. The reasons for these variations are not known, but may be related to the initial infecting dose of HIV, the route of infection and individual factors.

Decisions on prenatal screening practices will undoubtedly change in accordance with updated information on the natural history of AIDS, as well as the availability of more practical and cost-effective tests.

DIAGNOSING AIDS IN WOMEN AND CHILDREN

Making a diagnosis of AIDS in pregnant women may be difficult in developing countries which lack the facilities to diagnose the "AIDS indicator" diseases (primarily opportunistic infections). WHO has developed a clinical definition for areas where diagnostic resources are limited. According to this definition, AIDS in an adult is defined by the existence of at least two of the following major signs and associated with at least two of the following minor signs, and in the absence of known immunosuppression, such as cancer or severe malnutrition of other recognized etiologies.[5]

1. Major Signs
   a. weight loss $\geq$ 10% of body weight
   b. chronic diarrhea > 1 month
   c. prolonged fever > 1 month (intermittent or constant)

2. Minor Signs
   a. persistent cough for > 1 month
   b. generalized pruritic dermatitis
   c. recurrent herpes zoster
   d. oro-pharyngeal candidiasis
   e. chronic progressive and disseminated herpes simplex infection
   f. generalized lymphadenopathy

The presence of generalized Kaposi's sarcoma or cryptococcal meningitis is sufficient by itself for the diagnosis of AIDS.

The influences of pregnancy on the natural history of HIV infection are as yet unclear. Early studies, using small retrospective and biased samples, suggested that pregnancy accelerated the onset of AIDS in HIV-infected pregnant women. However, a more recent, large prospective study suggests no such effect.[6]

Serological testing for the presence of HIV infection in the newborn is fraught with difficulties. Testing cord blood for HIV infection in the newborn gives inconclusive results since maternal IgG antibodies cross the placenta. Follow-up studies have revealed that maternal antibody may be detectable for up to 18 months in some cases; however, 15 months has been suggested as a cutoff value. The slow clearance rate of maternal antibodies could explain the earlier high estimates of intrauterine infection rates reported in the literature. Testing for the newborn's IgM anti-HIV antibodies has not been helpful. It is presently estimated that between 12 and 65% of newborns acquire infection from HIV-infected mothers. It is estimated that worldwide more than 80% of pediatric AIDS cases are a result of perinatal transmission and as blood transfusions become safer this percentage will increase.

Diagnosing pediatric AIDS in both developed and developing countries has met with the same difficulties as described for adults in developing countries. A case definition for pediatric AIDS was established for developing countries. AIDS should be suspected in an infant or child presenting with at least two of the following major signs and associated with at least two of the following minor signs and in the absence of known immunosuppression such as cancer or severe malnutrition of other recognized etiologies.

1. Major Signs
   a. weight loss or abnormally slow growth
   b. chronic diarrhea > 1 month
   c. prolonged fever > 1 month

2. Minor Signs
   a. generalized lymphadenopathy
   b. oro-pharyngeal candidiasis
   c. repeated common infections (otitis, pharyngitis, etc.)
   d. persistent cough
   e. generalized dermatitis
   f. confirmed maternal HIV infection

DELIVERY PRACTICES

The transmission of HIV infection via blood has special meaning for MCH workers, midwives and home birth attendants. Obstetric patients receive more blood transfusions than other patients and every effort should be made to ensure safety. Health workers have a responsibility to ensure than any transfusion is clearly indicated and that its benefits outweigh its risks. Birth attendants are also exposed to relatively large quantities of blood during a delivery and should be diligent in following, as far as possible, universal precautions to protect themselves from HIV infection.[7]

In obstetrics a blood transfusion is usually given to a woman if she has lost greater than 500 ml of blood. Guidelines on transfusion requirements should be made locally and will be influenced by the overall health status of the population (prevalence of anemia, malaria, malnutrition, etc.). Acute blood loss must be dealt with urgently. Plasma expanders (crystalloids or colloids) are often preferable to the use of whole blood since volume replacement is often more urgent than red cell replacement, delay is inevitable with blood transfusion, and there are unavoidable dangers associated with blood transfusions. The critical decision involves the use of plasma expanders over blood; any transfusion which is not indicated is contraindicated.[8]

Prevention of hemorrhage is of primary importance in obstetrics and can be achieved in many cases. For example, a woman will almost never have a fatal hemorrhage due to a placenta previa if health workers treat all third trimester antepartum bleeding as a possible placenta previa, making sure that no vaginal exams are done and referring the patient immediately.

Use of partographs, the manual removal of retained placentas together with the judicious use of oxytocics could prevent a large number of postpartum hemorrhages.

There have been many incidents of blood spillage involving HIV, but only a few incidents have so far resulted in infection; it is estimated that less than one-half of one percent (<0.5%) of needlestick injuries involving confirmed HIV-infected patients and health workers have been documented to result in HIV infection. This is a low risk of infection compared to a similar exposure to hepatitis B virus.

Sterilization of all instruments used for delivery is important to prevent HIV transmission. HIV is readily inactivated by standard methods of sterilization and high-level disinfection. Methods used to inactivate other virus (e.g., hepatitis B virus) will also inactivate HIV.[9]

POST-PARTUM CARE

Following the birth of a baby from an HIV-infected mother, the health worker will be faced with three important aspects of MCH care: breast-feeding, contraception and child immunization.

Breast-Feeding

Although there are documented cases of HIV infection via breast milk, the current WHO recommendation is that breast-feeding by the biological mother, irrespective of her HIV-infection status, should be the feeding method of choice in areas where safe alternatives are not reliably available.[10]

Given present knowledge, the immunological, nutritional, psychosocial and child-spacing benefits of breast-feeding outweigh the little understood and possibly infrequent transmission of HIV through this method. Furthermore, the beneficial effects that breast-feeding provides in preventing intercurrent infections in children already exposed to HIV in utero should be considered. Further research is needed to clarify the risks of HIV transmission through breast milk and its potential benefits in situations where infants have been exposed to HIV or are already infected. Until this information is available, health workers in areas where safe effective use of alternatives is not possible should encourage mothers to breast-feed.

Use of Contraceptives

The possibility that there may be an interaction of oral contraceptives with HIV infection has caused some concern among MCH health workers. Oral contraceptives induce subtle changes in the vaginal and cervical epithelium (cervix ectropion), and it has been speculated that these changes may enhance susceptibility to HIV infection. The two studies which had shown an association between HIV and oral contraceptives had serious defects in research methodology.[11] Until adequate studies are conducted, the interaction between oral contraceptives and HIV infection is theoretical speculation. Intrauterine devices can also cause cervical irritation providing a portal of entry for infections which could have serious consequences in an HIV-infected woman. No epidemiological data, however, are currently available on the relationship between HIV infection and the use of IUDs.

Latex condoms have been documented to be impermeable to HIV in *in vitro* studies and an increasing number of studies (heterosexual couples, prostitutes) have demonstrated a reduction in HIV transmission when condoms are properly used. A woman must be informed that in addition to her current contraceptive practice, condoms should also be used when prevention of HIV infection is also required.

The choice of contraceptive methods for an individual/couple should continue to take into account the risks and benefits of each method, and the particular lifestyle of the individuals concerned.

CHILDHOOD IMMUNIZATION

Concern regarding the safety of routine child immunization in HIV-infected children led to a review of available information by the WHO Expanded Programme on Immunization (EPI) Global Advisory Group, who in turn made the following recommendations regarding the use of immunizing antigens:

"In countries where human immunodeficiency virus (HIV) is considered a problem, individuals should be immunized with the EPI antigens according to standard schedules. This also applies to individuals with asymptomatic HIV infection. Non-immunized individuals with clinical AIDS in countries where the EPI target disease remain serious risks should not receive BCG, but should receive the other vaccines."[12]

In addition, the group recommended the use of inactivated poliomyelitis vaccine as an alternative to OPV (live virus vaccine) in children with symptomatic HIV infection, and that BCG may be withheld from individuals known or suspected to be infected with HIV in areas where the risk of tuberculosis is known to be low.

Irrespective of HIV status, pregnant women should receive tetanus toxoid as prescribed.

OTHER SEXUALLY TRANSMITTED DISEASES

On a worldwide basis, sexual transmission is the most important route of HIV spread. Recent studies have suggested that sexually transmitted diseases (STD) may facilitate the transmission of HIV. While HIV is transmitted sexually in the absence of other STD, the weight of the evidence for genital ulcer disease (GUD) as a risk factor for HIV transmission is strong.[13] Since it is biologically plausible that any ulcer or inflammation caused by STD can increase infectiousness to HIV infection, health workers should institute appropriate therapy in any person with clinical symptoms of STD. Furthermore, the person must be counseled as to the increased risk of acquiring HIV infection and the association with genital ulcers.

THE FUTURE

There is no vaccine at present for the prevention of AIDS and most virologists agree that a vaccine is at least five years away and will not be easily developed. Presently, physicians treat the opportunistic infections or provide symptomatic relief for some of the conditions that develop due to the altered immune state of a patient with AIDS. These infections are usually difficult to treat and require long-term therapy. There are no antiviral drugs that permanently rid the body of HIV. At the present time, Zidovudine (also known as AZT) is the only anti-retroviral agent. AZT has not yet been evaluated in pregnant women. However, Zidovudine is expensive and has a relatively high level of toxicity.

Barring a dramatic medical breakthrough, the only effective weapon we presently have against the AIDS pandemic is educating people to avoid becoming infected. In many ways, MCH workers are in the front line in the battle against AIDS. A woman visiting an MCH clinic may represent the first contact point with the health system. It is at this contact where information and education could help prevent AIDS, and where questions concerning AIDS could be answered. With this in mind, the MCH health workers must be updated periodically on new knowledge of AIDS which will affect their work in the prevention, diagnosis and management of HIV-infected persons. The role of MCH services in the efforts against HIV/AIDS should be emphasized at the national and international level.

REFERENCES

1. Chin, J., and G. Sankaran, et al. Mother-to-infant transmission of HIV: an increasing global problem. In: Maternal and Child Care in Developing Countries. E. Kessel and A.K. Awan (eds.). Thun, Switzerland: Ott Publisher, 1989.

2. Mann, J.M., and J. Chin, et al. The international epidemiology of AIDS. Scientific American October: 60-69,1988.

3. Cuckle, H.S., and N. J. Wald. Principles of screening. In: Wald, N. (ed). Antenatal and Neonatal Screening for Disease. Oxford University Press. 1984.

4. Gordon, G., and T. Klouda. Some facts (Chpt. 1). In: Preventing a Crisis: AIDS and Family Planning Work. London: International Planned Parenthood Federation, pp. 7-24, June 1988.

5. World Health Organization. Acquired immunodeficiency syndrome. Weekly Epidemiology Record, 10:72-73 Geneva: WHO, 1986.

6. Selwyn, P.A., and E.E. Schoenbaum, et al. Prospective study of human immunodeficiency virus infection and pregnancy outcomes in intravenous drug users. Journal of the American Medical Association, vol 261, No 9:1289-1294, Mar 3, 1989.

7. Peckham, C.S., and Y.D. Senturia, et al. Mother-to-child transmission of HIV infection. The European Collaborative Study. Lancet:1039-1042, Nov 1988.

8. World Health Organization. Global programme on AIDS (GPA) guidelines for treatment of acute blood loss. Geneva: WHO, 1988.

9. World Health Organization. WHO AIDS Series No 2 (2d Ed). Guidelines on sterilization and high-level disinfection methods against human immunodeficiency virus (HIV). Geneva: WHO, 1989.

10. World Health Organization. Special Programme on AIDS (SPA) statement from the consultation on breast-feeding/breast milk and human immunodeficiency virus (HIV). Geneva: WHO,1987.

11. Meirik, O., and T. Farley. Special programme on research, development and research training in human reproduction. Evidence that contraceptives such as OCs affect HIV transmission. Geneva, Switzerland: WHO. (In press.)

12. World Health Organization. Special programme on AIDS (SPA) statement from the consultation on human immunodeficiency virus (HIV) and routine childhood immunization. Geneva: WHO, 1987.

13. World Health Organization. Global programme on AIDS (GPA) and programme of STD. Consensus statement from consultation on sexually transmitted diseases as a risk factor for HIV transmission. Geneva: WHO, 1989.

7

PRIMARY HEALTH CARE

Helen M. Wallace, M.D., M.P.H.
Kanti Giri, M.B.B.S., DG.O., F.I.C.S., F.R.C.O.G.

INTRODUCTION

All countries of the world are concerned about the problem of primary health care for their people. This concern includes such aspects as how to provide it; how to achieve coverage for all of the people; how to provide primary health care of some quality; how to make the maximum use of the country's and community's existing resources, both personnel, equipment, and supplies; and how to link up primary health care at the local community level with secondary and tertiary health resources. In 1978, it was estimated that four-fifths of the world's population lacked access to primary health care, mostly disadvantaged people.

It is for these reasons that the International Conference on Primary Health Care was held by the World Health Organization in Alma-Ata, USSR, 6-12 September 1978.[1]

DEFINITION OF PRIMARY HEALTH CARE (PHC)[1]

Primary Health Care is essential health care made universally accessible to individuals and families in the community by means acceptable to them, through their full participation and at a cost that the community and country can afford. It forms an integral part both of the country's health system of which it is the nucleus and of the overall social and economic development of the community.

CONTENT OF PRIMARY HEALTH CARE (PHC)[1]

Primary Health Care addresses the main health problem in the community, providing promotive, preventive, curative and rehabilitative services accordingly. Since these services reflect and evolve from the economic conditions and social values of the country and its communities, they will vary by country and community, but will include at least: Promotion of proper nutrition and an adequate supply of safe water; basic sanitation; maternal and child care, including family planning; immunization against the major infectious diseases; prevention and control of locally endemic diseases; education concerning prevailing health problems and the methods of preventing and controlling them; and appropriate treatment for common diseases and injuries.

GENERAL PRINCIPLES OF PRIMARY HEALTH CARE (PHC)

General principles of PHC include the following:

1. PHC should be shaped around the life styles of the people to be served.
2. PHC should be an integral part of the national health system and other services, in particular supplies, supervision, and referral and technical, should be designed to support the needs at the peripheral level.
3. PHC activities should be fully integrated with the activities of the other sectors involved in community development (agriculture, education, public works, housing, communications).
4. The local population should be actively involved in planning health care, so that it suits their needs and priorities. Decisions on what are the community needs requiring solution should be based upon a continuing dialogue between the people and the services.
5. The health care offered should make use of the available community resources, especially those which have hitherto remained untapped, and should remain within the limits of the funds available.
6. PHC should use an integrated approach of preventive, promotive, curative, and rehabilitative services for individual, family, and community. The balance among these services should vary according to community needs and may well change over time.
7. The majority of health interventions should take place in or as near as possible to the patient's home and be carried out by the worker most simply (but adequately) trained to give the treatment in question.

WHO PROVIDES PRIMARY HEALTH CARE?

Primary health care is usually delivered by community health workers. These are generalized public health workers, usually from the local villages which they serve. They may be full time or part time; they are usually paid. The PHC worker needs to understand and be knowledgeable about the major health problems and needs in his community. For primary health care of women, infants, and children, the traditional birth attendant (TBA) has been the person providing primary health care in the villages. Thus, in developing plans to provide PHC at village level, the TBAs represent a major resource to be called upon and utilized.

TRAINING OF PRIMARY HEALTH CARE WORKERS

In order to provide safe basic PHC, one of the early steps required is to define the roles, duties, and functions the PHC worker is expected to carry out. This "job description" for the community health worker then needs to form the basis, at the very least, for the content of the training program for the PHC worker. That is, the basic training program and its periodic refresher courses need to include content to make it possible for the PHC worker to carry out those tasks expected of them, in order to safeguard the health of the people in the community. This also means that the workers/trainers of the PHC need to be prepared in the appropriate content expected of the PHC staff.

Not only is appropriate teaching/training of the PHC staff essential. Careful supervision of the PHC staff is also essential on the job. Responsibility for their supervision needs to be clearly delineated. The supervisors need to be familiar with the job description of the PHC staff, and with the content necessary to supervise them, as well as methods of supervision.

In a similar fashion, there needs to be a job description of traditional birth attendants (TBAs). Courses for TBAs need to contain content to enable them to provide good safe basic prenatal, labor and delivery, and postpartum care for the mother. They need to be able to teach and carry out principles of safe hygiene, and health education for mother and baby. They need to be taught the principles and content of safe care of the newborn, of observation of the infant, and of breast feeding, and carefully timed supplementary food and weaning. They need to be trained in family planning education, and in well-child supervision of the infants and children. Training courses for TBAs need to contain this content; trainers and supervisors need to be well versed in this content.

Even with the presence and utilization of traditional birth attendants, all PHC staff need to be well prepared in the content of prenatal, intrapartum, postpartum, family planning, and child health care, because of the importance of the health of women and children in the community.

THE UNIQUE ROLE OF FAMILY MEMBERS, ESPECIALLY THE MOTHER

Family members, especially the mother, are often the main providers of health care for the family. It is the mother who raises and cares for the children, as well as other family members. It is the mother who usually raises the food and feeds the family. It is the mother who observes the condition of the children, and who notices and attempts to treat illness in the children. This means that women of the family need to have a good working knowledge of health care, including hygiene, feeding, family planning, and how to follow the child's development and recognize the signs of early illness. Health education, as well as general education of women is essential. Womens' organizations can play an important role.

THE RISK APPROACH

PHC workers need to be taught and be able to utilize the risk approach. This consists of the ability to follow carefully and observe family members, especially pregnant women, infants, and children, for symptoms/signs/risk factors which might lead to suspect the presence of a potential health problem requiring special care and referral. The concept of high risk at a simple basic level needs to be taught to PHC workers. Risk factors recognizable by the PHC worker need to be included in the training of PHC staff. Patients suspected of being potentially of high risk need to be observed and followed more carefully. Arrangements for quick referral of high-risk patients are essential.

LINKAGES TO SECONDARY AND TERTIARY CARE, REFERRAL SYSTEM, AND TRANSPORT

Patients suspected of high risk need to be referred to a resource in or available to the community, able to provide special diagnostic, treatment, and management service and care, especially a health center or local/district hospital. A referral system needs to be established so that easy, smooth, quick, and efficient referrals may be made through a pre-arranged system. Quick safe transport is an important aspect of such a referral system.

INDICATORS OF CARE AND OUTCOME

As with any activity in public health practice, evaluation of results is essential for primary health care. Record keeping is essential. The use of home-based mothers' health records is being tested.[2] The development of a system and of indicators is an important aspect. Basic indicators such as accessibility to health care; births attended by a trained health person; access to safe drinking water; level of immunization; contraceptive prevalence are frequently utilized to evaluate outcome of PHC.

REFERENCES

1. World Health Organization. Primary Health Care. Geneva: WHO, 1978. 49 pages.

2. Kumar, V., and N. Datta. Home-based mothers' health records. World Health Forum 9: 107-110, 1988.

8

PROMOTING MATERNAL AND CHILD HEALTH THROUGH PRIMARY HEALTH CARE

JOHN H. BRYANT,M.D., KAUSER S. KHAN,M.D.,
INAYAT THAVER,M.D.

Bringing about meaningful improvements in the health of mothers and children in Third World countries is an immense and complex undertaking. It is reasonable to think that a strong epidemiological base of understanding about the health problems, and a well designed and managed primary health care (PHC) system should ensure a substantial impact on health of a population. But that may not be the case. When people live in the conditions of severe underdevelopment – deep in poverty, without education, in contaminated environments, under conditions of social fragmentation and political instability – the technologies of health and management alone are not enough.

Here we will examine these issues, beginning with brief observations about the nature of the health problems of mothers and children in Third World countries, and select a few of those problems to serve as paradigms for discussing these larger issues. Then we will look at some approaches to the design, management and evaluation of PHC systems. In the context of such operating systems, we will turn to some of the social, economic and political factors that are strong and disturbing determinants of health outcomes.

PATTERNS OF HEALTH AND ILLNESS IN THIRD WORLD COUNTRIES

The health problems of mothers and children in Third World countries are quite consistent.

In children, the leading causes of ill health and death are malnutrition, immunizable diseases, diarrheal diseases and acute respiratory infections, with further additions depending on local disease endemnicity, such as malaria, schistosomiasis, traffic accidents, etc.

For mothers, the leading threats to health are associated with pregnancy and child birth. Too many pregnancies, spaced too closely together, without adequate antenatal and delivery care contribute to high risks of death and disability. Mothers, too, are vulnerable to locally endemic diseases such as dysentery, tuberculosis, malaria, parasitic infestations, etc. Commonly used indicators of these conditions include:

Infant Mortality Rate (IMR)...annual number of deaths of infants in the first year of life, per 1000 live births.

Under-5 Mortality Rate (U5MR)...annual number of deaths of children under 5 years of age per 1000 live births. (NOTE: this is UNICEF's definition used in *The State of the World's Children, 1989*.)

Maternal Mortality Rate (MMR)...annual number of deaths of women from pregnancy related causes per 100,000 live births.

Applying these indicators to the developed and developing countries of the world reveals the extreme differences in the impact of states of development on the health of mothers and children.

Selected Health and Social Indicators*					
	U5MR Median	IMR Median	MMR Median	%Children malnour. mod/ser	Literacy M/F	Per Capita GNP $/yr
Very High U5MR >170	209	129	420	30/6	43/22	265
High U5MR 95-170	123	84	140	25/5	68/49	740
Mid U5MR 31-94	60	45	91	—	87/80	1230
Low U5MR 30 and under	13	13	11	—	97/90	7295

*From *The State of the World's Children 1989, UNICEF*

The mortality rates quoted above illustrate the striking differences according to levels of socioeconomic development. Generally speaking the mortality indicators correlate inversely with per capita income. There are important exceptions: Some countries have poorer health indicators than expected on the basis of their per capita income, whereas others have achieved a more favorable health status. Caldwell has analyzed situations where there are favorable departures from this relationship and points out that there are usually three explanatory factors. In those countries:

- women have high rates of literacy and cultural autonomy;
- primary health care reaches to the household level; and
- a political system is responsive to public demand.

This study helps to explain the key roles of mothers, primary health care, and political systems as determinants of health, particularly of mothers and children.

While the leading causes of infant and young child mortality can be listed, it is important to understand the ways in which those causes interact with one another, often augmenting or reinforcing one another. Thus, malnutrition renders children more susceptible to infectious diseases, such as diarrhea and respiratory infection. Diarrhea and other infections, in turn, exacerbate the malnutrition, and a child can thereby cycle downward in a deterioration of health. Counteracting such disease complexes often requires dealing simultaneously with more than one condition. These interactions of the causes of death are so common among children who live in poverty and isolation as to give rise to the expression "the road to death." Not only is death commonplace, but efforts to limit mortality are often thwarted. For example, even though one-fourth of under-5 deaths might be due to immunizable diseases, immunizing the children might not decrease mortality by that amount. Even if protected by immunizations, the children would remain vulnerable to the other claims on their lives, and malnutrition and diarrhea or respiratory infection could carry them away.

It is useful to compare the impact of PHC systems on the threats to mortality of children and mothers, as there are important differences. The leading causes of infant and young child mortality can be effectively combated through primary health care. Health services that reach every community, preferably to the household level, where children at risk are identified, and remedial steps taken, including especially involving their mothers; where children are immunized, their growth is monitored, mothers become sensitive to the nutritional status of their children, learn to use oral rehydration salts (ORS) and strive to improve hygienic conditions of the household. There will be children whose illnesses are serious and complex and require referral to more elaborate health facilities, but generally speaking, the greatest part of the burden of childhood illness can be handled through effective PHC systems.

A somewhat different picture emerges for women. Given the major threats to maternal health, namely complications of pregnancy and childbirth, some of those can be dealt with effectively at the PHC level, but others cannot. Training of traditional birth attendants and care at the level of the health post can help to protect the mother against anemia, malnutrition and postpartum infection and tetanus but onward referral is required for more serious problems such as eclampsia, obstructed labor and severe hemorrhage. Here, it is worth noting that obstetrical death in the more developed countries is now a rarity, because the causes are so widely preventable and treatable, given access to an effective health care system with both primary and secondary health care (secondary care would include the possibility of operative intervention, as in obstructed labor). The problem in Third World countries is not that the technology is not known; rather it is that health services are underdeveloped. PHC does not reach the social and geographic periphery to identify women at risk, and referral channels to life-saving secondary care facilities are seriously inadequate.

Much more could be said about patterns of health and disease of mothers and children in Third World countries, but a general outline has been presented, together with emphasis on the interactions among the health problems, e.g., how one illness can render a child more vulnerable to others, how interactive they are with social and economic factors, and their differential susceptibility to PHC and other levels of health services. Let us now consider how PHC systems can be developed to deal with these problems.

PRIMARY HEALTH CARE FOR POOR AND REMOTE POPULATIONS

Here, we will focus on developing PHC systems for poor and remote populations because both the problems and opportunities are somewhat special in those settings. The challenge is to achieve some semblance of equity in the face of scarcity – that is, to reach everyone, or nearly everyone, with care that matches their need, with resources that are seriously constrained. Let us begin with principles, those associated with WHO's Goal of Health for All. Five cardinal ideas are essential:

- universal coverage, with care according to need (or risk)
- effective, affordable, accessible, culturally acceptable
- promotive, preventive, curative, rehabilitative

- community participation so as to promote self-reliance
- interaction with other sectors of development.

Let us describe a PHC system that has the potential for incorporating those principles. Later, we can look at problems of implementation. The key initial step in PHC system development is dialogue with the community, and engaging their interest, knowledge, and participatory support. It is imperative that they be involved in actual decisions about what will be done, and not simply expected to cooperate in implementing decisions made by health care providers.

A population can be identified in dialogue with community, usually defined by its geographic boundaries. This is the often mentioned "denominator" concept, the population whose numbers serve as the denominator in calculating rates of coverage or of morbidity or mortality that apply to that population. Thus, one is able to go beyond saying that a certain number of children were immunized to say what number or proportion of children in the denominator population can be characterized through a household survey, and priorities decided for health care.

A PHC infrastructure can be built around community health workers (CHWs), local men and women recruited from the community and trained in the community. The CHWs can be assigned households which they visit on a monthly or quarterly basis. During those visits, they look to priority problems, such as monitoring the growth of children under five, ensuring that immunizations are carried out and that mothers understand the proper use of oral rehydration therapy, and screening pregnant mothers for risk factors. In these actions, the CHWs are supervised by community health nurses (CHNs), community health doctors (CHDs) or other personnel who can continue their training and who can also make decisions about the needs for care locally or through further referral. The supervisory personnel usually work out of a local health center, and have access to a front-line hospital, possibly called a district hospital. Such a PHC infrastructure provides a service framework through which various PHC programs can be introduced, such as control of diarrhea, health education, antenatal care, etc., and is seen as being infrastructure, personnel, vehicles, etc.

A medical or health information system (MIS) is built on information collected by the CHWs, which is aggregated and assessed by the CHNs or CHDs, and used for management decisions about the care of individual patients and the community as a whole. As examples, growth monitoring may reveal that a child is proceeding more deeply into malnutrition and requires special attention, or the number of childhood deaths may be in excess of what is expected and require investigation.

Such a PHC system must be affordable, and indeed PHC systems such as this one can be implemented at costs of $2 to $3 per person per year. An important question is whether the community shares in the costs of these services – on a fee-for-service basis, on a pre-paid basis, or through contributions, such as of land, cash crops or volunteer services.

In dialogue with the community, non-health factors, such as lack of potable water, lack of sewerage, illiteracy, or severe unemployment may emerge as high priority concerns. The PHC teams must then assess their capacity for assisting the community in pursuing these problems across other sectors of development.

Let us review briefly how such a system meets the principles of Health for All through PHC:

- Universal coverage with care according to need– every household is visited on a monthly or quarterly basis, and those in the household who are in need are thereby identified and cared for or referred onward for care.

- Effective, affordable, accessible, culturally acceptable. Of these, effectiveness can be achieved by focusing on those problems that are identifiable and manageable, but active use of an MIS is necessary to ensure that objectives, such as reduction of the Infant Mortality Rate or increase coverage with immunizations, are being met. Sadly, many PHC systems do not have even the simplest MIS and they are blind to either success or failure of their programs. Affordability may or not be self evident: Costs can be monitored through the MIS, and dialogue with the community can reveal whether such costs are within their resources.

  Similarly, accessibility (which may have social and economic as well as geographic aspects) and acceptability can be monitored through the MIS and dialogue with the community.

- Promotive and preventive as well as curative and rehabilitative – the household-based services are designed to identify people at risk and to intervene before disease strikes, as in immunizable diseases (primary prevention), or to catch a disease early in its course, as in childhood malnutrition (secondary prevention), or to prevent its serious advance as in the management of diarrhea (tertiary prevention). Community-based rehabilitation is a field of its own, in which community people learn to care for the disabled, including fashioning crutches, walkers and various prostheses of simple, locally available materials.

- Community participation so as to promote self-reliance – the range of relationship the PHC system can have with community is very great, from community people cooperating with the PHC team to having the community actually in charge of the PHC system, making management decisions guided by the health personnel. Community involvement in health system management can be an important route to community empowerment and development. The role of the health team changes dramatically, depending on how much decision-making control is given over to the community.

- Interaction with other sectors of development – possibly the most difficult task for the health team, but often the most important for the community. The PHC team may be able to contribute across sectors by simply joining the community in trying to unravel a particular problem, such as how to divert a contaminated stream of water, or by serving as advocates of the community in dealing with a governmental or industrial bureaucracy.

Probably the most important of these principles are universal coverage and effectiveness, and they go hand-in-hand. Universal coverage with irrelevant and ineffective services, or effective services available only to a few, makes a mockery of the goal of health for all.

What about conditions in which it is not possible to have such thorough coverage as described above, as in remote rural areas with underdeveloped health services? It should first be acknowledged that it should be possible to develop community-based services, even under conditions of extreme poverty, given the patience and willingness to work largely with community resources. Nonetheless, the question is important. Let us examine some ways of stepping down from a full coverage, comprehensive PHC system.

It is possible to shift from house-to-house surveillance, as described above, to community-based surveillance. Cross-sectional surveys can be done periodically, say each year or every other year, to monitor impacts of programs, and the surveys could be of so-called sentinel sites, rather than of entire populations. Using growth monitoring of children under five as an example, instead of monitoring individual children on a monthly basis, communities could be monitored on a quarterly, semiannual or annual basis. Obviously, individual children who were faltering in their growth might be missed in this process, but this approach would make it possible to assess the impact of a program intended to promote improved childhood nutrition.

The focus could be on selected PHC programs, instead of a full range, and a minimal MIS could be used, in which a few indicators were followed that could serve as proxies for others. For example, immunization coverage, nutritional status, and mortality rates of children under five would provide substantial information on which to base PHC management decisions.

A general and practical observation can be made about developing and managing PHC systems. While international guidelines are helpful in getting PHC systems started, and in setting up parameters for planning and evaluation, there is no substitute for on-the-ground experience in a given setting. Inevitably, some things will not work locally that worked elsewhere, and successful ideas will emerge in the local setting that have not been described elsewhere. It is essential that local people – health personnel and community – come to know and guide their own PHC system, so that problem solving is done in local terms with local resources. One of the more difficult areas will be to determine the extent of impact of the PHC systems on local conditions. Here, international guidelines can help in determining changes in health status, which will require epidemiological and statistical methods, but determining impacts on social indicators, such as community participation and roles of women in development, will be more dependent on local insights and methods.

SOCIAL, CULTURAL, ECONOMIC, AND BUREAUCRATIC OBSTACLES TO HEALTH FOR ALL

The obstacles to Health for All go beyond those that are addressed through epidemiological analysis of patterns of disease, and beyond the design of PHC systems that have the potential of reaching all of the people in a given population. The obstacles involve social, cultural, economic, political and environmental factors. Let us examine some of these problematic areas. Two large sets of factors can be identified. One we will refer to as the social-cultural-environmental complex. The other is the health services-bureaucratic complex.

THE SOCIAL–CULTURAL–ENVIRONMENTAL COMPLEX

The burden of poverty is not easy to appreciate. Families who live in the conditions of poverty – unemployed, illiterate, socially unstable, in the midst of contaminated environments – have very limited chances of rising out of their circumstances.

The roles of women can be used to illustrate. Women may be born into poverty, often into a family that is illiterate and where educational opportunities are lacking, into a culture in which education of women may not be seen as appropriate or necessary, into a community where women have no voice as to what the priorities of development should be.

Women are often caught in a cycle of despair: They enter the world as low birth-weight girl babies, born of mothers who themselves are undernourished; stunted and wasted at birth, they never catch up with their growth potential, and remain physically and intellectually handicapped. Undernourished and immersed in poverty, they are vulnerable to diseases and hazards of underdevelopment – diseases of infection and deficiency, early marriage with too many pregnancies too close together – and they are likely to complete the cycle by giving birth to low birth-weight babies, some of whom will be girls.

Women are not only caught in such traps of underdevelopment, they helplessly contribute to perpetuating them. So much of the health and well being of the family rests with the mother – pregnancy and childbirth, child rearing, feeding the family, maintaining a household with a semblance of hygiene, and maintaining a social cultural milieu in which life values are built and from which family members can move out and take advantage of opportunities for individual and community development. But if she, herself, is trapped in poverty and illiteracy, and has little voice that might help to bring about change, the prospects for herself and her family are indeed grim.

This bleak picture is not universal, to be sure, but it must be recognized as the contemporary starting place for many women in the poorer countries of the Third World. There are bright exceptions, by country, and by community, and there are many progressive individuals and agencies who are working to overcome these problems. Strengthening the role of women in development should be seen as a priority item on the agenda of Third World development for the 1990s.

THE HEALTH SERVICES – BUREAUCRATIC COMPLEX

The political commitment at the national level to WHO's Goal of Health for All has been widespread, and policies, budgets and administrative support have been put in place in many countries, including the poorest. WHO and other international agencies, as well as donor countries aiding through bilateral channels, have made extensive contributions in both resources and technical assistance. But progress has been slow in many countries. It has become apparent that a network of health facilities does not ensure effective services, nor does the placement of health personnel with assignments to serve the rural and urban poor ensure that those people will be reached with services.

The conditions of severe national under-development too often include a syndrome of severe administrative under-development. Health services may be under-planned, under-staffed, under-financed, and under-managed by personnel who, themselves, are under-trained, under-supported, under-paid and often demoralized.

One sees pockets or even large areas of health services in which such administrative weakness is in place, and there the picture is familiar; the physical structure of PHC may be in place but effective programs are lacking; health services are out of touch with communities; there is little or no outreach to communities; communities have little confidence in the health services; there is not an effective information system that might tell them that mortality rates are high and not being diminished by existing services – the classical story of services under-used and communities under-served.

CONCLUDING OBSERVATIONS

In conclusion, three important points can be summarized:

For PHC systems to be effective in addressing the needs of mothers and children in Third World settings, careful attention must be given to patterns of disease and design and management of PHC systems, taking into account socioeconomic and environmental determinants of health, that will carry the potential of universal coverage with care according to need.

But carefully developed policies, plans, budgets and even a PHC infrastructure do not ensure effective services. Health systems are often under-managed, under-used, and communities are often under-served. Attention must be given to each level of implementation, from national to provincial to district to local, where patience and persistence are required to ferret out and remedy the shortfalls, identify and spread the strengths, and encourage and support health workers and communities who have found the way toward PHC systems in which services and community interact in socially sensitive and effective ways.

Beyond or behind PHC services, there are powerful determinants of health and response to services that are imbedded in the social structures of a society. Using the dilemmas of women to illustrate, when women live in deep conflicts with a near-impenetrable patriarchal system supported by archaic socio-economic and political structures, then simply bringing PHC programs into existence may have little effect on their health, and when a society has a dilapidated service infrastructure, and where women are either powerless or rendered helpless by lack of options and clogged or non-existent services, then the health status of women and children is not likely to change.

SELECTED REFERENCES

1. Walsh, J. A. Establishing Health Priorities in the Developing World. New York: UNDP, 1988.

2. UNICEF. The State of the World's Children 1989. New York: UNICEF, 1989.

3. World Health Organization. From Alma Ata to the year 2000 – a midpoint perspective. Geneva: WHO, 1988.

9

MCH IN THE CONTEXT OF
PRIMARY HEALTH CARE:
THE WHO PERSPECTIVE

U KO KO, M.B.B.S., D.P.H., D.T.M.&H., F.R.C.O.P.

Throughout the history of medicine, since the days of Hippocrates in 460 B.C., the focus of medicine was on the case management though thoughts were given in aphorisms on the importance of environment and food and style of living as contributory factors. After the Renaissance and along with industrial reforms and scientific discoveries when hygiene and public health were evolved, the new focus in those days was on hygiene and sanitation followed by epidemiology and disease prevention and control. It was towards the end of the eighteenth century and beginning of the nineteenth century that there was a tremendous awakening, particularly in Europe and the UK, on the plight of mother's pregnancy, infants and children. One may refer to the works of Thomas Turner (1793-1873), William Farr, and William Ballantyne (1861-1923) to have an insight on such developments. At the turn of last century, Maternal and Child Health became an accepted discipline in the frame of public health as a result of various enactments in the UK, Europe, USA and through efforts of various voluntary and non-governmental organizations on MCH, child care and family planning. The concept of MCH spread to Africa, Asia and other developing countries but the MCH programs were conceived more as philanthropic voluntary work rather than as national or governmental activities. During the early twentieth century until the end of World War II, governmental efforts of health departments focused on treatment of clinical cases as they came to the hospital and public health, mainly to control epidemics with some attempts to prevent them. MCH was done exclusively by voluntary organizations, particularly patronized by wives and daughters of royalties, senior government officers and rich people.

After the end of World War II, the newly independent countries took upon themselves the responsibility to take care of health of the people. This sense of awakening prompted the politicians and policy makers to seriously consider how they should provide service for the child and the mother. In many countries – Burma, Mongolia, and DPR Korea – the importance of health of the child and mother was reflected in the Constitution itself. In many others, they are included as observations and recommendations in the reports of enquiry commissions or planning commissions such as Bhores Commission of India. With the growing of interest in family planning and the overwhelming support from all developing agencies on this subject, the MCH division of developing countries undertook the additional task of family planning. In practice, however, the emphasis on family planning, driven by the tremendous population pressure, outgrew MCH and in some countries MCH work relapsed if not totally pushing out MCH from the center of the health arena.

With the growing interest of the people themselves coupled with new discoveries in medical sciences, the inadequacy of health services in the developing countries also became very evident gradually and a search for a solution went around in 1960s and 1970s. Needless to say, MCH services suffered most from the inadequacies of health services compounded by the tremendous pressure from the targeted approach of FP.

It is therefore no accident or chance that when the International Conference on Primary Health Care took place in Alma Ata in 1978, MCH received great attention. Out of eight essential elements of primary health care which are to be taken as minimal, MCH is included as "maternal and child health care, including family planning." In practice, one has to take note of the other seven elements like education for health, environmental health and sanitation and availability of essential drugs and food. Some others like nutrition, immunization, control of endemic diseases and treatment of common ailments may be understood as technical components to be delivered by the health system – and in this case as an integral part of MCH.

Indeed the interlinkages of other elements to MCH is too strong and obvious so that all can be taken and should be implemented as an integrated approach. The main essence of PHC approach in MCH would be to plan and implement MCH – along with individual components as an integral part of the health science system and delivered in totality in a holistic manner. Based on experiences in South-East Asia, most effective MCH programs are seen in countries where health care is taken as a package without fragmentation. To identify one or two important components – whether nutrition or immunization, growth monitoring or family planning, ORT or ARI, and implement each of them with vigor, but in isolation, in the long run will be defeating the purpose. The main objective of MCH is for child development in totality as the integral part of health development which must be conceived within the context of a national development plan. The sole purpose of MCH is to take care of the child and prepare him/her to become a healthy productive citizen of the future and not just to prevent for surviving and prevent mortality. In South-East Asia, the integrated approach for MCH is accepted by all countries but with various systems of implementation and varying degree of success. The totally integrated approach to MCH with base in the hospital with outreach programs for the community and two-way referral systems are seen in DPR Korea and Mongolia. In Indonesia, Sri Lanka and Thailand, the departments/sections responsible for different PHC elements try to collaborate and work together in the form of Posyandu of Indonesia and BMN program of Thailand. The Sri Lanka MCH Division is responsible for many technologies needed for MCH, such as nutrition, immunization, diarrheal disease control, ARI and so on. The five pillars of PHC approach are well-known and need not be elaborated repeatedly but may just be mentioned, viz., equity, community involvement, intersectoral coordination, appropriate technology and focus on prevention. Needless to say, MCH as part of health systems is delivered more efficiently and effectively in the countries where these five pillars of PHC are solid and strong. One has to realize that PHC approach when applied successfully will promote a strong and effective MCH program.

Apart from seeing MCH as a service, as an integral part of health service system, MCH demands an effective, technically sound and affordable technology. Since MCH covers "M" for mother component and "C" for child component, the health technology is needed for both the mothers, children and expectant mothers who form the link between the mother and the child. Since PHC approach depends heavily on the outreach program and the community, the need for technologies which are simple yet safe and effective cannot be overemphasized. The development of the growth chart for monitoring children, simple indicators and tests for monitoring nutrition of mother and child, and the system of growth charts for pregnant women to monitor and prevent low birth-weight (LBW) are extremely useful and important. Simple diagnostic technologies for testing anemia, PEM, urine and blood tests, throat swabs and immunological exams – all will contribute to effective identification of risk groups among pregnant women and children. The relatively new intervention technologies which can be applied safely in an outreach program have revolutionized the MCH service. Just to quote a few examples, one may mention weighing of pregnant women and children, use of arm circumference for children, ORT in diarrheal diseases control, simple antibiotic treatment based on classification of serious ARI cases, supplementary feeding with locally available foodstuff, and EPI immunization schedules.

The required manpower for MCH as such had to be trained in a balanced mix of administration, clinical technology, and preventive medicine in addition to health education and communication skills. The clinical background of necessity must include general medicine with a focus on pediatrics/child health, obstetrics and gynecology. Those who are in the periphery amidst the community should be women with nursing/midwifery skills but with a strong sense of socio-epidemiology with a flair for the community approach. The level of competency in different disciplines and the predominance of one or the other will of course depend upon where he or she is working. While ANM and CHW or BHW in the field preferably should be women with strong nursing/midwifery skills, those at the intermediary level or the center should be medical doctors who may be classified as health developmentalists, whose training and skills should include, apart from medical sciences, socio-economics, administration and management. One of the problems at intermediary level is the officers who act more as supervisors/administrators spend much of their time in inspection and policing of the junior colleagues with little or no interest in clinical or technical work. In order to counterbalance, the Government of India with technical support from WHO, has developed a handbook on MCH which is used as practical handbook and training manual for MCH officers at primary health center (PHC) and district level. The manual, with coordinated inputs from pediatrics, obstetrics and gynecology, PSM and nursing offers a balanced guideline for practical MCH work. The approach here is to stimulate and train intermediate level MCH Officers with supervisory role to take leadership role in technical aspect of clinical management of the program and not limiting themselves to pure policing and inspection role.

Health as defined by WHO Constitution is physical, mental and social well-being and not merely the absence of disease or infirmity. Alma Ata Conference on PHC also concerns health care in an integrated approach covering promotive, preventive, curative and rehabilitative phases. The delivery system also should be planned as a package, covering all levels – from family to community, voluntary health workers to health center, and field hospitals, including apex bodies with proper referral services. These principles of service delivery in the health system are very much essential for an effective maternal and child care program in any country.

The current obstacles in the MCH program are due mostly to inadequacy in establishment of a viable effective delivery system with MCH as an integral part of the health care system manned by appropriately trained health workers at all levels, and functioning as a team. Many a situation is seen where linkages are broken among health workers at a particular level or between different levels. These are the reasons why antenatal care, growth charts of infants or school medical inspections implemented efficiently in their own activity become ineffective as a program. Attempts should be made to develop a system, viable and active, so that an undernourished infant, an abnormal pregnancy or a school child with potential for serious situations like otitis media or impaired vision can be attended to and the condition rectified by supportive services which function as part of the MCH package.

One very positive development during recent years is the closer intersectoral involvement and effective participation of NGOs, voluntary organizations and through their leadership, enlightened village leaders, community and family themselves in the horizontal place of MCH at the community level. The days of socialite ladies condescending to do social work for poor mothers and children are now being replaced by meaningful effective field work of NGOs and voluntary organizations. There are hundreds of such examples in India – some organized by individual missions or philanthropic organizations but many coordinated by VHAI. The Thai BMN program with built-in voluntary work by VHV or Activists is well-known. The Indonesian PKK movement with six of their ten major activities focusing on health of the infant and child attracts so much attention that PKK was recognized internationally through the Morris Pate award of UNICEF and Sasakawa Prize of WHO recently. Quoting the above as illustrations, the recognition of role of NGOs, VHO for MCH in the field is seen all over the world including South-East Asia. With improved income and better living standards for the general population, with better literacy rate and higher education among women, it is expected that health of the people will be the responsibility as well as the right of all people. Since mothers and children form the majority of the population, estimated generally around 60-75%, there is no doubt that MCH will have the benefit from this intersectoral approach. Public awareness, self-care and healthy life styles should permeate the mind and behavior of the general population. Looking at these community approaches in the context of 10-point recommendations of Riga Conference – "midpoint to HFA"; the approach fits in very well with many recommendations – leadership development, empowering people, intersectoral collaboration, etc.

Since MCH, as an integral part of health care, is basically an application of medical sciences with socio-epidemiology stance, all research activities to solve problems of MCH are being encouraged. Generally speaking, all research geared towards solving MCH problems, whether basic or applied, should be undertaken by countries commensurate with the available resources, financial or otherwise. The developing countries with adequate resources may undertake research to solve basic problems – development of new diagnostic tools or drugs and vaccines or new intervention technologies for case management. However, due to limitations in resources, most of the developing countries, except those with adequate manpower and finance, are encouraged to undertake operational research type of applied research. The stress therefore is on KAP studies, feasibility studies, operationalization of known scientific knowledge, manpower needs, setting criteria and evaluation. Socio-anthropological studies on acceptance and application of known effective technologies in MCH are to be encouraged. In South-East Asia, apart from general practice as above, countries have undertaken low birthweight studies for babies, risk approach for intervention of infant deaths and safe mother-hood, operationalization of EPI, CDD, ARI, supplementary feeding, and so on. The major thrust in the near future would be research into adopting or changing health life styles, promotive health, minimizing risk-taking behavior of older children and adolescents.

Due to general socio-economic developments with accompanying demo-graphic changes and epidemiological patterns, the technical contents and focus on MCH may change in the future. Though in many countries, nutri-tional disorders and communicable diseases are still major health problems, the degree and type of problems are not the same. For instance, frank third degree malnutrition with frank PEM or deficiency disorders are not so com-mon but still under-nutrition and subclinical cases of nutritional disorders are rampant. Massive outbreaks of poliomyelitis or diarrhea with high mortality rates are being replaced by subclinical or mild cases with negative results on nutrition and growth. In the better developed countries among developing world IMR is now below 20/1000 live births where in place of nutrition and communicable diseases, congenital and genetic disorders or problems of low birth weight and post-obstetrics, pediatric problems are emerging. Though not yet common the developing countries need to be prepared for tackling MCH problems of affluence – over-nutrition, potential for hypercholesterol-emia, mental stress, etc. The MCH organizers therefore of necessity should be prepared to undertake modern sensitive clinical and diagnostic technologies and also broaden their scope to have closer collaboration with other sectors like education, social welfare, etc.

Extending the care of the infant to the child, then to school-going age and adolescents and youth, the responsibilities of MCH divisions must now in-clude such far-sighted programs. The pressing problems of modernization – risk-taking behavior, tobacco and abuse of addictive substances, promiscuous sex, teenage pregnancies, and exposure to AIDS, are now looming in the horizon of the MCH program.

While preparing to meet these challenges, attempts should be made to instill in the minds of children and young adults the joy of healthy living. Coordinating with other agencies, culture, physical fitness and sports, volun-tary work and community activities need to be encouraged. It is being conceptualized in SEARO that an effective integrated MCH school health program would be able to give protection to young adults from many avoidable disabilities. To illustrate, we may mention prevention of impairment of eyesight, IDD and other deficiency nutrition disorders, dental and mental diseases – just to quote a few.

The future MCH program, therefore, must be conceived and implemented as an integral part of health systems based on PHC approach which must also be planned in the context of national general development. Fragmented approaches to push one component or another will not do. This must be a holistic approach taking general development as a base, if MCH programs are to be effective and successful.

10

PRIMARY HEALTH CARE: RELATIONSHIP TO MATERNAL AND CHILD HEALTH: THE MINISTRY OF HEALTH PERSPECTIVE

Somsak Varakamin, M.D., M.P.H.

I. CONCEPTS OF PRIMARY HEALTH CARE

Long before the advent of the 1978 WHO Declaration of Primary Health Care[1] as the program approach to Health for All by the Year 2000 at the historic Alma Ata Conference, Thailand had very quietly crept into the concept of revolutionary community movements, commitments and participation towards self-care and self-help.

Primary health care (PHC) concept and principles were not new to Thailand. Health development activities based on people participation had long been taking place in rural Thai communities. "Moh Tum Yae" or traditional birth attendants (TBAs) in Central, Northwestern and Southern Thailand and "Mae Jang" in the North had played significant roles in the promotion of maternal and child health particularly in home deliveries.[2] With technical and financial support from WHO and UNICEF, Thailand had embarked upon full community participation in health development through village volunteer workers. In 1975, this successful experiment resulted in the creation of a nationwide village health volunteer system to form the backbone of the National Primary Health Care Program.[3]

There were two groups of health volunteers being utilized. The first group was trained to undertake preventive and promotive services including first aid and simple curative treatment and the provision of essential drugs in case of minor illnesses. They were known as village health volunteers (VHVs).

The second group was responsible for health information dissemination, e.g., health education and transmission of information in case of communicable diseases or epidemics. They were called village health communicators (VHCs).

In 1977 at the 36th meeting of the World Health Assembly, the policy of Health for All by the Year 2000 was unanimously adopted. WHO in 1978 organized a meeting of health leaders of the member countries at Alma Ata. Following resolutions of the meeting, in 1978 General Kriangsak Chomanan,[4] then the Prime Minister of Thailand, endorsed the Charter agreeing to adopt primary health care as the key strategy for health development. Shortly after this, the National Primary Health Care Programme was developed and incorporated as a part of the Fourth Five-Year National Economic and Social Development Plan (1977-1981).

There are 10 essential elements of PHC in the Thai context;[5] health education concerning prevailing health problems and the methods of preventing and controlling them; promotion of food supply and proper nutrition; MCH/FP; safe water supply and sanitation; immunization prevention and control of endemic diseases; appropriate treatment of common diseases and injuries; provision of essential drugs; mental health and dental health.

The working concepts of PHC program in Thailand are as follows:

- PHC cannot function as a vertical program, rather it needs to be integrated with other development activities aiming to achieve better quality of life.
- PHC is possible only when the community recognizes and accepts its problems and cooperates in finding appropriate means to tackle such problems.
- Community involvement and self-reliance constitute the heart and soul of PHC activities.
- PHC activities must be in harmony with existing socio-behavioral community norms and other health-related institutions.
- Effective intersectoral collaboration is mandatory to support village-based, self-managed development projects.
- Program/policies on health and social development activities should be need-based, priority-oriented and community recognized.[6]
- Appropriate technology should be developed and community resources maximally utilized.

II. IMPLEMENTATION OF PRIMARY HEALTH CARE PROGRAM WITH EMPHASIS ON MCH AND FAMILY PLANNING

Typical to the rest of health program activities, the MCH/FP program thrust is in an integrated village approach utilizing locally existing village resources. The following pyramid, Figure 1, reflects the different levels of care in the integrated MCH/FP program approach:[7]

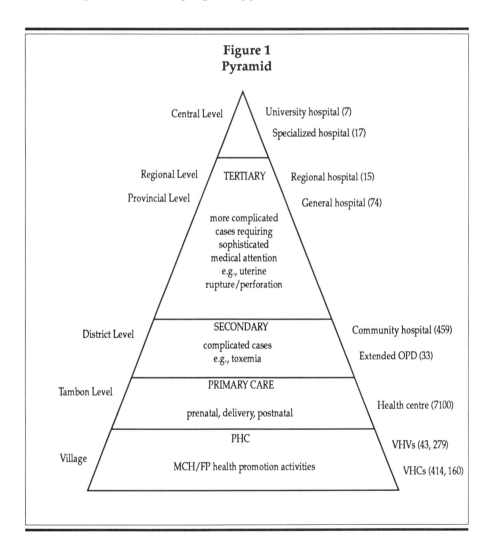

Figure 1
Pyramid

Central Level — University hospital (7)
Specialized hospital (17)

Regional Level — TERTIARY — Regional hospital (15)
Provincial Level — General hospital (74)

more complicated cases requiring sophisticated medical attention e.g., uterine rupture/perforation

District Level — SECONDARY — Community hospital (459)
complicated cases e.g., toxemia — Extended OPD (33)

Tambon Level — PRIMARY CARE — Health centre (7100)
prenatal, delivery, postnatal

Village — PHC — VHVs (43, 279)
MCH/FP health promotion activities — VHCs (414, 160)

Four major implementation approaches were underlined to ascertain the efficiency and effectiveness of the PHC activities:[8]

- Community involvement
- Utilization of appropriate technology
- Intersectoral collaboration
- Improvement of the government support services

COMMUNITY INVOLVEMENT

MCH/FP activities were given high priority in the implementation of PHCs' program activities to the effect that existing community organizations and human resources were mobilized at the village level for MCH/FP service delivery. At first the VHVs and VHCs were trained to disseminate MCH/FP information and motivate the target groups to accept the services. The VHVs had additional responsibilities for the resupply of condoms as well as oral contraceptives to family planning acceptors after physical examination by physicians. The VHCs' major tasks were to disseminate health information, serve as contact points for local health personnel and collect basic data on MCH/FP and report through the VHVs to the health personnel at the Tambon level.

The Ministry of Public Health recognized the potential of the TBAs in augmenting MCH/FP health service. They were widely respected and well-accepted by mothers and the community at large. Training courses were organized to familiarize TBAs with aseptic techniques in child delivery, identify their role as service providers to prenatal and postnatal cases, and stress their linkage with existing health service infrastructure. TBAs were also trained on condom and oral contraceptive distribution.

As an additional measure to strengthen community participation and generate community involvement, the Model Mother Project was launched. A set of criteria was established in the identification of candidate mothers in order to ensure that those selected were conversant of, and subscribed to MCH/FP program activities.

The model mothers were given the role of local change agents for promotion of MCH/FP activities with specific goals to improve the health behavior and lifestyle of mothers in the village. Such an innovative step has initiated the mothers as prime entry point to health promotion at the village level.

Another initiative in MCH promotion was the development of Health Care Project[9] or a prepaid health insurance system through a very simple mechanism. Under this project the villagers would use their own money to buy health cards which were available in two types – one for MCH services and the other for medical care services. The health card holders were entitled to free MCH services covering antenatal care, delivery, postnatal care, immunization and medical care services.

APPROPRIATE TECHNOLOGY

Two pilot projects were initiated: the Low Birth Weight (LBW) Surveillance Project and the Screening of High-Risk Mothers and Children Project.

In the LBW Surveillance Project, the TBAs, model mothers, VHVs and VHCs were trained to use spring scales as a tool to measure the infant's birthweight and identify the low birthweight cases. They also learned to measure chest and mid-arm circumference of infants, utilizing a tape measure which was a simplified and low-price tool for estimating the infants' birth weight. VHVs and TBAs were trained to employ a pictorial check chart for simple screening of high-risk mothers and children for proper case referral to appropriate health authorities.

INTERSECTORAL COLLABORATION

In 1981, the National Rural Development Committee was established under the chairmanship of the Prime Minister, General Prem Tinsulanon. Under this mechanism, all the Ministries which were responsible for rural development closely collaborated in supporting people's activities at the village level.

IMPROVEMENT OF THE GOVERNMENT SUPPORT SERVICE

Before the initiation of the PHC project, the health infrastructure was underutilized and could cover only 15 per cent of the population. After the people were mobilized to be active partners in health development, there has been an increasing demand for health services. More mothers were referred for MCH/FP services, and more children for immunization.

III. SELF–MANAGED PRIMARY HEALTH CARE AND TCDV[10]

It was considered a fundamental premise in Thailand that with the right support from the government health infrastructure, particularly at the peripheral level, the people can successfully plan, manage, and to a large extent finance, their own micro-PHC village program. Furthermore, it was proposed that having reached a mutually agreed level of "excellence" in their own PHC development, a certain number of villages could efficiently and effectively contribute to improve the quality of life. This process was known in Thailand as "TCDV" or "Technical Cooperation among Developing Villages."[11]

IV. EVALUATION

Taking into consideration that evaluation should reflect the effectiveness, efficiency and equity of all the achievements that the MCH program made, the MOPH had formulated the following set of evaluation indicators: Access of mothers and children to local health care, birth attendance by trained personnel, percentage of children at risk immunized against the major infectious diseases of childhood, percentage of newborn infants with birthweight of at least 2500g, infant mortality rate, child mortality rate, under-5-year mortality rate and maternal mortality rate.

The following are the Key Health Indicators[12] in particular reference to MCH.

Key Health Status Index	Previous Data (1980)	Latest Data (1987)
1. Infant death rate (per 1,000 live births)	48.6	37.5 (Adjusted rate)
2. Maternal death rate (per 1,000 live births)	1.0	0.4
3. Morbidity rate (Per 100,000/ 0-14 years population) from common childhood diseases		
Diphtheria	10.0	2.7
Tetanus in Newborn (per 100,000 newborn)	61.6	46.8
Other types of tetanus	6.6	1.3
Whooping cough	25.6	7.6
Poliomyelitis	1.6	0.1
T.B. in children	-	0.1
Measles	86.8	215.2

V. CONCLUSION

The MCH program activities in Thailand have made great progress in terms of program viability and program implementation over the short span of time. Service delivery has been strengthened at all levels of the health care infrastructure. Accessibility and acceptability of health care to the population at large have shown marked improvement based on the number of evaluation parameters set by the MOPH. To be credited are: The PHC approach, the formulated innovative strategies, the employ of appropriate technology, the maximization of existing health resources, the intersectoral collaborative activities and the continuing community participation and involvement; altogether paving the way towards a more efficient and effective program delivery. However, at this stage it became imperative to take note that all efforts to reach the MCH program goals would have been elusive if not for the strong commitment and unrelenting support that the pooled interministerial program approach has continuously generated from the Royal Thai Government.

REFERENCES

1. World Health Organization. Alma Ata 1978 Primary Health Care.Geneva: WHO/UNICEF, 1978, pp.1-5.

2. The Ministry of Public Health. The Realization of Primary Health Care in Thailand. Bangkok, Thailand, 1988, pp.9-12.

3. Ningsanonda, P. Targeting for Health for All andQuality of Life: The Care of Thailand. Ministry of Public Health, 1987, pp.1-67.

4. The Ministry of Public Health. The Realization of Primary Health Care in Thailand. Bangkok, Thailand, 1988, pp.12-13.

5. Leekpai, C. Minister of Public Health. Thailand Health Development Policy and Strategies. Ministry of Public Health. Bangkok, Thailand, 1988, pp.165ff.

6. Chanawongse, K., S. Wongkhomthong, and R.C.F. Cosico. Primary Health Care: A Continuing Challenge. Mahidol University, Thailand: ASEAN Institute for PHC, 1986, pp.1-10.

7. The Ministry of Public Health. The Realization of Primary Health Care in Thailand. Bangkok, Thailand, 1988, pp.100.

8. World Health Organization. Global Strategy for Health forAll by the Year 2000. Geneva: WHO, 1981, pp.51-59.

9. Ministry of Public Health: Thailand Mini-Health Profile 1988. Bangkok, Thailand, 1988, pp.49-50.

10. Royal Thai Government. Health and Social Development in Thailand. Bangkok, Thailand: Royal Thai Government, 1988, pp.31-32.

11. The Ministry of Public Health. The Realization of Primary Health Care in Thailand. Bangkok, Thailand, 1988, p. 91.

12. Leekpai, C. Minister of Public Health. Thailand Health Development Policy and Strategies. Ministry of Public Health. Bangkok, Thailand, 1988,pp.29-31.

11

TRENDS OF WOMEN AS PROVIDERS OF HEALTH CARE

Trinidad A. Gomez, M.D.,M.P.H.

Women have always been known and considered all over the world as the first providers of health care in the home. Whether in an urban or rural area, it is the mother that first notices a cold, a cough, a rise in temperature or any gastrointestinal condition (diarrhea or vomiting) that may arise from any member of the family. It is therefore the woman who more easily administers the care that is needed for any physical condition observed.

It is a fact that doctors and other health personnel are not available in all places. Not only that health departments may not have the adequate and badly needed personnel due to budgetary constraints or due to lack of trained staff, but sometimes rural areas are inaccessible. Bad roads and inadequate facilities for transportation make the situation more difficult and added to this is the insufficient travel allowance that inhibits health personnel from making more frequent visits to the villages. With the ushering in of Primary Health Care, so conceived for people especially in countries of the Third World to benefit from it, women all the more had been thought of to be the crucial members of society that could help in health care delivery. They could promote awareness on the importance of health, on the need to identify health and community problems that could call for the involvement of people and which could in turn lead to self-reliance and to health development programs.

In some countries with a dearth of resources and inadequate health facilities, different strategies are used.

All over the world, in Asia, Latin America and Africa, women undergo training that not only enables them to provide health care especially in underserved areas but also in developed countries. As an example to this we have the so-called CARERs in the United Kingdom who are charged with the responsibility of delivering health care after the necessary orientation. There are 3-5 million women carers, eleven percent of whom are single women, and are involved in a variety of tasks.

THE PHILIPPINE EXPERIENCE

In the Philippines a good number of traditional birth attendants in the provinces have been given the necessary orientation so that they could render aseptic services to parturient women and learn the proper care that they must give to the newborn. For more than 30 years now, TBAs who are mostly women had been given an orientation on how to manage simple cases of illness in the home. Starting with the assistance of the World Health Organization and the Department of Health and later followed suit by some NGOs such as the League of Puericulture Centers, the Institute of Community and Family Health and the Institute of Maternal and Child Health (both outreach arms of the Children's Medical Center) conducted training programs for women. With the subsidy granted by the International Development Research Centre, TBAs' capabilities in a province had been strengthened, thus enabling them to render services to mothers including family planning and child care that would help in promoting child survival including rehydration.

It is interesting to note that after the training of Volunteer Women Health Workers in our project area in the Philippines, one may go to the health center and find that there is always a volunteer who is scheduled to be in the center to wait for those who may come for some minor ailment. This shows how committed the women are to serve the health needs of the community.

In the Philippines the health care delivery system is made possible with volunteer workers which are generally of two types:

1. Volunteers for specific programs such as those recruited to assist in the implementation of a program. There are the Barangay (village) Health Workers who deliver services especially to mothers and children. The population program also has its women volunteers, as does the nutrition program which has trained women to help in the implementation of the nutrition programs and services all over the country.
2. Women as individual workers or as members of women's organizations. These organizations have undertaken different activities and programs in support mainly of maternal and child health, nutrition, population and environmental sanitation. Financial and administrative support of these programs is borne by the organizations themselves, or in coordination with other community resources.

WOMEN PERSONNEL IN THE DEPARTMENT OF HEALTH (PHILIPPINES)

Women constitute the majority force in the Department of Health. Female employees greatly outnumber their male counterparts. Of the total employees (numbering 65,000), females make up 66%. While men dominate the top posts in the Department of Health, women comprise the bulk of the work force.

WOMEN IN THE PROFESSIONS

In Medicine during the last 10 years, women compose about half of the medical graduates.

In the Nursing, Midwifery and Pharmacy groups women are predominant. In the Dental profession and Medical Technology groups a good proportion are women (75%) while among Nutritionists and Dieticians almost all are women. The same is true with social workers. All-in-all this makes a good corps of women potential for health care delivery.

Of interest is the fact that of five medical schools in Metro Manila four deans are women and for the first time the Institute of Public Health has a woman for its dean.

IN THE PUBLIC SCHOOLS

About 95% of public school teachers are women and to date all of the primary school teachers had been trained with the help of UNICEF and are called "health guardians." They are able to handle simple cases of children's illnesses, cough, colds, fever, diarrhea, parasitism, skin lesions as scabies, burns, etc. The Department of Education provides school clinics and for lack of nurses or other health personnel, the teachers are the ones (the women) handling the clinics, and are designated as Teacher Nurses.

THE PHILIPPINE DEVELOPMENT PLAN FOR WOMEN

During the Women's Day (March 8, 1989) President Corazon C. Aquino signed the Philippine Development Plan for Women which has been designed to be a major instrument for integrating women in development. The plan aims to operationalize the constitutional provision on women: "The State recognizes the role of women in nation building, and shall ensure the fundamental equality before the law of women and men." It favors women such that it aims to eliminate the limited participation of women in different endeavors. Within the framework of the plan, there are sectoral targets that include the lowering of the crude birth rate from 30.8 to 28.6/1000 population, as well as the reduction of the crude death rate from 7.5 to 7/1000 from 1988 to 1992. One important target is the fall in infant mortality rate from 52.9 in 1988 to 47.8 in 1992 which is considered as an index of progress in health development.

Provided in the Development Plan for Women is the training of 2,500 Traditional Birth Attendants every year, in order to reach 90% of the remaining untrained TBAs by the year 1992. This is a significant step for women providing health care. In this kind of training emphasis is given to safe motherhood, childhood survival, breastfeeding, immunization, management of diarrhea, environmental sanitation and child spacing. TBAs are everywhere, especially in the rural areas where in the absence of health personnel, they could be the best providers of health care.

The Women's Role

It is common knowledge and observation that women have by avocation the innate feeling of caring for the sick and the infirm, whether within the family, among neighbors and anyone in the community.

In the Philippines where half of its population are women, one can proudly say that the health providers are mostly women. With 76 women's organizations all affiliated to the umbrella organization of the Civic Assembly of Women of the Philippines, which is the National Council of Women, the membership of which organizations reaches 10 million women from the whole country. It can be safely said all over the world women are assets that compose the instrumentality which could help promote the health and well being of people.

As providers of health care one may say that women contribute largely to the attainment of the World Health Organization's goal of having "health for all by the year 2000." Not being far away, it calls for everyone's participation so that there would be fewer people dying every year, mothers need not die from maternal causes, and the newborns to survive through childhood – all these help to create a healthy and happy citizenry for the world of tomorrow.

12

APPROPRIATE TECHNOLOGY IN MATERNAL AND CHILD HEALTH AND FAMILY PLANNING

Kanti Giri, M.B.B.S., DG.O., F.I.C.S., F.R.C.O.G.

INTRODUCTION

At the International Conference on Primary Health Care held in Alma-Ata, USSR (1978), the word "technology" was defined as "association of methods, techniques and equipment which, together with the people using them, can contribute significantly to solving a health problem." "Appropriate" means that besides being scientifically sound the technology is also acceptable to those who apply it and to those for whom it is used. This implies that technology should be in keeping with the local culture. It must be capable of being adapted and further developed if necessary. In addition, it should preferably be easily understood and applied by community health workers, and in some instances even by individuals in the community; although different forms of technology are appropriate at different stages of development, their simplicity is always desirable. The most productive approach for ensuring that appropriate technology is available is to start with the problem and then to seek, or if necessary develop, a technology which is relevant to local conditions and resources. The principle that technology should be appropriate in the sense described above applies not only to primary health care in the community, but also to all the supportive levels, and especially to those closest to the community such as health centers or district hospitals. An important factor for the success of primary health care is the use of appropriate health technology.[1]

Maternal and Child Health, including Family Planning, is one of the eight elements of primary health care and for the successful implementation of the program, especially in the developing countries, it is vital to have appropriate technology in MCH/FP. There exist many traditional practices and beliefs in regard to care during pregnancy, child birth, puerperium, care of newborn, infants and children which are being practiced in many developing countries, as they are readily available, acceptable and of low cost. All those need to be reviewed and evaluated, as many which are appropriate need to be retained and those harmful need to be discouraged. Some developing countries import advanced medical technologies from the developed countries which are sometimes inappropriate and expensive. There are other problems as well associated with lack of proper training of manpower to handle such technologies in regard to safety and maintenance of equipment. The developing countries need first to review the existing local technology and identify and assess the relevance, cost and acceptability to national and local needs before importing technology from developed countries.

APPROPRIATE TECHNOLOGY

1. APPROPRIATE TRAINING OF PERSONNEL INVOLVED IN MATERNAL AND CHILD CARE TRAINING AND SUPERVISION OF TRADITIONAL BIRTH ATTENDANTS (TBAS)

In many developing countries, over 70% of women still deliver at home assisted by TBAs, hence the cheapest and quickest way to reduce the appallingly high maternal and infant mortality is to train and reorient this already existing and available category of workers in:

- Identifying risk factors in pregnancy and referral,
- Safe delivery by practicing 3C methods (clean hands, clean surface for delivery and clean cutting and dressing of umbilical cord),
- Taking proper care of the newborn, and
- Promotion of family planning, nutrition and immunization also should be included.

2. STAFF AT THE FIRST REFERRAL LEVEL

Other health workers, mostly women such as midwives, assistant nurse midwives, public health midwives, family health workers, family welfare visitors who deal with maternal and child health care including family planning and who are posted at the clinics need reorientation training on risk factors, referral and supervision of TBAs. The medical doctors at the first referral center who are not specialists should be trained to handle obstetrical emergencies which according to WHO include caesarean section, giving anesthesia, giving blood transfusion, performing vacuum extraction, carry out suction curettage for incomplete abortion, inserting intrauterine devices and performing tubal ligation or vasectomy.[2]

3. COMMUNITY INVOLVEMENT

Information on risk factors in pregnancy, safe delivery, child care and family planning should be disseminated to the community, family members and the mothers themselves. In some countries female community volunteers who are identified by the community are being trained for the promotion of maternal health, nutrition, childcare, immunization and family planning. This gives added status to women and allows them to be useful to the community and generate income for themselves as well.

APPROPRIATE TOOLS OR EQUIPMENT

1. ANTE–NATAL PERIOD — IDENTIFICATION OF RISK FACTORS

Home-Based Mothers' Record (HBMR)

In recent years, a Home-Based Mothers' Record has been developed which is a useful tool for intervention as it indicates risk factors and helps in early intervention. Many countries have produced the card in national languages and, for the use of non-literate TBAs, pictorial symbols depicting danger, edema, anemia, etc., are given for easy recognition. In India, such HBMR for TBAs has been successfully field tested and tried in Vellore and Chandigarh. Proper training is required to fill in the card. WHO has prepared a prototype of HBMR which is being field tested in 14 countries after being translated in the respective national languages.[3]

Advantages of HBMR

- It gives risk characteristics with cut-off point for BP, hemoglobin.
- It records the antenatal period, intrapartum period, outcome of baby, postnatal period for three subsequent pregnancies and also interpregnancy periods if any family planning methods have been used or not.
- It shows immunization status of the mother, referral and feedback from referral centers on action taken.
- It remains with the mother.

Height

In developing countries young girls are married at an early age and become pregnant soon after marriage. Due to poor nutritional status they usually have stunted growth and undeveloped pelvic bones. Height is an important indicator and 145 cms is given as the cut-off point. In order to measure the height, a stick measuring 145 cms is given to the TBAs or, in some cases, the TBA herself is measured to give an idea of 145 cms.

Hemoglobin

Hemoglobin is an indicator of anemia. Although in the developed countries the cut-off point for anemia is 10 gms per 100 ml, it is 8 gm per 100 ml in the developing countries. To determine hemoglobin, many methods have been tested for reliability and ease of operation for peripheral workers at the field. The Jamaica study of various methods (i.e., Copper Sulphate method, the Dare hemoglobinometer, the Lovibond comparator, the A.O. Spencer hemoglobinometer, the Talqvist and the new device, Carib hemoglobin comparator) found the Copper Sulphate method and Carib hemoglobin comparator to be accurate, easy to use and cheap.[4]

i.   Talqvist Method – Logistically the method is easy and needs only a strip of blotting paper with a range of standard colors printed on a paper. A drop of blood is put on a strip of blotting paper and compared with the various standards of color supplied; the range of error is great.

ii. The Copper Sulphate ($CuSO_4$) Method – This method has been successfully tried in a study on "Risk Approach and Intervention Strategy" (1981-1984) in a rural training center Sirur, 65 kms from Pune (Maharashtra), India, consisting of 22 villages. Female community health workers/guide (CHW/CHG) performed the test while doing antenatal care for identification of risk factors after one month training. This copper sulphate method is based on the fact that the specific gravity of the blood depends on erythrocyte volume. The cut-off point of anemia was set at 8 gm/100 ml of blood. A copper sulphate solution with a specific gravity equivalent to that of blood with a hemoglobin content of 8 gm/100 ml was prepared and supplied to the CHWs. A drop of blood of the pregnant mother from the finger tip is dropped in a test tube containing the $CuSO_4$ solution. The reading is taken after 10 seconds and if the drop of blood sinks, it shows that the hemoglobin content is above 8 gm% and if it floats it is less, showing the woman is definitely anemic needing treatment.[5] The advantage with copper sulphate solution is its stability. When kept in a closed glass or a plastic container, the specific gravity showed no change over a period of a year and when kept in open vessels in various environments it showed negligible change in an eight-hour period. The copper sulphate solution needs to be made in a central point and distributed.[6]

iii. Carib Hemoglobin Comparator – was developed by Caribbean Nutrition and Food Institute (CNFI) of Jamaica. It is found to be reasonably accurate and simple, requiring no reagent, electricity or batteries and using undiluted blood. It needs standard gray filters. This is still being modified for simplicity and cost.

Detection of Albumin in Urine

This can be done easily by means of Albustick, and similarly, sugar for diabetes can be detected by means of the dipstick. This is an easy technology but expensive. The presence of albumin in urine, complaint of headaches and weight gain can easily alert the peripheral worker to refer the mother to the health clinic where her blood pressure can be measured. Program for Appropriate Technology in Health (PATH) has developed PATH strips which are dipstrips to detect albumin. The urine changes color from yellow to green to blue with increasing amounts of protein in urine.[7]

Weight

Excessive weight gain indicates retention of fluid and can be suggestive of pre-eclamptic toxemia if accompanied by headache in the absence of BP recording. No gain in weight can be suggestive of poor fetal growth leading to a low birthweight baby. Weighing at regular intervals is necessary.

Fundal height and girth of abdomen can be indicative of fetal growth and of low birth weight baby.

Use of Ultrasound

In many institutions it is being used antenatally to assess the gestational age of the fetus if in doubt, to monitor the fetal growth, suspected intrauterine death, site of placenta and congenital defects. It is a useful diagnostic tool but as yet no long-term effects of ultrasound on the fetus are known by the exposure even in the first trimester.

2. INTRAPARTUM PERIOD — CHILDBIRTH

Ambulation and human support during the first stage of labor help a woman by giving her moral support. Many women of developing countries in labor refuse to come to the institutions because they are left alone in the first-stage room or in the labor room whereas at home, they have other women around to comfort them. Recently this human support factor is receiving attention. Randomized controlled studies in Guatemala on continuous maternal support during labor have shown the reduction in the length of labor (14 to 8 hours) and reduction in the incidence of Caesarean section from 17.2% to 6.2% and pitocin 13% to 2%.[8,6]

Position During Delivery

In all the institutions, women are delivered in lithotomy and sometimes in left lateral position (Dublin method) as propagated by the Western world. But in home delivery conducted by TBAs/family assistants, women sit with a slight recline supported by a female relative, or in some cultures, women squat for delivery. The sitting position facilitates the woman to push down the baby along the force of gravity. In Bali (Indonesia) the male TBA kneels/stands behind the woman and delivers her supporting her back with his body. It has been shown radiographically that the sitting position increases the transverse and the anteroposterior diameters of the pelvic outlet of the pregnant woman.[6] However, WHO's collaborating centers have been recommended to undertake control trials to ascertain the effects of mobility and sitting position during labor on the mother and the newborn.

Use of Partograph

It is a managerial tool for the prevention of prolonged labor and its hazards. It is a record of all observations of a woman in labor and the dilatation of the cervix is recorded every four hours by a vaginal examination unless contraindicated.[9]

The Three Cleans (3C)

The 3 CLEAN PRACTICES not only prevent neonatal tetanus but also reduce the incidence of maternal sepsis during the postpartum period as well as mortality and morbidity rates. This can be achieved by training the TBAs in this method and providing them with the delivery kit consisting of soap, handbrush, nail stick or file, a plastic sheet (1m x 1m) to spread on the floor for the woman in labor, cotton wool, four lengths of boiled string, a new razor blade, clean towels, rectified spirit and a small tinted polyethylene vial containing 1% silver nitrate solution. In some countries a "Cord Pack" consisting of a razor blade, a few boiled cord ties, cotton wool and rectified spirit are commercially sold at a reasonable price which can be bought by expecting mothers and kept at home. A delivery kit should be given to all TBAs after the reorientation training which should contain simple, manageable items, which have been demonstrated during the training. Items as described above can be carried in a light plastic or vinyl bag. Additional items can be a pair of scissors, tape measure, weighing scale, and plastic apron.[10]

3. PostPartum Period — Third Stage

The least interference, no pulling of cord and pushing of the uterus is advocated. Putting the baby to the mother's breast induces the uterus to contract and helps in the separation of the placenta and initiates early lactation.

4. Child Care

Weight

Birth weight is an important indicator of the chance of survival of a newborn. Low birth weight (LBW) is the cause of more than half of the neonatal deaths in developing countries. A simple color-coded spring scale to detect a low birth-weight baby has been developed by PATH. Yellow in the window of the scale handle indicates a weight less than 2500 gms, i.e., low birth-weight baby, and blue indicates a weight above 2500 gms. The baby is put in a sling made of strong cloth.[7] This device can be easily used by illiterate TBAs to detect low birth weight for immediate special care.

Surrogate for Birth Weight

In the absence of weighing scales, in order to determine the baby's weight, many studies have been carried out to find a correlation with mid-arm, chest circumference and foot length. A study from the Guatemala Social Security Institute shows that mid-arm circumference at birth is a useful measure for predicting risk of death during the first 14 days of life. Infants with low arm circumference at birth (LACB) equal to or less than 9.0 cms have a 10-17 times higher risk of death during the first 14 days of life than infants with a larger arm circumference. This indicator is cheap, simple, quick and reliable and may be used whenever it is not feasible to weigh babies at birth. But, as any other field indicator, appropriate supervision and standardization are essential for its usefulness.[11] Tapes for measuring the mid-arm and chest circumference of newborn babies have been tested and the final prototype will be made of plasticized color-coded paper showing three situations corresponding to the above 2500 gms, 2000-2500 gms and under 2000 gms.[6] This can be used by peripheral health workers and will enable them to refer babies under 2500 gms for intensive care.

Eye Care of Newborn

The prophylactic treatment of all newborns by putting a drop or two of silver nitrate solution in the eyes immediately after birth is inexpensive and effective against gonococcal infection in case the mother has gonorrhea which is untreated. In developing countries the incidence of gonorrhea among pregnant women ranges from 0.7% in Malaysia to 20% in some areas of Africa.[8] A tinted polyethylene vial containing 1% silver nitrate solution can be added to the TBAs delivery kit. A single application immediately after birth is sufficient.

Rooming-in the Babies and Early Breast Feeding

Traditionally, in many cultures, babies are not put to breast immediately after birth as colostrum is supposed to harm the baby. Early feeding is beneficial and the suckling induces contraction of the uterus and allows the placenta to separate. In the postnatal period it helps in early involution of the uterus and good drainage of lochia.

The baby should not be kept away from the mother as is the practice in many institutions. Keeping the mother and infant together (rooming-in) allows the mother to breast feed whenever she feels like, and on demand, which increases the milk secretion and benefits the health of the baby and prolongs the contraceptive effect. For females in developing countries it has several benefits: It meets the nutritional needs of infants and provides them with some immunological protection from infection and other diseases and diarrhea; it reduces maternal mortality rates by providing birth spacing through the delay of ovulation and it reduces infant health care costs and money spent on infant formula.[12]

Warmth to the Newborn

Warmth is necessary for a newborn as he/she comes into a cooler atmosphere than the womb of a mother which is at 37°C. Warmth is needed more by LBW babies with little or no subcutaneous fat. It is better for such a baby to be cleaned with warm oil, dried and wrapped in material of three layers of cotton which is softer and warm and doesn't irritate the soft skin as woolen or knitted materials sometimes do. The head should be covered by a cap made of the same three layer cotton. The best way to keep the baby warm is for the baby to be with the mother. Besides this the room can be heated.

5. IMMUNIZATION

This is one of the most powerful public health weapons available today. In the developing world annually 5 million children die and another 5 million are disabled by the six dreaded and preventable childhood diseases. Pregnant women must be given two doses of tetanus toxoid during pregnancy to protect the babies from neonatal tetanus as nearly 100% of newborn babies born with neonatal tetanus die. The clean delivery method also protects the newborn especially the clean cutting and clean dressing of the umbilical cord. All babies must receive the complete doses of immunization as advocated by the EPI programs of WHO and UNICEF. For transportation of vaccines to the peripheral level, maintenance of cold chain is essential.

Use of Oral Rehydration Salt (ORS) in Diarrhea

Diarrhea accounts for the highest number of deaths in children under 5 in the developing countries. Nearly 5 million children die annually due to diarrhea, mostly because of acute dehydration.

- The introduction of ORS has revolutionized the treatment of diarrhea in combating acute dehydration. Ready-made ORS in packets is easy to dissolve in water but the water used as <u>solvent must be clean and potable</u>. In the absence of ready-made ORS packets, mothers must be provided the knowledge to prepare the fluid at home.
- Breast feeding protects babies from diarrhea as many mothers do not carry out proper sterilization of bottles. Proper weaning of babies between 4-6 months with supplements of home-made easily digestible food is advocated.
- Maintenance of hygienic conditions at home and in personal hygiene. Mothers must be given health education because after discharge from the hospital, the same child gets readmitted repeatedly due to carelessness at home.
- Diarrhea is a common and fatal complication of measles so children must be immunized against measles.

Prevention and Treatment of Acute Respiratory Diseases (ARI)

This accounts for 20-25% of all child deaths in the developing world.

- Peripheral health workers and parents must be taught to recognize the danger signs of severe respiratory infection for referral, such as rise of temperature and pulse, in-drawing of chest during inspiration and inability to swallow, etc.
- Training of peripheral health workers in proper management of cases and use of antibiotics is to be encouraged.

Mid-arm Circumference Measurement in Diagnosis of Malnutrition

Between the first and fifth birthdays, the mid-arm circumference remains fairly constant at about 16 to 17 cms. A measurement below 80% of normal, i.e., 12.4 cms, indicates severe malnutrition and between 12.5 cms and 13.5 cms indicates moderate malnutrition. A simple color-coded tape has been developed for peripheral health workers to diagnose malnutrition in children – red, yellow and green indicating severe malnutrition, moderate malnutrition and normal. Even illiterate workers can use it after training to place the tape at the midpoint of the arm. A bangle with an internal diameter of 4 cms can be used in the child's upper arm to diagnose quickly a severely malnourished child. If it goes over the child's upper arm, the child is severely malnourished.

Growth Chart

Growth charts have been introduced by many developing countries in their national languages to monitor the growth of children and other prophylactic health measures taken such as immunization, etc. This is a sensitive indicator of faltering growth, needing the attention of parents and health workers regarding the nutritional needs of the child. The cards are kept by the mothers and they take keen interest in the weighing activities.

Control of the Specific Nutritional Deficiencies

Vitamin A deficiency not only causes nutritional blindness but also affects the immune system and increases the risk of death from diarrhea and respiratory diseases. Administration of oral Vit. A 200,000 IU at 6 months intervals and intake of carotene-rich foods, e.g., carrots and green leafy vegetables which are well within the reach of the poor, has reduced the incidence of xerophthalmia.[14]

Birth–Spacing Methods

- Family planning is beneficial to both mother and child. Through birth spacing, both maternal and infant mortality rates can be reduced.
- Information on family planning and contraceptives must be available at the community level.
- Family planning services should be integrated with maternal and child health services and not provided in isolation.

CONCLUSION

The application and adaptation of the current knowledge of appropriate technologies and making them readily accessible to the community are of special concern to health services. Neither knowledge nor technology is lacking for the solution of the majority of health problems of mothers and children. What is lacking is the application and adaptation of the existing knowledge. A major obstacle at the national and local levels is the lack of understanding of the technical content of MCH/FP care and how such an understanding is essential to the process of adaptation and appropriate application of MCH/FP technologies through Primary Health Care.[15]

REFERENCES

1. Primary health care – Alma Ata, report of the international conference on primary health care.6-12 Sep 1978, p.59 (para 72), p.61 (para 75).

2. World Health Organization. Essential obstetric functions at first referral level. Report of the Technical Discussion Group, FHE/l86.4.Geneva: 23-27 June 1986.

3. World Health Organization. Prototype home-based mother's record – guidelines for its use and adaptation in maternal and child health/family planning programme. MCH/85.13. Geneva: WHO, 1985.

4. Stone,J.E., W.K. Simmons, P.J. Jutsum and J.M. Gurney. An evaluation of methods of screening for anaemia. Bull WHO 62 (1): 115-120, 1984.

5. Pratinidhi, A., U. Shah, A. Shrotri, P.V. Bhatlavande, H.H. Chavan, and N. Bodani. Risk Approach and Intervention Strategy in MCH Care. Project Report, 1981-1984.

6. Appropriate Technology for Maternal and Newborn Care. Progress Report on Activities of WHO and WHO Collaborating Institutions. WHO/MCH/86.9.

7. Health Technology Directions. PATH, vol. 8, no. 2, 1988.

8. World Health Organization. Primary Health Care - 7 Years After Alma-Ata. Mother's Children's Care. Newsletter 17, 1985.

9. The Partograph — Section II. A User's Manual. WHO/MCH/88.4.

10. World Health Organization. Guidelines for Introducing Simple Delivery Kits at the Community Level. MCH/87.4.

11. De Vaquera, M.V., J.W. Lechtig Townsend, J. Arroyo and A. Lachtig. The relationship between arm circumference at birth and early mortality. J. Trop. Paed.,vol. 29, June 1983.

12. Network, Family Health International. vol. 7, no. 1 Autumn 1985.

13. Ghosh, S. The feeding and care of infants and young children. VHAI (rev. ed.), 1985.

14. Information Kit of SEARO on "Banish Malnutrition," Sep. 1988.

15. Traditional Birth Practices: Annotated Bibliography. WHO/MCH/85.11.

13

EVALUATION OF MATERNAL AND CHILD HEALTH PROGRAMS

Stephen A. Sapirie, Dr.P.H.

BACKGROUND

In the decades of the 1960s, 1970s and 1980s, national health administrations of developing countries made tremendous progress in expanding the infrastructure of their health services. This service expansion is best reflected through the rapidly growing number of staff and service points particularly in the "periphery." For a variety of reasons governments focused this expansion on achieving high coverage with selected technologies, most of which are directed toward preserving the health of children, and for establishing the ability to provide support and supervision to primary health care in the villages.

Managerially, during this period national health administrations most developed their planning systems and abilities. Social/economic, and health development plans, major programs and projects were widely produced with and without the support of external agencies. More recently in this period managerial attention began to shift from planning to program implementation and evaluation. Particularly in the 1980s health administrations have expanded their activity in evaluation with a variety of approaches, most of which were aimed at determining the coverage being achieved with important primary health care activities such as immunization, diarrheal disease control and water supply. Many of these evaluations were focused on single elements of primary health care such as family planning or immunization, fostered by the international agencies supporting the development of these services.

These evaluations proved the effect of the heavy investment being made in the infrastructure on the specially targeted services in terms of continual growth of coverage. They have also identified a rather consistent series of service problems and needs, many of which have proven difficult to solve. Often the issues identified relate to insufficient support such as supplies, logistics, supervision and operating budget. Other factors felt to be lacking are sound management and good information. Occasionally the quality of staff performance was questioned.

With the achievement of higher levels of coverage with important services, many health administrations are now seeing the opportunity to further develop service efficiency, quality and effectiveness. Generally, improvement in efficiency is seen possible through the integration of services which are often delivered in specialized clinic sessions by specialized staff. Integration is also likely to lead to further expansion of coverage and improved service quality, but underlying quality is the central question of whether and how well staff are performing the tasks that are supposed to be delivered during important services such as antenatal care, delivery, postnatal care and child care. These services involve a variety of diagnostic and therapeutic tasks which are not as easily measured as family planning or immunization services.

THE MCH/FP RAPID EVALUATION METHOD (REM)

For this reason the Family Health Division of the World Health Organization is further developing the cluster sample program review technique used so successfully by the Expanded Program of Immunization and in evaluating Primary Health Care. However, for MCH/FP, the evaluation method is being developed for use by national health administrations in studying quality of care and client satisfaction in addition to confirming the coverage being achieved with the broad range of MCH services while giving much deserved emphasis to maternal care.

The rapid evaluation of MCH/FP is being designed with several clear principles in mind:

1. Purpose and Problem Orientation – It is expected that the information obtained through this type of evaluation is to be used immediately by service providers, administrators, and the communities to further develop the delivery and acceptability of MCH/FP services. Thus a rapid MCH evaluation could lead to:

    • improvement of clinical and outreach service procedures
    • development of supply and logistics systems
    • more effective education of the clients

- improved staff performance, technical and managerial
- strengthened staff supervision
- relocation of staff and facilities
- improved linkage and coordination between government, non-government, and private service providers.

2. Sponsorship and Direction by National Program Managers – It is strongly felt that such evaluations should be requested, designed and managed by the national program directors (rather than instigated from outside) in order to insure that the results are used. This implies that the national managers must necessarily choose the central issues or problems to be studied.

3. National Staff Participation – Further, that all phases of the evaluation design, planning, conduct and analysis be carried out by a working group of national program management, service and training staff. This insures their appreciation for the findings and helps them develop ideas for problem resolution.

4. Local Design – The evaluation must be locally designed to obtain the most critical information needed. This argues against using existing evaluation instruments produced by international agencies or other countries. (This principle should not inhibit the sharing of experience from past evaluations.)

5. Need for Innovation – Because of the emphasis on client satisfaction, quality and effectiveness of care, there will necessarily be a need for innovative approaches to the design and conduct of the evaluation, and for the use of several data collection methods.

6. Truly Rapid – Finally it is intended that such evaluations be designed, conducted and completed quickly. This implies that the scope of subject areas and size of the sample be kept modest, and focused on the questions and levels of the service of most concern.

The MCH rapid evaluation method described here is being applied by national health administrations to study selected portions of their MCH/FP services at all or selected levels of their health system depending on the issue or questions being addressed. There is built into this method a concept called the program hypothesis which helps in determining the types of information and the levels of the health system which need to be studied. The hypothesis states that desired impact in health or social-economic conditions is related to a chain of cause-and-effect relationships which extend across a number of levels of program characteristics. These characteristics normally include:

Relevance – of policies, programs, activities and services in terms of their response to essential human needs.

Adequacy – in terms of sufficient attention, resources and effort having been paid to the problem, the responding program and the necessary courses of action for its implementation.

Progress (implementation) – in terms of the actual activity carried out as compared with that which was planned and scheduled, and the actual results of that activity (facilities constructed, staff trained, equipment procured, laws enacted, etc.) compared with the expected results.

Efficiency – the results achieved from an activity in relation to the resources, effort and time expended, often in comparison with stated service norms or targets.

Effectiveness – the extent to which a specific desired health improvement or problem reduction is achieved, often in comparison with a stated objective.

Impact – the overall effect of a program or service on health and related social-economic development.

Program hypotheses can be constructed using these program characteristics both when designing a program and subsequently when developing questions and indicators for use in evaluating the priorities. An example of this is presented in Annex 1 in which the hypothetical cause-and-effect relationships are stated for the decision to add long-acting injectable contraceptives to a national family planning program. These statements lead naturally to the levels of inquiry and to indicators or types of information that would be sought when evaluating the success and effects of implementing such a service. Annex 2 illustrates questions and indicators derived from the hypotheses.

While the MCH/FP REM can be used to evaluate only one service or intervention, normally program managers have several overriding issues in mind when deciding to undertake an evaluation. Generally a particular problem, such as maternal health (or mortality), or a particular aspect of MCH services, such as antenatal care or delivery services will be addressed as a whole. This normally requires that several levels of the health system be studied using several types of data collection methods. Most evaluations include the main service facilities (provincial and district hospitals, health centers and posts, community health workers and traditional birth attendants), administrative and supervisory offices at central, provincial and district levels, and the community, including the household.

Data collection methods often include all of the following:

- client questionnaires (in household, or on exit from service)
- focal group discussions (clients in communities or waiting rooms, staff in facilities)
- review, sampling and extraction of data from records in facilities
- observation of service procedures
- check of facilities, supplies and equipment

THE MCH/FP RAPID EVALUATION PROCESS

The key to the successful completion and use of this type of evaluation is to manage it very well in order that it be completed in a relatively short period of time, thereby providing the required data to program planners and decision-makers when they need it. Ideally the entire process from conception to production of the final report should be completed within six months.

The following phases and steps are recommended when undertaking rapid evaluations:

A. INITIATION

1. Confirming the need for the evaluation, including confirming the interest and concerns of the national program managers, and what they have in mind to do to improve the services, once the detailed problems are better understood. This first step should produce a clear statement of the objectives of the evaluation and the issues of central concern placed within an evaluation and the issues of central concern placed within an evaluation "Terms of Reference." (Annex 3 is a list of questions, the answers to which can constitute such a "terms of reference.")

B. PREPARATION

2. Identify the types of information needed to explore the issues, using the program hypothesis.
3. Review existing data to determine additional data needed.
4. Identify the programs and services to be included in the evaluation.
5. Identify the necessary participants in the evaluation, those that

will be within the core design and working group, those that will support the field data collection and other support required (data analysis, report preparation, etc.).

6. Design dummy tables and formats for presenting the results of data analysis.
7. Identify the preferred sources of the needed data (types and levels of service).
8. Choose data collection methods.
9. Design the questions, formats and instruments to be used at each level and type of service.
10. Test and revise the instruments in actual service situations.
11. Prepare the field evaluation procedures manual and print the instruments.
12. Determine the required sample size for each level of the service.
13. Draw the sample (identify the districts, communities and facilities to be studied).
14. Plan and arrange the field work.
15. Train the field teams with actual use of the instruments.

C. CONDUCT THE EVALUATION IN THE FIELD

16. Conduct the data collection at each level of the service.
17. Begin the preliminary analysis (initial tallies are prepared in the field in order to find and correct mistakes).

D. ANALYSIS AND REPORTING

18. Complete the preliminary analysis and prepare the initial report.
19. Present and discuss the findings (to decision-makers and service staff and trainers).

E. FOLLOW-UP

20. Prepare a plan of action for addressing the problems found.
21. Conduct secondary analysis (such as multi-variate analysis) to determine unanticipated associations.
22. Prepare the final report (containing the description of the evaluation, its methods, initial findings, secondary findings and the plan of action for problem resolution).

While the time required for completing the process will vary depending on the scope and size of the evaluation, the initiation and preparation phases have been completed in a month, the field work is normally completed in 10 days, the analysis and completion of the initial report should not take more than a week. The initial report should focus on the issues of central concern and not attempt to present all the findings of the evaluation. Seminars for presenting the findings and the final report are produced within several weeks.

The step that often is forgotten is to plan the follow-up actions that are needed to address some of the problems found. In most cases it is possible to identify immediate actions that can begin to address some of the problems found, such as inadequate supplies of certain important supply items, or inoperative equipment. Performance problems are more difficult and require consideration of a range of options usually including revising operating procedures, improving supervision, providing in-service training, developing improved procedures manuals and recording formats. Such actions may have to be placed within a project for strengthening MCH/FP throughout the country.

In recent years great emphasis has been placed by the international health community on identifying standard indicators for monitoring and evaluating health and health services, including MCH and family planning. These efforts are worthwhile because progress can be made in identifying which few pieces of information are most sensitive and reliable in determining how the health of women and children is changing and how well the services are caring for them. Such indicators are most needed within the recording and reporting systems of the health services in order to reduce the often burdensome reporting requirements placed on service staff.

While progress in indicator development continues it will be necessary to rely on rapid field evaluations of health status and service to provide the best possible picture of the current situation. As described earlier, this approach to the design of each evaluation stresses the need for responding to each situation with tailor-made evaluation questions and instruments. In a way, standardized indicators are not recommended in this approach for fear of violating this principle of local relevance. However, as more experience is gained with REM it is possible that some of the data collection and analytical methods will prove to be commonly useful as have some of the indicators used in service reporting.

SUMMARY OF RAPID EVALUATION OF MCH AND FAMILY PLANNING

A method for evaluating MCH and family planning is proposed which enables program managers to focus their attention on issues of current concern and then quickly capture selected information at all relevant levels of the service necessary to study those issues.

This is done with a rapid cluster sample survey designed to obtain data from several levels of the health services and in the community through a variety of data collection techniques. The results are quickly analyzed, discussed and used to prepare a plan of action for resolving the problems found. The types of information developed from the REM can help determine the extent of selected health problems, family health practice and knowledge, service utilization and client satisfaction, service performance in terms of output and coverage, quality of care, cost-efficiency, and effectiveness. Selected operational difficulties can be analyzed in detail to determine the underlying causes.

A number of features of this approach include the fact that the heavy involvement in the choice of issue and method of evaluation helps insure the interest and confidence in the resulting information by the decision-maker. While the need to design the evaluation specifically for the local situation prevents the use of imported evaluation instruments, the experience from other evaluations will be made available to interested health administrations by WHO in the form of question catalogues which present in disaggregated and categorized form questions used in a large number of past evaluations.

In addition to capturing important information, this approach insures that health program managers and service staff at many levels will gain through direct involvement valuable capabilities in the design and conduct of evaluation and how to use the information to take corrective action.

ANNEX 1 – PROGRAM HYPOTHESES RELATED TO THE INTRODUCTION OF LONG-ACTING INJECTABLE CONTRACEPTIVES

A hierarchy of hypotheses normally exists within any new program which might be explicitly stated as a series of cause-and-effect relationships and targets such as the following:

Impact:

1. As overall family planning prevalence increases, the overall fertility rate and population growth rate will decrease.

2. Overall contraceptive prevalence will increase if clients are offered one or more additional methods, particularly, if these methods have unique advantages.

Effectiveness:

3. Fertility of some high-risk groups (women over 35) can be reduced through the use of long-acting contraceptives, thereby reducing the complications and mortality associated with pregnancy in these groups.

Efficiency:

4. If staff in government clinics is given the ability (training and supplies) to administer injectable contraceptives, and if potential clients are given information about injectables, (__)% of women in childbearing age will choose injectables for contraceptive practice and will continue to use the method for at least two years.

Progress:

5a. MDs, nurses and nurse-midwives can be given appropriate training to enable them to administer injectable contraceptives, and to inform and counsel their clients adequately about this method and its side effects with (__) half-days of in-service training.

5b. In-service training for (__) government and non-government clinic staff can be administered through the efforts of (__) trainers in (__) training institutions, over a period of (__) months at a cost not to exceed (__)/trainee.

6. (__) service facilities can be provided with the required extra equipment (syringes, needles, sterilizers) and a continuous supply of consumable items (doses of hormonal injectable contraceptives, gauze, disinfectant, record forms) to supply the expected demand for this method at the equilibrium level of usage.

7. A public information program can be implemented which creates awareness of the availability of injectable contraceptives in 80% of women in childbearing age in (__) months.

8. An appropriate, in-service training course of (__) one-half days for preparing clinic staff to deliver injectable contraceptives and informing clients about the method can be designed, tested and initiated in selected training institutions in a (__)-month period.

9. A revamped medical supply system capable of procuring and maintaining the required supply of hormonal injectable contra-

ceptives at (___) clinics can be designed and initiated in a nine-month period.

10. Appropriate public information messages and methods for informing women about injectable contraceptives can be designed, tested and initiated in a (___)-month period.

Adequacy:

11. The overall additional resources required to implement an injectable program (supplies, training, information) can be adequately budgeted and successfully appropriated, donated or recovered from clinics.

Relevance:

12. A policy and plan for introducing an injectable contraceptive program progressively throughout the health system can be formulated in order to convince policy-makers and collaborating agencies of its relevance to national social-economic and health goals, and of its technical, financial, organizational and cultural feasibility.

ANNEX 2 – POSSIBLE LEVELS OF INQUIRY AND INDICATORS FOR USE WITHIN THE EVALUATION OF LONG-ACTING CONTRACEPTIVES

Adequacy:
- of the planning for this type of service
- of the design of the support systems and procedures
- of the preparation of staff, the training programs and methods
- of allocation of funds for supplies, equipment, training costs
- of other inputs, such as technical collaboration, time and attention by service staff to set up the new service, and the cooperation of various institutions and agencies, national and international

Progress:
- training, numbers of courses, staff
- supply system, facilities served
- procurement of supplies, amounts
- facilities and staff actually introducing the new methods

Efficiency:
- the number of clients served with the new methods
- the proportion of communities receiving such services
- the amount of staff time devoted to these activities
- the amount of supplies consumed as compared to the client served
- the overall cost per client

Effectiveness:
- the number of pregnancies per 100 clients
- the nature and amount of side effects experienced by clients
- the expressed satisfaction of clients with these methods, causes of dissatisfaction
- the proportion of clients continuing with the method after various time periods (6, 12, 18, 24 months)
- the overall level of family planning practice with all methods, and the proportion using each, by various age groups

Impact:
- the effect of the introduction/expansion of the long-acting methods on specific health indicators such as:
  - birth interval
  - pregnancy rate in high-risk groups (under 18, over 35, grand multiparas)
- maternal anemia

ANNEX 3 – TERMS OF REFERENCE FOR HEALTH PROGRAM EVALUATION

The following questions are felt important to be raised and answered before undertaking the design and conduct of a health program evaluation:

1. Who wants the evaluation? (Clearly indicate the office or officer who has requested that the evaluation be undertaken.)

2. Why is the evaluation being requested? (Indicate how the findings of the evaluation will be used and the nature of the decisions which will be taken on the basis of the evaluation results.)

3. Are there additional purposes for undertaking the evaluation and will other than the requesting office be using the evaluation results?

4. Who does the requesting office want to participate in the evaluation and why?

5. What specific questions or topics should the evaluation address?

6. Are there any topics which the evaluation should avoid?

7. Are there notable issues of current concern to the requesting office or to other decision-making levels which must be addressed? (Examples include how to confront increasing budgetary pressure, how to proceed more rapidly to integrate special program activities into the basic health services, how to deal with staff shortages, how to respond to political pressures for quick results.)

8. In what format should the evaluation results be presented and should there be both findings and recommendations?

9. Are the results of the evaluation to be representative of the country as a whole or are they to be selective and focused on certain population groups or geographic areas?

10. What bases are to be used against which to assess performance and change? (Possible reference could be made to previous baseline situation, change from a previously defined problem level, progress toward a desirable state such as an amount of problem reduction, or adherence to specified policies, regulations or norms.)

11. Are there existing program objective statements which are so unrealistic as to not be useful for judging performance or progress?

12. Are there implicit objectives which, although unwritten, should be measured?

13. Is the subject program to be evaluated over a specific time frame? (For example, to review the performance of the MCH over the last five years.)

14. What sources of information are recommended for use in the evaluation and are there any information sources which should not be used?

15. Is there any particular evaluation method which the requesting office prefers to be used? (Obvious available evaluation methods include existing monitoring system, case studies, survey research, experimental designs. In addition, typical data collection methods could include observation, direct measurement, open-ended interview, focal group discussion, structured interview, review of existing records.)

16. Is there any evaluation approach which the requesting office prefers not be employed?

17. What are the sources and limits of staff and financial resources to be used in carrying out the evaluation?

Once these points are clarified they should be presented in a brief "Terms of Reference" to enable the common understanding of all persons supporting or utilizing the evaluation.

14

MEASURING THE IMPACT OF FAMILY PLANNING PROGRAMS

Jacqueline D. Sherris, Ph.D. and Phyllis T. Piotrow, Ph.D.

Family planning programs have been more carefully evaluated than most other types of health service. There are several reasons for this:

1. The concept of reducing fertility and population growth through organized service programs was a new one, when first introduced in the 1960s. Even the strongest advocates could not produce evidence of previous successes since declines in fertility to date had occurred in the absence of – and even in the face of opposition from – government policies.

2. The major methods of family planning introduced in the 1960s, oral contraceptives and intrauterine devices, were new methods, requiring careful evaluation of safety, efficacy, and appropriateness within various contexts and programs. These evaluations of specific methods set a pattern for continued evaluation of programs.

3. Substantial international support was required from the start for family planning programs. International donors, including especially the U.S. Agency for International Development, emphasized the need for evaluation to determine whether both the concept of reducing fertility in this way and the particular program applications were effective.

4. Finally, ideological opposition to contraception produced a continuing debate over the social and health implications of family planning. Assertions were frequently made that fertility decline occurred only as a result of individual motivation or as a result of broad social and economic changes which led to changes in indi-

vidual motivation. Thus there was constant pressure on family planning programs to demonstrate that they were indeed effective.

To meet sophisticated arguments that questioned the demographic impact of family planning programs, it was necessary to develop complex approaches to evaluation. These approaches had to take account of all the other factors that might also cause lower fertility and assess how much family planning programs reduced fertility, at what pace, in what circumstances, and among which segments of the population. Particularly, evaluation of family planning programs had to demonstrate that declines in fertility would not have taken place to the same extent simply as a result of economic and social development and in the absence of organized family planning programs.

The first step in any evaluation focuses on process, that is, whether a program actually delivers the supplies and services projected on paper. This type of output evaluation is essentially no different from output evaluation in other programs. It involves primarily assessment of manpower, training, supplies, and facilities to be sure that all program elements are in place and functioning. In family planning programs, assessment of availability of services has received particular emphasis since programs that exist on paper do not necessarily exist in the field.

To measure the demographic impact of family planning programs, at least eight different methods of analysis have been used. These eight methods are:

- standardization,
- trend analysis,
- standard couple-years of protection (SCYP),
- reproductive process analysis,
- component projection,
- prevalence model,
- experimental design, and
- multivariate areal analysis.

Each utilizes different types of data, seeks to answer a different question, and evaluates different aspects of fertility change. Some evaluate the net impact of a family planning program: That is, the impact due to use of contraception supplied by the program minus the effect of substitution (when couples using contraceptives from the private sector switch to program sources). Others evaluate the gross effect, not taking substitution into account.[1-11] None actually measures the extent of substitution or of the countervailing "spill-over effect," in which family planning programs stimulate people to use methods not provided by the program.[12]

A **standardization analysis** – often called decomposition – generally determines how much of an observed decline in fertility is due to lower fertility among married couples and how much is due to other changes such as a rising age at marriage or a decrease in the number of married couples in their peak reproductive years.[10,13] It usually is assumed that virtually all change in marital fertility is caused by contraception, including voluntary sterilization, whether provided by a program or other source. Thus standardization provides a rough estimate of the gross effect of a family planning program plus the effect of contraception available through the private sector.

Another type of standardization analysis more specifically examines the impact of contraception. It uses John Bongaarts' model of proximate fertility determinants based on an earlier model by Kingsley Davis and Judith Blake of 11 intermediate variables that determine fertility.[14] Standardization using Bongaarts' model assesses how much of an observed fertility decline was due to changes in each of four factors: Use of contraception, proportion married, use of induced abortion, and postpartum infecundability due to breastfeeding.[12,15,16]

Trend analysis compares trends in birthrates or fertility before family planning programs began and after they are underway. Any difference in the trends – specifically any speeding up in fertility – is considered a rough measure of new program impact.[12,17,18] Figures 1, 2 (next page), and Figure 3 (page 144) illustrate trends in the crude birthrate in Thailand, Mexico, and Tunisia.

Three methods use family planning program statistics. These three – **standard couple-years of protection** (SCYP), **reproductive process analysis,** and **component projection** – all estimate how many births will be averted through the supplies and services provided by the family planning program. The estimate is produced by comparing the expected fertility of contraceptive users to their fertility if the program did not exist – a hypothetical projection. These methods generally produce an estimate of gross program impact.[12,19-23] Reproductive process analysis is usually used to evaluate only the impact of IUD use.

The **prevalence model,** a fairly new method, uses contraceptive prevalence survey data to estimate the number of births averted by contraceptive use. If the surveys include questions about source of supply, the prevalence model can distinguish the effect of the program from the effect of contraception obtained from other sources.[12,24,25,26]

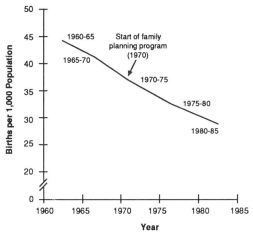

Figure 1
Trends in Crude Birthrate in Thailand, 1960 to 1980s

Source: United Nations (UN) Department of International Economic and Social Affairs. Population Division. Demographic indicators of countries: estimates and projections as assessed in 1980. New York, UN, 1982 (ST/ESA/SER.A/82)

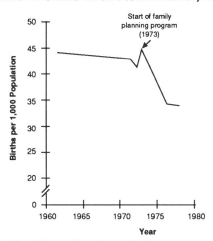

Figure 2
Trends in Crude Birthrate in Mexico, 1962 to 1978

Source: Cabrera YP and Navarro LM: Application of methods of measuring the impact of family planning programmes on fertility: the case of Mexico. In:United Nations (UN) Department of International Economic and Social Affairs. Population Division. Evaluation of the impact of family planning programmes on fertility: source of variance. New York, UN, 1982 (Population Studies No. 76; ST/ESA/SER.A/76) p 114-150

A study using an **experimental design** compares fertility in a situation with a program to fertility in other, similar situations where there is a different program or no program. Ideally, which areas, groups, or individuals will receive program services and which will not should be selected at random, but this is rarely possible. When it is not, the study is called quasi-experimental. Quasi-experimental studies often involve matching: Program clients and others are paired on the basis of similar characteristics such as age and socioeconomic status; then their fertility is compared. Fertility differences indicate the net program effect.[12,27,28]

Multivariate areal analysis compares data from different geographic areas where program strength, socioeconomic status, and fertility differ. Multiple regression techniques (using a variety of quantified indicators of program strength and socioeconomic setting) are used to evaluate the relative influence on fertility of the family planning program effect.[12]

This technique can be used to compare regions within a country or to compare different countries.

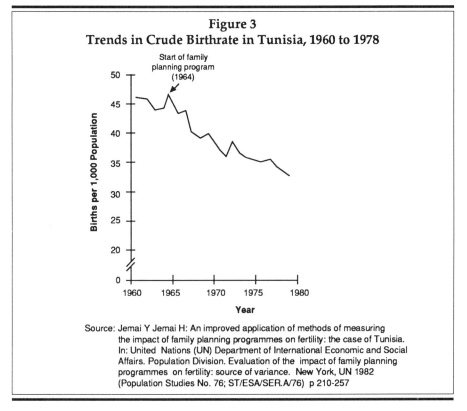

Figure 3
Trends in Crude Birthrate in Tunisia, 1960 to 1978

Source: Jemai Y Jemai H: An improved application of methods of measuring the impact of family planning programmes on fertility: the case of Tunisia. In: United Nations (UN) Department of International Economic and Social Affairs. Population Division. Evaluation of the impact of family planning programmes on fertility: source of variance. New York, UN 1982 (Population Studies No. 76; ST/ESA/SER.A/76) p 210-257

Other methods besides these eight have been used to estimate the impact of family planning programs on fertility. These other methods range from correlation analyses of the simple relationships between specific indicators and fertility changes to complex, computerized simulations that project the response of fertility to hypothetical changes in various family planning and sociodemographic indicators. For example, the Coale-Trussell "m" calculation is a technique frequently used to indicate how a given pattern of age-specific marital fertility differs from the standard age pattern of natural fertility.[30,31] This technique thus indirectly gauges the extent of contraceptive use.

METHODOLOGICAL ISSUES

Methodological issues arise with every method for analyzing the fertility impact of family planning programs. Each method may encounter specific difficulties involving the validity of assumptions; the availability accuracy, and comparability of data; and the complexity of calculations. More broadly, a variety of general issues apply to most or all of the methods.

Each method relies on specific assumptions about the variables used in the analyses. The validity of the results of course depends on whether the various assumptions are met. For example, the standardization method generally assumes that the factors analyzed are independent of each other; trend analyses assume that non-program factors do not change during the period under analysis; and areal regression techniques generally assume that there is a linear relationship between fertility on one hand and various socioeconomic and program factors on the other.

ESTIMATING POTENTIAL FERTILITY

One especially important methodological issue is how to estimate potential fertility – the fertility expected in the absence of family planning programs.[6,8,25,32] All eight methods discussed above can be used to estimate births averted, a useful approach when comparing results of various studies. Estimates of births averted require an assumption of potential fertility. Potential fertility can be estimated from previous fertility levels of program clients, fertility levels of the general population, or estimates of natural fertility. Each type of estimate has its problems. For instance, the previous fertility of program clients may be inappropriate since, even after controlling for such factors as age, parity, marital status, and socioeconomic status, these users may differ from the general population with respect to other factors – most importantly, the strength of the desire to limit childbearing. Using natural fertility (fertility in the absence of any deliberate attempt to control fertility) fails to take account of traditional contraceptive methods, contraception available through the private sector, and abortion, any of which may be widely used. Using natural fertility as an approximation of potential fertility leads to an estimate of the gross program effect. Using the other two approximations leads to a rough estimate of net program effect. Recent work on the issue of potential fertility provides up-to-date guidelines for researchers.[11,25]

Procedural and technical problems also can affect study results. Most methods require substantial demographic and/or program data, many of which may be impossible to find or of uncertain accuracy.[3,12,33,34] Finding comparable demographic data from various regions almost always poses problems. Measures of program effort often must be developed anew for each study depending on the data available.[9,12,33] Even for a single program, obtaining comparable, accurate statistics on acceptance, use, and continuation for a period of years may be difficult.[3,12]

A number of the methods – most notably experimental design and some component projection approaches – are technically difficult to carry out.[33] Statistical assumptions must be met, and extensive calculations often are necessary.[12] Some technical problems can be partially overcome by the use of computerized models.[33]

EVALUATION ISSUES AFFECTING ALL PROGRAMS

In addition to the problems of assumptions, data quality, and exhaustive calculations, a number of more general questions arise when planning and evaluating studies of family planning program effects.

These questions apply to most or all methods of analysis. The most important are:

- How should a family planning program be defined? Should privately run programs be considered along with public programs? Should relatively new projects, such as some social marketing programs, be included as family planning programs?[9,33]

- When does a program really begin – on the date it was officially established or at some later time when services are being provided to a substantial proportion of the population?[3] How should analyses take into account private family planning programs that operated before a national program began?

- How can substitution effects be separated from the overall effect? How many program clients actually substituted program sources for non-program sources? Similarly, how can the spillover effect be gauged – the number who begin using contraception because the program makes them more receptive to family planning but who obtain contraception elsewhere?

- Can program and non-program factors be separated? How much of a fertility decline is due to non-program factors? How much is due to the effect of socioeconomic conditions, such as improved health status, educational opportunities, and standard of living, on program function?[12,21,33]

- Finally, when should a family planning program be considered successful? Should the level of contraceptive prevalence increase by 10, 20 or 30 percentage points? Or should fertility drop by a specific amount,[34] or fall to a predetermined level? How should differences in the impact of a program in rural and urban areas or among ethnic groups be considered?

Each method of analysis has problems, and every study needs scrutiny. Nevertheless, in a number of countries, a variety of methods has been used to assess the demographic impact of a family planning program, and most have reached similar conclusions. These similar results strengthen the overall conclusion that organized family planning efforts can contribute significantly to fertility declines.

CONDITIONS FOR A SUCCESSFUL PROGRAM

On the basis of the available data and the observations of family planning experts, some preliminary generalizations can be made about the elements crucial to the success of family planning programs.

AVAILABILITY AND ACCESSIBILITY

The most successful programs generally provide a variety of contraceptive methods, including OCs, IUDs, condoms, barrier methods, and voluntary sterilization[35,36,37,33,39] although a few programs have been successful while emphasizing only one or two methods. Different methods appeal to different couples, and people's needs change during their reproductive years. Thus, offering the widest range of methods appeals to the most users. The availability of abortion also has contributed substantially to fertility declines in some countries, most notably China, South Korea, and Tunisia[35,40,41] – even though it is not generally promoted as a family planning method.

FLEXIBILITY OF SERVICE DELIVERY

Successful family planning programs often provide contraceptive services and supplies through various delivery systems. These delivery systems include stationary clinics, village outreach workers, community-based distribution, mobile clinics, and social marketing. Certain delivery systems may suit cultural preferences in specific areas and overcome supply problems that could limit other systems. While a separate family planning program may be easier to organize and implement initially, integration of family planning with other family health services helps to attract and keep users once the program is established. A variety of program delivery systems combined with widespread sales of contraceptives almost always leads to increasing contraceptive use and declining fertility.[35,39]

LOCAL INVOLVEMENT IN MANAGEMENT DECISIONS

The involvement of regional and local family planning personnel in decision-making characterizes a number of successful programs. Such decisions include what types of contraceptives to provide, what types of delivery systems to use, and how to follow up acceptors. Local involvement probably contributes to success for three reasons: (1) Information campaigns, delivery approaches, and services provided are more likely to be appropriate; (2) local personnel are likely to be more effective when they can see that their decisions and actions make a difference to program achievements; and (3) activities are more likely to be implemented when local rather than distant national leaders direct them.[39]

APPROPRIATE MANAGEMENT

Appropriate management at all levels clearly is essential to all program elements and thus is crucial for success. Supervisors who are trained in management are particularly important. Physicians are sometimes poor supervisors since they usually are not trained in management and have too many medical responsibilities. Effective, well-trained managers at the local level who respond to information from clients and workers may be most valuable.[39] Indeed, among the program elements identified by Mauldin and Lapham as having the greatest impact on fertility are these management elements:

- adequacy of supervision at all levels,
- extent to which staff carry our required tasks,
- extent to which evaluation is used to improve the program.[38]

INFORMATION, EDUCATION AND COMMUNICATION (IEC) ACTIVITIES

IEC campaigns, if they are backed by good service delivery and good management, among other factors, contribute to program success. IEC activities that use mass media to convey appropriate messages can be especially useful, largely because they reach so many people. They tend to have a legitimizing effect if people have doubts about family planning. Also, messages for the mass media are more likely to be developed by professionals who have the technical and communications expertise to prepare and present effective messages.[35,38,39]

Today researchers' attention is focusing increasingly on why family planning programs are successful in reducing fertility and less on whether they can reduce fertility. This new emphasis reflects the fact that over the last two decades family planning programs have proved themselves. Research has shown that family planning programs can reduce fertility as well as protect the health of mothers and children. These benefits are increasingly recognized. At the same time, it has become clear that socioeconomic conditions are closely linked both with people's desire to limit their family size and with the efficiency of family planning programs. Family planning programs of varying strength are currently underway with government support in more than 130 countries worldwide. Organized volunteer efforts are underway in these countries and more. Thus the key issue now is how family planning programs should be designed, implemented, and managed so that they can best accomplish their objectives and achieve both improved health and lower fertility at a reasonable cost and in a manner acceptable to each society.

REFERENCES

1. Chandrasekaran, C., and A.I. Hermalin (eds). Measuring the effect of family planning program on fertility. Dolhain, Belgium: Ordina Editions, 1975.

2. Forrest, J.D., and J.A. Ross. Fertility effects of family planning programs: A methodological review. Social Biology 25(2): 145-163, Summer, 1978.

3. Hermalin, A.I. Issues in the comparative analysis of techniques for evaluating family planning programmes. In: United Nations (UN) Department of International Economic and Social Affairs. Population Division. Evaluation of the impact of family planning programs on fertility: sources of variance. New York: UN, 1982 (Population Studies No. 75; ST/ESA/ser.A/76), pp. 29-40.

4. Hermalin, A.I., and B. Entwisle (eds). The role of surveys in the analysis of family planning programs. (Proceedings of a Seminar, Bogota, Colombia, October 28-31, 1980) Liege, Belgium: Ordina Editions, 1980.

5. International Union for the Scientific Study of Population (IUSSP). Vol 1. International Population Conference, Manila 1981. Liege, Belgium: IUSSP, 1981.

6. Potter R.G. The analysis of cross-method variance in assessing family planning programme effects on fertility. In International Union for the Scientific Study of Population (IUSSP). Vol 1. International Population Conference, Manila 1981. Liege, Belgium: IUSSP, 1981, pp. 261-272.

7. Ross, J.A., and J.D. Forrest. The demographic assessment of family planning programs: a bibliographic essay. Population Index 44(1): 8-27, Jan 1978.

8. United Nations (UN) Department of Economic and Social Affairs. Methods of measuring the impact of family planning programmes on fertility: problems and issues. New York: UN, 1978 (Population Studies No. 61; ST/ESA/ser.A/61).

9. United Nations (UN) Department of International Economic and Social Affairs. Population Division. Evaluation of the impact of family programmes on fertility: sources of variance. New York: UN, 1982 (Population Studies No. 76; ST/ESA/ser.A/76).

10. United Nations (UN) Department of International Economic and Social Affairs. Manual 9. Methodology of measuring the impact of family programmes on fertility. New York: UN, 1979 (Population Studies No. 66; ST/ESA/ser.A/66).

11. United Nations (UN) Department of International Economic and Social Affairs. Population Division. Studies to enhance the evaluation of family planning programmes. (Draft) New York: UN, 1984 (Population Studies No. 87; ST/ESA/ser.A/87).

12. Nortman, D.L. A critique of the methodologies to measure the demographic impact of family planning programmes. In: United Nations (UN) Department of International Economic and Social Affairs. Population Division. Studies to enhance the evaluation of family planning programmes. (Draft) New York: UN, 1984 (Population Studies No. 87; ST/ESA/ser.A/87) pp. 101-132.

13. Cho, L-J., and R.D. Retherford. Comparative analysis of recent fertility trends in East Asia. In: International Union for the Scientific Study of

Population (IUSSP). International Population Conference: Liege, Belgium: IUSSP, 1973, pp. 163-181.

14. Davis, K., and J. Blake. Social structure and fertility: an analytic framework. Economic Development and Cultural Change 4(4): 211-235 July 1956.

15. Bongaarts, J. A framework for analyzing the proximate determinants of fertility. Population and Development Review 4(1): 105-132, March 1978.

16. Bongaarts, J. The fertility-inhibiting effects of the intermediate fertility variables. Studies in Family Planning 13 (6-7): 179-189, June-July 1982.

17. Jemai, Y., and H. Jemai. Fertility projection/trend analysis. In: United Nations (UN) Department of International Economic and Social Affairs. Manual 9. The methodology of measuring the impact of family planning programmes on fertility. New York: UN, 1979 (Population Studies No. 66; ST/ESA/ser.A/66) p 150-152.

18. Mauldin, W.P. Fertility projection/trend analysis. In: United Nations (UN) Department of International Economic and Social Affairs. Manual 9. The Methodology of measuring the impact of family planning programmes on fertility. New York: UN, 1979 (Population Studies No. 66 ST/ESA/ ser.A/66) p. 149.

19. Gorosh, M., and D. Wolders. Standard couple-years of protection. In: United Nations (UN) Department of International Economic and Social Affairs. Manual 9. Methodology of measuring the impact of family planning programmes on fertility. New York: UN, 1979 (Population Studies No. 66; ST/ESA/ser.A/66) pp. 34-47.

20. Lee, B.M., and J. Isbister. The impact of birth control programs on fertility. In: Family planning and population programs (proceedings of the International Conference on Family Planning Programs, Geneva August 1975). Chicago: University of Chicago Press, 1966, pp. 737-758.

21. Ross, J.A. Births averted methods: a guide. 1984 (Unpublished).

22. Wishik, S.M., and K-H Chen. Couple-years of protection: a measure of family planning program output. New York, International Institute for the study of Human Reproduction (manuals for Evaluation of Family Planning and Population Programs No. 7), 1973.

23. Wolfers, D. The demographic effects of a contraceptive programme. Population Studies 23 111-140. London, 1969.

24. Bongaarts, J. A prevalence model for evaluating the fertility effect of family planning programmes: age-specific and method-specific results. In: United Nations (UN) Department of International Economic and Social Affairs. Population Division. Studies to enhance the evaluation of family planning programmes. (Draft) New York: UN, 1984 (Population Studies No. 87: ST/ESA/ser.A/87) pp. 331-339.

25. Bongaarts. J. The concept of potential fertility in evaluation of the fertility impact of family planning programmes. In: United Nations (UN) Department of International Economic and Social Affairs. Population Division. Studies to enhance the evaluation of family planning programmes. (Draft) New York: UN, 1984 (Population Studies No. 87: ST/ESA/ser.A/87) pp. 133-170.

26. Bongaarts, J., and S. Kirmeyer. Estimating the impact of contraceptive prevalence on fertility: aggregate and age-specific versions of a model. In: Hermalin, A.I., and B. Entwisle (eds). The role of surveys in the analysis of family planning programs (Proceedings of a Seminar, Bogota, Colombia, October 28-31, 1980) Liege, Belgium: Ordina Editions, 1980, pp. 381-408.

27. Fisher, A.A., J. Laing, and J. Stoeckel. Research designs for family planning field studies. Bangkok: Population Council (Regional Research Papers), 1984.

28. Wells, H.B. Matching studies. In: Changrasekaran, C., and A.I.Hermalin (eds). Measuring the effect of family planning programs on fertility. Dolhain, Belgium: Ordina Editions, 1975, pp. 215-244.

29. Hermalin, A.I. Multivariate areal analysis. In: United Nations (UN) Department of International Economic and Social Affairs. Manual 9. Methodology of measuring the impact of family planning programmes on fertility New York, UN, 1979 (Population Studies No. 66; ST/ESA /ser.A/ 66) pp. 97-111.

30. Coale, A.J., and T.J. Trussel. Model fertility schedules: Variations in the age structure of childbearing in human populations. Population Index 40(2): 185-258, April 1974.

31. Knodel, J. National fertility: Age patterns, levels, and trends. In: Bulatao, R.A., R.D. Lee, P.E. Hollerbach, and J. Bongaarts (eds), vol. 1 Determinants of fertility in developing countries: Supply and demand for children. New York: Academic Press 1983, pp. 61-102.

32. Bongaarts, J. A note on the concept of potential fertility and its application in the estimation of the fertility impact of family planning programmes. In: United Nations (UN) Department of International Economic and So-

cial Affairs. Population Division. Evaluation of the impact of family planning programmes on fertility: Sources of variance. New York: UN, 1982 (Population Studies No. 76; ST/ESA/ser.A/76) pp. 261-262.

33. Ross, J.A. Overview. In: United Nations (UN) Department of International Economic and Social Affairs. Population Division. Studies to enhance the evaluation of family planning programmes. (Draft) New York: UN, 1984 (Population Studies No. 87: ST/ESA/ser.A/87) pp. 797-820.

34. Srinivasan, K. Recent developments in the evaluation of the demographic impact of family planning programmes. In: International Union for the Scientific Study of Population (IUSSP). Vol. 3. International population conference, Mexico 1977. Liege, Belgium: IUSSP, 1977, pp. 187-207.

35. Clinton, J. An assessment of family planning service programs in 21 selected countries: The family health care report. Washington DC: Family Health Care, Inc., April 1976 (Contract AID/AFR-C-1138).

36. Donaldson, P.J., D.J. Nichols, and E.H. Choe. Abortion and contraception in the Korean fertility transition. Population Studies 36(2): 227-235, July 1982.

37. Mauldin, W.P., and B. Berelson. Reply to R.B. Dixon on drawing policy and conclusions from multiple regressions: Some queries and dilemmas. Studies in Family Planning 9(10-11): 288, Oct-Nov 1978.

38. Mauldin, W.P., and R.J. Lapham. Conditions of fertility decline in LDCs: 1965-1980. Presented at the Annual Meeting of the Population Association of America, Minneapolis, Minnesota, May 3-5, 1984.

39. World Bank. World development report 1984. New York: Oxford University Press, 1984.

40. Jemai, Y., and H. Jemai. An improved application of methods of measuring the impact of family planning on fertility: The case of Tunisia, 1956-1979. In: United Nations (UN) Department of Economic and Social Affairs. Population Division. Evaluation of the impact of family planning programmes of fertility: Sources of variance. New York: UN, 1982 (Population Studies No. 76; ST/ESA/ser.A/76) pp. 210-257.

41. Mumford, S.D., and E. Kessel. Is wide availability of abortion essential to national population growth-control programs? Experiences of 116 countries. Am J Ob Gyn 149(6): 639-645, July 15, 1984.

15

EVALUATION OF CHILD SURVIVAL PROGRAMS

Jack Reynolds, Ph.D.

Evaluation of child survival programs can be complicated because there are many interventions to consider, including oral rehydration therapy (ORT), immunization, growth monitoring, and maternal care. This chapter describes and illustrates a systematic approach to this problem that can be applied by program staff as well as professional evaluators.

THE PURPOSE AND SCOPE OF PROGRAM EVALUATION

Evaluation is sometimes defined as a: **Process** (how it is done; the steps and procedures involved in designing and conducting an evaluation); as a **product** (the findings or judgments that result from an evaluation); or in terms of its **purpose** (the end use of evaluation, for example, for planning or policymaking).

The evaluation process is essentially the same as that used in research. Both use the same techniques – sampling, data collection, analysis, quasi-experimental designs, etc. What distinguishes them is the product. Whereas research is conducted to gain knowledge, evaluation is conducted to produce judgments. Evaluators want to know not only what a program is doing, but also whether it is doing well, whether it is effective, whether it is efficient.

Many evaluations stop at that point. Having made a judgment, many evaluation reports are then filed away. To ensure that evaluation has some utility, the product should be linked to a specific purpose, the reason for conducting the evaluation in the first place. Experience has shown that evaluation can be most useful when it is designed to provide information that managers need to help them make decisions. Typical decisions are whether to continue a program, whether to modify it, and whether to replicate or expand it. If evaluation is seen as an information tool for managers of child survival programs, then it can be defined as: A process for making judgments about part or all of a child survival program for the purpose of deciding among alternative courses of action. Evaluation can be conducted at several stages in a child survival program's life cycle (Figure 1):

- Evaluation of Need: Often called "needs assessments" or "situation analyses" to determine the relative need of a population for various child survival services.

- Evaluation of Program Plans or Design: Evaluation of the feasibility and adequacy of a child survival program plan or proposal to meet a population's needs.

- Evaluation of Processes or Operations: Assessment of the conformity of an ongoing child survival program to its plan, the adequacy of the expected services, in both quantity and quality.

- Evaluation of Effects: Evaluation of the immediate effects of a child survival program on mothers' knowledge, attitudes, and behavior (similar to KAP studies).

- Evaluation of Impact: Assessment of the child survival program's impact on health, especially infant and child morbidity and mortality.

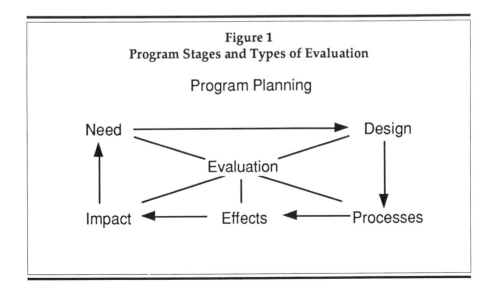

Figure 1
Program Stages and Types of Evaluation

Ideally, evaluation of child survival programs should include all of the above, to ensure that evaluation is an ongoing and comprehensive process. And to enhance utilization, all program evaluation should be designed from the outset to provide child survival managers with information that they need to make judgments and decisions about their programs.

THE EVALUATION PROCESS

Figure 2 summarizes a set of steps for designing and conducting a child survival evaluation. The steps in Phase I are designed to help the evaluator and decision maker specify what is to be evaluated, who is going to use the findings, why the evaluation is to be conducted, when it is to be carried out, and whether it is feasible. The steps in Phase II are to help the evaluator design the procedures for collecting information and analyzing it to produce evaluative judgments about the topic. Phase III steps are to help the evaluator organize and manage the evaluation.

Figure 2
Phases and Steps in the Evaluation Process

Phase I: Specify the Evaluation Topic

    1. Specify the evaluation subject
    2. Determine program stage to evaluate
    3. Specify the purpose of the evaluation

Phase II: Develop the Evaluation Plan

    1. Select a study design
    2. Select indicators
    3. Select standards of comparison
    4. Develop analysis procedures
    5. Specify sampling procedures
    6. Specify data collection procedures
    7. Develop a reporting plan

Phase III: Conduct and Manage the Evaluation

    1. Develop a management plan
    2. Develop, test, refine procedures
    3. Collect, analyze, report data
    4. Implement utilization strategies

Phase I: Specify the Evaluation Topic

Step 1-Specify the subject of the evaluation:

- Decide what child survival service(s) (immunization, ORT, growth monitoring, all, etc.) and/or support service(s) (training, supervision, planning, etc.) are to be evaluated.

- Decide what object(s) (growth charts, syringes, etc.) and/or events (weighing sessions, counseling, record-keeping) and/or people (community health workers [CHWs], supervisors, clinicians) are to be assessed.

- Decide how many of the above are to be evaluated at this time: one, two, several, all?

- If there are several subjects, decide whether they are to be evaluated independently (each CHW), collectively (all CHWs), or as alternatives to one another (volunteer vs. paid CHWs).

- Do a feasibility check: Can this subject be evaluated?

Step 2- Determine the stage of the subject to be evaluated:

- Determine if this is to be an evaluation of the need for the subject; its plan (design); its operation (implementation, processes); its effects on knowledge, attitudes, or behavior or its impact on health.

- If more than one stage is to be evaluated, the first two stages (needs and design) can often be combined into a single evaluation, as can the last three (operations, effects and impact).

Step 3 - Specify the purpose of the evaluation:

- Define the program objectives of the subject to be evaluated. For example, if immunization services are to be evaluated, the objective is probably to increase coverage of children under 2 or 5 years of age to X percent.

- Identify the user(s) of the evaluation (manager, administrator, board, committee, etc.).

- Specify the purpose the users have in mind for the evaluation (knowledge or information only, judgment, decision-making).

- If the use is decision-making, identify the specific decisions the evaluation should address (e.g., whether to modify the immunization services).

PHASE II: DEVELOP THE EVALUATION PLAN

1. Select a study design (experimental, quasi-experimental, non-experimental).
2. Select the indicators that will be used to evaluate the subject (see following section on indicators) and assign weights to indicate the relative importance of each indicator.
3. Select the standards of comparison (for example, actual performance can be compared with that of a control group, the program plan, last year's performance, etc.).
4. Develop the data analysis procedures (data categories, coding instructions, tabulation procedures, statistical analyses).
5. Specify the sampling procedures for each population from which data will be collected (children under age 2, mothers, health workers, etc.).
6. Specify the data collection procedures for each sample (observation, interviews, service statistics, etc.).
7. Develop a reporting plan for each audience (including the timing, frequency, medium – oral, visual, or both).

PHASE III: CONDUCT AND MANAGE THE EVALUATION

1. Develop a management plan (organization, staffing, tasking schedule, budget, monitoring procedures).
2. Develop, test, and refine the evaluation procedures.
3. Collect and analyze the data; report the results.
4. Implement strategies for using the evaluation findings.

INDICATORS FOR EVALUATION OF CHILD SURVIVAL PROGRAMS

The heart of evaluation is the set of indicators used to make judgments about a program's effectiveness (whether it does what it is supposed to do) and its efficiency (whether it does it inexpensively). Three steps are involved in this process:

1. deciding which criteria to use,
2. developing specific measures for those criteria, and
3. selecting standards of comparison for those measures.

A criterion is a characteristic, or variable, that decision-makers use to make judgments about a program. A measure is a number assigned to a criterion according to certain rules that the evaluator must follow. There can be a variety of measures of any criterion. The following example should illustrate this:

Criteria	Measures
Children immunized	Number of children immunized.
	Number of children under 2 years immunized.
	Number of children under 2 years fully immunized against 6 vaccine-preventable diseases/total number of children under 2 years of age.

When data are collected on actual program performance, they need to be compared with some standard, for example:

	No.	Actual	Standard
No. children under age 2 fully immunized	345	53.1%	80%
Total No. children under age 2	650	Immunized	Immunized
For an indicator of efficiency:			
Cost of immunizing children under 2 years	$825	$2.38	$3.00
No. of children under age fully immunized	345	child	child

A standard is a norm, or expected value, to which actual performance can be compared. Without it there can be no evaluation, no meaningful judgment. Immunizing 53.1 percent of the children may be poor performance in a middle-class urban area but exceptional performance in a jungle. Thus, not only are standards necessary for evaluation, but they must also be program-specific.

A SYSTEMS FRAMEWORK FOR SELECTING EVALUATION INDICATORS

It is useful to select evaluation criteria from a systems framework, which is a way to organize criteria according to a logical continuum. The continuum starts with key resources (inputs) that are processed to produce desired services (outputs), which are expected to result in changes in mothers' knowledge, attitudes and behavior (effects), which should ultimately lead to improved child survival (impact). Figure 3 illustrates this systems framework.

Ideally, child survival programs should be evaluated in terms of their impact on health. But it is difficult and expensive to measure impacts. Most child survival managers would like to assess impact occasionally, but they tend to be more interested in evaluating the parts of the program they can control (inputs and processes) and the immediate results of program effort (outputs and effects). Typically, they want to know whether their health workers are skilled in growth monitoring (input); whether they are enrolling children in growth monitoring programs (process); whether most children have been weighed (output); and whether mothers have learned how to interpret growth monitoring charts (effect). If all this is happening, the chances are that the children will benefit and their health will improve (impact).

SELECTED CHILD SURVIVAL INDICATORS

Figure 4 (pages 162-163) is a list of selected child survival evaluation indicators for immunization (IMM), oral rehydration therapy (ORT), maternal care (MC), and growth monitoring and nutrition (GMN), arranged by the systems categories. These indicators are drawn from the recent experience of the PRICOR (Primary Health Care Operations Research) project* in over 40 developing countries.

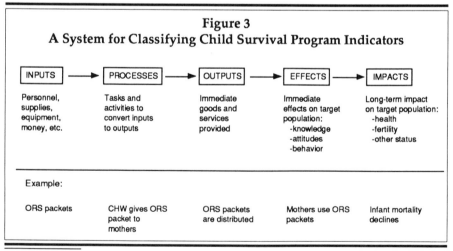

Figure 3
A System for Classifying Child Survival Program Indicators

INPUTS	PROCESSES	OUTPUTS	EFFECTS	IMPACTS
Personnel, supplies, equipment, money, etc.	Tasks and activities to convert inputs to outputs	Immediate goods and services provided	Immediate effects on target population: -knowledge -attitudes -behavior	Long-term impact on target population: -health -fertility -other status

Example:

| ORS packets | CHW gives ORS packet to mothers | ORS packets are distributed | Mothers use ORS packets | Infant mortality declines |

* PRICOR began in 1981 with funding from the U.S. Agency for International Development to find and test ways to improve the effectiveness and efficiency of primary health care programs in the developing world.

EXAMPLES OF CHILD SURVIVAL
EVALUATION IN THAILAND

EVALUATION OF COMMUNITY NEEDS

A primary health care (PHC) demonstration project in a northeast province of Thailand included a community-needs assessment to determine what mothers of young children knew and did about ORT, immunization, growth monitoring and nutrition, and maternal care. The purpose of the assessment was to evaluate current knowledge and practices so that the provincial health office could identify ways to help mothers take better care of their children.

A "Mothers Survey" was designed to gather information on many of the knowledge and behavior indicators shown in Figure 4. A sample of 630 mothers with children under age 2 was drawn from 210 of the province's 1,700 villages. Data were collected by three teams of five newly-graduated health workers. Data collection was completed in three weeks and the report presented to the provincial health staff a week later. The overall conclusion was that coverage levels for key aspects of the child survival program were low. For example:

- Immunization: 48 percent of children under age 1 were completely immunized;

- ORT: 28 percent of children received ORS (oral rehydration salts) during their last diarrhea episode;

- Antenatal Care: 40 percent of mothers received 2 or more prenatal exams during their last pregnancy;

- Growth monitoring: 11 percent of mothers had a growth chart for their child.

The health staff developed an intervention strategy to remedy these and other needs identified by the assessment. After one year they planned to repeat the Mothers' Survey to evaluate the effect of their efforts on these same indicators.

PROCESS EVALUATION OF HEALTH WORKER ACTIVITIES

Another evaluation component of this same project focused on service delivery processes. Checklists were developed to help the evaluators observe the interaction of health workers and mothers, again using many of the process indicators shown in Figure 4. Three teams of four evaluators visited 34

Figure 4
Selected Child Survival Evaluation Indicators

INPUTS	PROCESSES	OUTPUTS	EFFECTS	IMPACTS
IMMUNIZATION No. trained Hlth Wkrs No. vaccines (PC6, DPT Polio, measles, TT) No. needles No. syringes No. sterilizers No. vaccination cards No. cold boxes No. icepacks No. refrigerators No. ltrs fuel	No., % of Hlth Wkrs who: Check name on vial Check amount of vaccine in syringe Clean vaccination site Aspirate syringe Insert needle at correct angle Apply pressure/cotton Correctly record child's card Counsel mother correctly	No., % target population: Registered Attend IMM session with vaccination card	No., % Mothers who know: 6 immunizable diseases where & when to bring child for IMM Recommended age for 1st immunization No., % target pop: Vaccinated at least once 100 % vaccinated BCG DPT Polio Measles	No. cases of: Diphtheria Whooping cough Tetanus Tuberculosis Polio Measles No. deaths from: Diphtheria Whooping cough Tetanus Tuberculosis Polio Measles
ORAL REHYDRATION THERAPY No. trained Hlth Wkrs No. ORS packets No. spoons No. containers No. sets educational materials	No., % of Hlth Wkrs who: Take case history Conduct physical exam Assess hydration status Explain how to give ORS Explain how to feed child Counsel mother correctly	No.,% target population: Contacted about ORT Given ORS packet Taught how to mix ORS Taught how to give ORS	No., % Mothers who know: Purpose of ORT How to mix ORS How to give ORS When to give food No., % diarrhea cases Treated with ORT	No. cases of: Dehydration No. deaths from: Dehydration
GROWTH MONITORING No. trained Hlth Wkrs No. growth cards No. scales No. food supplements No. sets educational materials	No., % of Hlth Wkrs who: Do rapid appraisal of child Calibrate scale to 0 Test scale for accuracy Remove child's clothes Place child correctly Read weight correctly Record weight correctly Plot wt/age correctly Counsel mother correctly	No., % target population: Contacted about GM/N Given GM card Registered Weighed	No.,% Mothers who know: Purpose of GM/N How to weigh child How to read chart When to give supplementary food How long to breastfeed	No., % malnutrition 2nd degree 3rd degree No. malnutrition deaths

Figure 4 (continued)

MATERNAL CARE No. trained Hlth Wkrs No. trained TBAs No. Drugs (iron, folic acid, ergonovine, anti-microbial drugs, anti-convulsant drugs, IV crystalloids) No. needles, syringes, scissors/razor blades, sutures, specula, cord ties, MH cards, IV set-ups) No. vaccines (TT, BCG) No. sets educational materials	(ANC only) No.,% of Hlth Wrkers who: Take pregnancy history Assess risk factors Conduct physical exam Give TT immunization Counsel women correctly Record findings correctly Make appropriate referrals	No.,% target population: Contacted about MC Registered in MC	No.,% target population: Had antenatal care Had TT injection Had supervised delivery Had postnatal care	No. maternal deaths No. complications Pregnancy Abortion Obstetrical No. Stillbirths No. Abortions No. Perinatal deaths No. Neonatal deaths No. low birthweight

subdistrict health centers in the province. They made a total of 1,400 observations among 87 children covering 12 immunization tasks, 19 growth monitoring tasks, and 22 ORT tasks. The evaluators observed actual immunization and growth monitoring sessions; for ORT they asked health workers and mothers to role-play treatment of a child with diarrhea. The results showed that in immunization sessions staff rarely replaced the syringe after injection, as they should have; that all drew and measured the vaccine correctly; and that they recorded all required information correctly on the proper EPI form. In ORT role plays, health education for the mother was thorough; but only half of the cases included a complete history, few physical examinations were conducted, and there was little recording of findings. In growth monitoring sessions no staff did rapid appraisals of the child's health status, they rarely asked about recent illnesses or eating habits and the child's clothes were never removed for weighing; but the staff almost always read and recorded the weight correctly.

The results of the process evaluation were presented to the provincial health staff for discussion. The result was a revised operational plan to increase support for needed equipment and supplies, refresher training in service delivery skills for health workers, and a revised supervision model. As with the Mothers' Survey a follow-up process evaluation was planned to assess improvements in the evaluation indicators.

GENERAL REFERENCES

1. Center for Human Services, PRICOR. Primary Health Care Thesaurus, vol II. A list of service and support indicators. Bethesda, MD, 1988.

2. World Health Organization. Evaluation of Family Planning in Health Services: Report of a WHO Expert Committee. Technical Report Series No. 569. Geneva, 1975.

Section II
MATERNAL
HEALTH

16

WOMEN'S HEALTH IN THE DEVELOPING COUNTRIES

BEVERLY WINIKOFF, M.D., M.P.H.

The intimate relationship between the physical and psychological well-being of a mother and her child has always been obvious. Less well recognized and less utilized in health programs is the fact that the linkages between mother and child are not linear but, rather, part of a continuous process in which health or ill health can be perpetuated from mother to child over decades. It is not very long before the four-year-old becomes the teenage bride who is likely to become a new mother within the first year or so of her marriage: The pre-schooler of today may be a mother in less than a dozen years.

The maintenance of ill health across generations results from a complex interplay of social, economic, cultural, and biological factors. (Figure 1, next page) This cycle can in theory be broken at any point. The complexity of the relationship provides many points at which the passage of ill health from generation to generation can be interrupted. Similarly, protecting the health of infants and young children also protects the health of the next generation of adult women.

Figure 1 illustrates the elements that go into the intergenerational perpetuation of ill health for women and girls in many poor societies. Starting arbitrarily with pregnancy, poor maternal health often results in a baby who is less than robust at birth. Such a baby has impaired chances for survival, and, if it does survive, may well continue in poor health.

In turn, the mother, suffering from ill health (primarily malnutrition in its broadest sense and acute and/or chronic infections), has less energy and personal resources for adequate child care. The child, if a girl, can suffer health, nutrition, socioeconomic, and educational discrimination, the lot of many young girls in developing countries. As a result, she is endowed with fewer resources for her own care, less knowledge, and if she grows up illiterate, less chance to acquire knowledge and less possibility for employment to improve her socioeconomic condition.

She may be anemic and have intestinal parasites or repeated bouts of malaria, which together with her poor nutrition, will sap her energy and undermine her ability to prevent a very early first birth, risky for herself and for her child; and she may not have reliable and adequate medical care during pregnancy and delivery. She may experience complications from pregnancy because her own small stature (due to inadequate early childhood nutrition) puts her at greater risk for obstructed labor, ruptured uterus, sepsis, and death. Her chances of receiving prenatal care are one-half to two-thirds compared to her industrialized country counterpart. If she lives in South Asia or Africa, her chances of having a trained health care attendant for childbirth are even slimmer: 20% to 35%. (Figure 2, next page) Even if she does obtain medical care, her marginal nutrition during pregnancy puts both her and her fetus at risk of continued poor health and development.

Though it is often obvious that the poor health of both women and children is closely intertwined with social and economic problems, the prob-

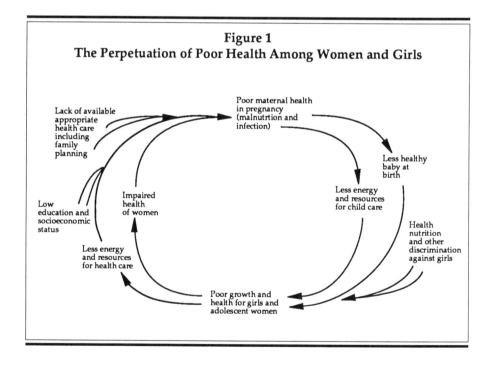

Figure 1
The Perpetuation of Poor Health Among Women and Girls

Lack of available appropriate health care including family planning

Poor maternal health in pregnancy (malnutrtion and infection)

Less healthy baby at birth

Less energy and resources for child care

Impaired health of women

Low education and socioeconomic status

Health nutrition and other discrimination against girls

Less energy and resources for health care

Poor growth and health for girls and adolescent women

lems of mothers and children are less frequently dealt with simultaneously. This chapter outlines the health problems of mothers and demonstrates that the attention to maternal health logically complements the international health community's long-standing involvement with the problems of children. Child health interventions have been relatively well studied. Now, attention should focus more clearly on the problems of women and the interventions that might be developed to help them.

In the past, the major health problems of the community were addressed in terms of their effects on children. Shifting the focus to women's health problems could inspire new and creative thinking about appropriate services at the community level and may, perhaps, generate new impetus for other types of interventions. Considering the recent enthusiasm and rapid adoption of interventions to address child health problems, a set of interventions and service provision packages designed to reach women would be an important complement.

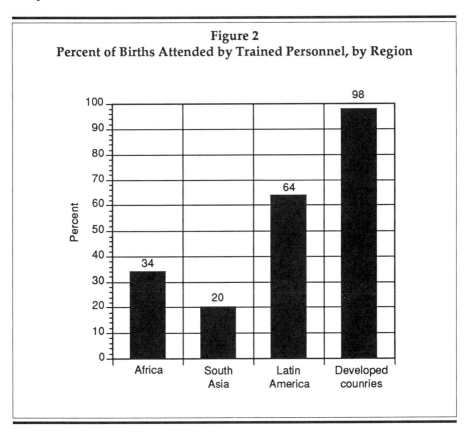

Figure 2
Percent of Births Attended by Trained Personnel, by Region

GIRLS AND WOMEN IN THE DEVELOPING WORLD

Poor health of women during pregnancy compromises the health of fetuses. Female children may suffer additional health problems due to unequal allocation of household resources resulting in excess mortality in infancy and childhood, which runs counter to basic biological tendencies.[1] A recent review of the health situation of women and children in developing countries indicates the excess female mortality among young children which was noted in 19 of 84 countries examined.[2]

As a result of poor health and lack of appropriate medical services (including lack of access to safe means of fertility control), women bear an enormous risk every time they become pregnant. More than 99% of maternal mortality occurs in developing countries. This means that, of the approximately 500,000 women who die each year as a result of pregnancy, only 6,000 or so die in the developed world. Where a child in the developing world suffers a risk of death approximately four to ten times that of a child in Western Europe or North America, a pregnant woman bears approximately 50-100-fold the risk of death of her counterpart in the developed world. Because of the higher fertility of developing country women, her lifetime risk of death from pregnancy may be 400 times greater than that for a woman in North America.

Access to maternity care is poor, particularly in relation to trained supervision of delivery, when life-threatening obstetric emergencies are most likely to occur. According to a World Health Organization (WHO) report, maternal mortality is the first or second cause of death to women 25 to 34 years of age in over half of the developing countries for which data were available.[3] Paradoxically, these are the women who, according to all epidemiological knowledge, are at the lowest risk from reproduction. Yet, because of the large number of women who have children during this age period, pregnancy-related mortality is often a major cause of death for young women in their prime reproductive years.

Because of a lack of available services, both for family planning and for termination of unwanted pregnancy, a substantial component of maternal mortality is the result of improperly performed abortion. The exact number of women who die from this cause is not known, in part because it is very difficult to obtain statistics on what is usually a clandestine procedure. An overview of studies on maternal morality suggests, however, that on the order of 25-50% of maternal deaths are the result of poorly performed abortion procedures.[4]

The toll may even be quite a bit higher, since most women in the developing world do not have access to safe services. Thirty-two percent of women in developing countries live under restrictive abortion laws, and 10% live in areas where abortion is not legal for any reason. Even where abortion is legal, safe procedures are not usually available. For example, in India, where abortion has been legal since 1972, only 250,000 legal abortions are performed each year, while an estimated four million illegal procedures are obtained annually.[5]

The cost of clandestine abortions to the community is high. Services that are necessary to treat complicated abortion cases demand the use of more intensive and costly medical care than most other maternity services. As much as 50% of some hospital maternity care budgets is spent on abortion patients. An estimated 20-50% of gynecology beds are occupied by abortion patients in developing countries.[6] In Nairobi, at one hospital, 60% of the beds used for gynecologic patients were occupied by women under treatment for abortion complications.[7,8]

In addition to the cost in dollars and hospital bed availability, abortion patients put a stress on surgical facilities and supplies of drugs and blood products. Where blood products themselves are not screened, and where the health of the community is poor, the necessity for extensive use of blood products means that women under treatment for abortion face the further risks of malaria, syphilis, hepatitis, and, in some communities, AIDS.

Maternal mortality generally has a devastating effect on families. Newborn infants fare particularly poorly when their mothers die. In one study, 95% of the children of such mothers had also died within a year of their mothers' death.[9] Not very much is known about the fate of older children when a mother dies, but all children probably suffer from poorer health and less medical attention than they would have had if their mother were alive. Where fostering of relatives' children is fairly common (as in parts of Africa), it is assumed that such children fall into the general foster care pattern. It is not known, however, whether such fostering results in less favorable health outcomes and less attentive child-rearing than for children who are raised by the biological parents. For some communities, this is an issue worthy of consideration of child health/child welfare program research.

Aside from acute medical problems encountered during pregnancy and childbirth, women suffer from two main types of morbidity, both of which may have their roots in childhood ill health: nutritional problems and infectious problems. (Figure 3, next page) Several major sources of morbidity fall into each category and, together, they impair women's health and may shorten their lives. In addition, they lead, variously, to pregnancy wastage, low birth weight, impaired child survival, difficult deliveries, and even to infertility. These problems in turn, operate to increase the health risks to the mother both directly and via the need to have more pregnancies in order to achieve a desired family size, given high rates of infant mortality. The balance of this paper gives a brief overview of the extent of these nutritional and infectious problems, highlighting the most important aspects of the relationship between the health of women and their children. Areas where further work could contribute to a greater understanding of the nature of the problems and possible programmatic interventions are emphasized.

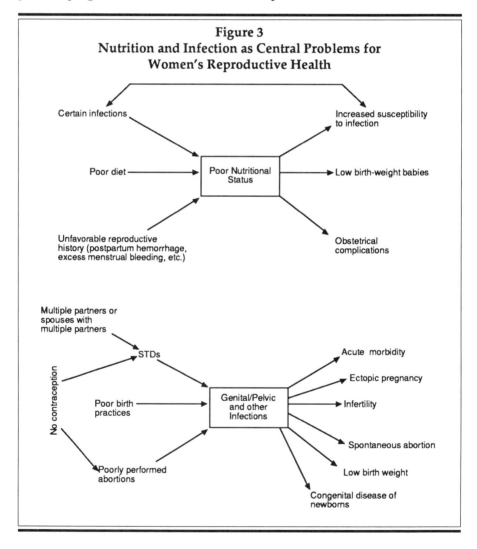

Figure 3
Nutrition and Infection as Central Problems for Women's Reproductive Health

Certain infections

Increased susceptibility to infection

Poor diet ⟶ Poor Nutritional Status ⟶ Low birth-weight babies

Unfavorable reproductive history (postpartum hemorrhage, excess menstrual bleeding, etc.)

Obstetrical complications

Multiple partners or spouses with multiple partners

No contraception

STDs

Poor birth practices

Genital/Pelvic and other Infections

Poorly performed abortions

Acute morbidity

Ectopic pregnancy

Infertility

Spontaneous abortion

Low birth weight

Congenital disease of newborns

NUTRITIONAL MORBIDITY

INADEQUATE CALORIC INTAKE

Inadequate energy intake, a problem throughout the developing world, affects women and children particularly severely. (Table 1) Most nutritional studies have focused on children, in part because their normal sequence of growth in weight and height makes it possible to measure with some accuracy the prevalence of malnutrition.

The situation may be similarly serious for adult women. This, in turn, may have serious implications for the health of all children: Prepregnancy weight and weight gain during pregnancy are two of the strongest determinants of birth weight, and good fetal growth depends on the mother's nutritional health at least as much as on any other known factors.[10,11] Low birth weight, in turn, presents one of the clearest and most universally apparent

Table 1
Prevalence of Energy-Deficient Diets in 87 Developing Countries, 1980

Developing countries[a]	Not enough calories for an active working life[b]		Not enough calories to prevent stunted growth and serious health risks[c]	
	Percent of population	Number of people affected (millions)	Percent of population	Number of people affected (millions)
Total (87)	34	730	16	340
By income				
Low income (30)	51	590	23	270
Middle income (57)	14	140	7	70
By region				
Sub-Saharan Africa (37)	44	150	25	90
East Asia and Pacific (8)	14	40	7	20
South Asia (7)	50	470	21	200
Middle East and North Africa (11)	10	20	4	10
Latin America and the Caribbean (24)	13	50	6	20

[a] Number of countries shown in parentheses [b] Below 90% of FAO/WHO
[c] Below 80% of FAO/WHO requirement
Source: Reference 11

risks for subsequent mortality in young infants.[12] Thus, aside from the stunted growth that makes pregnancy a hazard to the mother herself, early nutritional insults make it more likely that a woman will deliver a low birth-weight child, one who is more likely to die young.

It has been observed frequently that many perinatal problems, and particularly low birth weight, are more common among women who do not have prenatal care.[13,14,15] It appears, in fact, that most of the impact of prenatal care on neonatal and perinatal mortality has occurred through improved medical treatment of high-risk infants once they are born.

From a programmatic point of view, one of the key issues is how to get more calories to mothers both before and during pregnancy. Part of the answer may have to do with improving nutrition education and the utilization of energy-dense foods. Improving the production and consumption patterns of edible oils in developing countries would be an important intervention in this respect.[16] In addition, emphasis on food fats and oils might improve fat-soluble vitamins (for example, vitamin A) in nutrition. Improvement in dietary fat consumption might also improve energy density of mother's milk which might, in turn, improve the caloric intake of infants and make mother's milk adequate as a source of calories for a longer period in the infant's life.

Experience in developed countries may also bear on this issue. Recent evaluations show that a feeding program for women, infants, and children in the United States has dramatically reduced the incidence of early childhood anemia by providing subsidies for iron-enriched foods and also appears to have increased birth weight.[17,18]

NUTRITIONAL ANEMIA

Anemia describes a deficiency in either the quantity or quality of circulating red blood cells – the oxygen-carrying component of the blood. Nutritional anemia suggests that the condition is due not to metabolic defects, hemorrhage, or chronic blood loss, but to deficiencies in the diet that restrict the formation of new blood cells. Shortages of iron, folate, or B12 in the diet can all contribute to anemia. Because of dietary restriction and the increased iron needs of women of reproductive age, iron-deficiency anemia is common in women. Folate deficiency is also common, especially in areas of the world where cereal diets with very little animal protein, fruits, or vegetables are consumed.

Anemia has been associated with many problems of women and children. Severe anemia itself is often listed as a cause of maternal mortality.

Belsey and Royston cite an eight-fold risk of maternal death associated with hemoglobin of less than 8 grams per cc. during pregnancy. Low birth weight and perinatal mortality have also been described as related to low pregnancy hemoglobin, particularly those lower than 9 grams per cc.[19,20] Most studies do not distinguish the cause of anemia, and much of the anemia studied is due to a mix of causes.

Because anemia in poor populations may be caused by many factors, it is useful to have a good idea of the distribution of causes of anemia in a population before undertaking programmatic interventions. Fortunately, a good amount of general information is already available on this subject. Iron deficiency is almost universal in its prevalence but appears most common in South Asia and parts of Africa. In southern Africa, where maize meal diets are common, folate deficiency is relatively much more important.[21] Malaria is another frequent cause of anemia, especially in tropical Africa. Since it is common for women to have deficiencies of iron and folate and, at the same time, suffer from malarial infections, interventions must take into account the possibility of all three problems. Oral and parenteral supplementation of pregnant women, and fortification of food, as well as malaria prophylaxis for pregnant women, have been attempted as interventions to address the problem of anemia.

Recent observations suggest that zinc nutrient may also have an important effect on pregnancy outcome.[22] Interestingly, it appears that iron supplementation and possibly folic acid supplementation may impair maternal zinc nutrition. This issue needs to be resolved by clinical investigation to determine whether, indeed, any important compromise of zinc nutritional status may be caused by iron or folate for pregnant women and whether zinc ought to be included as a recommended supplement during pregnancy. The problems of reaching pregnant women with supplements, and the possibility that high doses of some supplements may not be without negative effects, raises the more general question of whether pregnancy is the best time for offering interventions to prevent anemia in women. Indeed, data on anemia in pregnant and non-pregnant women suggest that women continually bear an enormous burden of anemia. It would seem logical that interventions correcting anemia should be offered to all women, even before a first pregnancy. Such interventions would have the added benefit of protecting women from severe anemia during pregnancy and the deleterious consequences for themselves and their infants.

Waiting to treat anemia until pregnancy, when hemoglobin drops physiologically, ensures that more women will have more severe anemia and clinicians will feel pressed to improve iron status rapidly to ensure maximum hematocrit counts at delivery. There will be real impetus to resort to iron injections which may be painful and can stain the skin, or to very high doses of oral supplements, which may cause gastrointestinal distress.[23] The side effects of iron supplementation are particularly intolerable during pregnancy when women are much more sensitive to nausea, constipation, and heartburn, which they may also be experiencing from pregnancy itself. It would seem logical, and important, to explore alternative interventions and service delivery points that might be used more efficiently than the prenatal care vehicle to combat anemia in the community.

Since iron needs, for example, are not acute during pregnancy but are ongoing throughout a woman's reproductive life, and since iron is well stored in the body, why not supplement women when they are not pregnant as a form of insurance against additional demands of pregnancy?

Community-level fortification of food-stuffs with iron has often been resisted on the basis that iron overload can occur.[18,21] Interestingly, the concern in this instance is sometimes for males who may, for example, in some parts of southern Africa suffer from iron overload because of the iron containers in which their favorite alcoholic beverages are brewed.[18] Some foods, such as paps and weaning foods, might be appropriate items for fortification because they are eaten only by intended target groups. This strategy is only applicable, however, if such foods are centrally processed. Perhaps, indeed, communities exist in which more widespread iron fortification can be tried.

In some respects, anemia provides a useful model for testing interventions which assist mothers in a broader context than prenatal care alone. The low hemoglobin levels of most women throughout all their adult years, their generally hard physical labor, and their need to stay healthy to keep the family healthy, suggest that centering concern for anemia only on the months when a woman is pregnant is short-sighted indeed.

OTHER NUTRITIONAL DEFICIENCIES

Perhaps the nutritional deficit with the clearest link between maternal and child health is iodine deficiency. Populations affected by iodine deficiency are usually far from sea coasts in isolated areas, including the Himalayas and Andes, as well as in Indonesia, New Guinea, and Zaire.

When there is a high rate of iodine deficiency in the population, children may suffer from cretinism at birth. In its severest form, this syndrome includes profound mental retardation, deaf mutism and spasticity. A recent review estimates that, in Asia alone, 400 million people are living in iodine-deficient areas and are therefore at risk for clinical problems.[18] In areas in which deficiency is severe, studies have revealed 4% (India) to 10% (Zaire) of neonates with evidence of iodine deficiency. This compares with a frequency of .02% in developed countries.[24]

Iodine supplementation of food (bread, flour), as well as iodized oil administered by injection and orally have all been successful in improving iodine nutrition on a community level. Since iodine supplementation reduces the incidence of goitre, a readily visible and disfiguring marker for the deficiency, intervention programs are often well accepted on a community level. Such programs have value to the entire population, but particularly to women and to the children who will be born to them.

INFECTIOUS MORBIDITY

SEXUALLY TRANSMITTED DISEASES AND PELVIC INFECTIONS

Sexually transmitted diseases can have devastating consequences for mothers and their children. Serious genital and pelvic infections can result from diseases transmitted through sexual activity and can also be the outcome of poor obstetric and gynecologic practices, including those associated with induced abortion, spontaneous abortion, and childbirth. The effects, depending on the organism involved and the organs affected, can vary from self-limited local lesions to overwhelming pelvic infection resulting in sepsis and death. More limited infection can produce tubal scarring with subsequent infertility or ectopic pregnancy. In addition, spontaneous abortion, premature rupture of the membranes, and chorioamnionitis with infant sepsis and mortality may result from maternal infections. Other possible results of maternal genital infection for infants include congenital anomalies, blindness, pneumonia, and mental retardation.

Common genital and pelvic infections that are sexually transmitted include gonorrhea, syphilis, chlamydia infection, colonization with mycoplasma and ureaplasma, and genital herpes.

Gonorrhea is a highly infectious bacterial disease, which is easily contracted during sexual activity. It is well known to be a cause of upper-genital tract infection or pelvic inflammatory disease (PID), resulting in a subsequent elevated risk of infertility or ectopic pregnancy. Tubal occlusion has been reported to result in over 5% of women following gonococcal infection, and up to one-quarter of women who experience PID are reported to suffer sequelae such as infertility or ectopic pregnancy.[25] In addition, if present in the vagina during childbirth, the causative organism (*N. gonorrhoea*) may infect the newborn and cause an ophthalmitis, which can cause blindness. Gonococcal eye infections are more than 50 times as common in Africa as in industrialized countries.[26] Transmission rates from mother to baby are especially high if the mother is concomitantly infected by chlamydia.

Until recently gonorrhea was exquisitely sensitive to penicillin, but lately, penicillinase-producing antibiotic-resistant strains have become widespread. This has made therapy increasingly expensive and difficult, a particularly serious problem for developing country health services. On the other hand, the consequences of maternal infection for the newborn can be much reduced by the very inexpensive intervention of silver nitrate or antibiotics applied to the eyes at birth. It has also been suggested that colostrum may prevent serious conjunctivitis and ophthalmitis from gonorrhea and other organisms, but this possibility has not been studied adequately.[27]

Chlamydia trachomatis is an infectious agent that has recently come under closer scrutiny, as it has been more clearly implicated as a cause of substantial morbidity. It is a common cause of urethritis and is easily transmitted through sexual contact. Infections with chlamydia are apparent causes of PID and upper genital tract infections with a relatively high risk of producing permanent scarring and infertility. In fact, the risk of infertility following chlamydia infection appears to be even higher than the risk following gonorrheal PID. One study cites a rate of tubal occlusion approximately three times higher with chlamydial disease than with gonorrheal disease.[25]

Chlamydia can also cause ophthalmitis in the newborn, an infection that does not cause blindness as does gonorrheal ophthalmia. In addition, chlamydia may also cause a recently recognized pneumonia of the newborn. In general, this pneumonia is not life-threatening, but it can occasionally require intensive hospital treatment. Low birth weight and preterm delivery have both been associated with infection with this organism.[25] A recent onset of chlamydia infection appeared to increase the risk of low birth-weight babies in a population of American Indians.[28]

The difficulty with chlamydia is not so much in its treatment as in it identification. The infection generally causes no symptoms until later when tubal scarring or infertility is discovered. In addition, until recently it has been necessary to use relatively high-cost cultures to identify the organism. The availability of new less-expensive methods for diagnosis which may make possible the screening of more women for this infection, appears to be imminent.[29] As has long been known, barrier contraceptives appear to protect against PID and infection by sexually transmitted diseases generally. Recently, it has been shown that the commonly used spermicide nonoxynol-9 appears to reduce the risk of chlamydia infection by one-third and gonorrheal infection by two-thirds.[30]

Syphilis is still a problem for mothers and children, especially in the developing world. In the short term, syphilis is an infection with remarkably little morbidity, but, in the long term, it can cause severe symptoms, including neurological problems, incapacitation, and death. For the gestating infant, syphilis in the mother can be devastating. If a mother is infected with syphilis, she runs a high risk of suffering spontaneous abortion or late intrauterine death. Women with positive serology for syphilis have more than seven times the risk of fetal death as women who are not so infected.[25]

A recent WHO review calculates that between 35 and 50% of stillbirths in Ethiopia can be attributed to syphilis.[2] It has been estimated that 5 to 8% of all pregnancies surviving past 12 weeks in parts of Africa are affected by either fetal death or congenital syphilis of the newborn.[26] In a review of ten studies of pregnant women in six countries in Africa, from 4 to 15% of patients showed positive sero-reactivity for syphilis. In eight of these studies, over 10% of women were so affected.[31] In a hospital in Zambia, nearly 1% of the babies delivered had clinical signs of congenital syphilis infection and as many as 6.5% were sero-positive for the infection and at risk for further health problems.[32]

Infection with mycoplasma and ureaplasma also may have an effect on fetal development. Spontaneous abortion, fetal wastage, prematurity, and low birth weight have been associated in some studies with maternal colonization with these organisms.[25] Women with surgical deliveries have been linked to an increased risk of postpartum endometritis.[28]

A recent study of women with proven mycoplasma and/or ureaplasma vaginal infection showed a significant rise in birth weights among the infants of those women who took an antibiotic (erythromycin) for at least six weeks, starting in the third trimester.[33] These results have raised interest in the possibility of unselected treatment of groups of pregnant women with erythromycin where low birth weight and maternal ill health are common. The appeal of this strategy is understandable, since it eliminates the need for screening patients and since erythromycin is relatively inexpensive, of low toxicity, and active against many of the sexually transmitted pathogens, including ureaplasma, mycoplasma, chlamydia, and syphilis. The available information in this particular treatment is inadequate to advocate its routine use, however. The initial report of the treatment contains inconsistencies, suggesting that more work needs to be done to understand the potential efficacy of the intervention and the mechanism by which it works.

Genital herpes infections, apparently becoming more widespread currently in developed countries, are troublesome and symptomatic for women. The infection also may have catastrophic effects on the newborn, particularly if the mother has active lesions when the child is born. In such cases, brain infection, with high frequency of higher death or permanent and severe neurological damage, is possible. At present, although some drugs attenuate the symptoms, no cure is known for this infection, and once infected, a woman is continuously at risk for recurrent infections.

Another virus, human papilloma virus, which is transmitted by sexual contact, is widely thought to be responsible for cervical cancer. Over three-quarters of the world's cases of this disease are said to occur in developing countries.[2] The extent of the morbidity and mortality can be substantial. In the United States alone, in 1975, approximately 6,800 deaths from this cause were expected, more than from all others STDs.[34]

Urinary tract infections (UTIs) have also been linked strongly to unfavorable outcomes of pregnancy, especially for births taking place within two weeks following the onset of infection.[35] The low birth weight associated with urinary tract infections is due both to preterm delivery and to fetal growth retardation. Increased perinatal mortality is associated with UTIs in women with hypertension.

Very few community surveys have been done of vaginal or pelvic infections. This inhibits consideration of what might be reasonable interventions for these problems during pregnancy and among non-pregnant women. One of the few studies that attempts a community-wide look at the problem was conducted in rural Bangladesh. In this study, 22% of the women who were interviewed reported symptoms consistent with reproductive tract infection.[36] The most common complaint was chronic vaginal discharge. Almost two-thirds of the symptomatic women who were examined were infected, but the infection rate varied greatly by the method of contraception used. Non-users and hormonal method users had lower rates of infection than IUD users.

The results of the study in Bangladesh are strikingly different from the prevalence rates uncovered in studies of pregnant women in Africa. This suggests that rates and types of infection may be extremely different in different cultural groups and geographic locales. For this reason, it is important to generate a more secure factual base about the community prevalence of urinary and genital tract infections.

INFERTILITY AND ECTOPIC PREGNANCY

One of the major sequelae of sexually transmitted disease is tubal damage and the associated infertility and risk of ectopic pregnancy. These problems occur not only with sexually transmitted infection, but also with infection secondary to poor obstetric and gynecologic practices in childbirth or abortion. A WHO review notes that the risk of secondary infertility in one African country was twice as high among women delivered by an untrained birth attendant as among those delivered by a trained attendant or with no assistance.[3] The risk of infertility was tripled among women in Nigeria who had a previous abortion, either spontaneous or induced. The extent of the infectious problem may also be seen by the number of women diagnosed as primarily and secondarily infertile in WHO community surveys. Generally, the number of women with primary infertility is low. The rate increases markedly for secondary infertility (infertility after the birth of at least one child), suggesting an acquired and, frequently, an infectious cause of the infertility.

The incidence of infertility in some communities is alarmingly high, particularly in some regions of sub-Saharan Africa, where infertility rates may reach as high as 50% in comparison to 11% in the developed world, 14% in Asia, 15% in Latin America, and 20% in the Eastern Mediterranean (Tunisia, Egypt).[26] Similarly, pelvic adhesions were diagnosed in 24% of the women from Africa, and only 12-17% of women from other regions.[37] In addition, women from the African region reported more frequent histories of STDs and more frequent complications of abortions or childbirth than women in the other regions.[38] Finally, in Africa, even women with no live births were almost twice as likely to have a diagnosis of infection-related infertility as women in other regions.

The suggestion from these studies is that several types of interventions be explored. These include attempts to prevent STD occurrence (for example, by education and the wider use of contraceptive methods likely to diminish transmission), projects to treat STDs in both symptomatic and asymptomatic women through family planning programs and/or other maternal health services, and concerted efforts to prevent the poor obstetric/gynecologic practices that result in secondary infections after procedures for abortion and childbirth.

The programmatic questions raised are many and difficult. The question of how to design appropriate services to detect and/or treat pelvic and genital infections in women is not easy. The idea of mass prophylaxis with antibiotics, while appealing in its simplicity, deserves very critical thought and much more epidemiologic and programmatic investigation before it can be advocated. It is clear that using prenatal care as the sole focus for infection control will not be adequate to the needs of women and their children: Women may have symptoms when they are not pregnant, and fetuses may be injured very early in development by certain sexually transmitted diseases. Some types of contraceptives may be extremely useful in preventing the spread of sexually transmitted diseases, and other contraceptives appear, under some circumstances, to be associated with an increased risk of infection. These issues need to be studied further and taken into account when addressing program issues and the design of family planning services in different locations. Finally, improvements in obstetric care and abortion services clearly are needed urgently so that women who avail themselves of medical services are not placed at needlessly high risk of adverse outcomes.

OTHER INFECTIOUS DISEASES

VIRAL DISEASES

Two other infections, hepatitis B and human immunodeficiency virus (HIV, the virus that causes AIDS), can also be transmitted by sexual contact. These are not primarily infections of the genital/pelvic area, and are considered together with discussions of systemic infections. In addition, of course, both these diseases can be transmitted by sharing needles and by using contaminated blood products, although hepatitis appears to be much more easily transmitted and much more infectious than HIV. The geographic distribution of these diseases makes each a problem for maternal and child health in different parts of the world.

Hepatitis B constitutes a major problem primarily in Southeast Asia, although it is also a problem elsewhere. AIDS, on the other hand, has become a serious public health concern for mothers and children mostly in Central and East Africa, in Haiti, and in the United States. With time, however, it is generally predicted that AIDS may become a universal problem. Both these infections are caused by viruses with similar routes of transmission. Both infections are generally more prevalent among homosexuals, drug abusers, and sexually promiscuous groups, particularly prostitutes. There is no cure for either infection, but the implications for health of the two diseases are quite different.

AIDS, a new disease, has been known for less than a decade. As a result, the natural history of the infection and the biology of the virus that causes the syndrome have only recently been discovered. What is known, however, is that the disease, once it is present, is uniformly fatal, usually within less than two years. The percentage of infected individuals who ultimately develop symptoms of the disease is probably close to 100%, but the exact figure is not yet known. Hepatitis B is less often fatal, but is still a serious infection. Not only does it cause acute, sometimes severe, morbidity, but it also causes chronic hepatitis, cirrhosis of the liver, and carcinoma of the liver. Both hepatitis B and HIV may be passed from mother to infant, so that neonatal infection with these diseases is a problem wherever the carrier rates for the infections are high. Hepatitis B virus transmission is associated with the presence of specific antigen (HBsAg and HBeAg) in the mother's blood. Ninety-five percent of infants infected in the perinatal period become chronic carriers.

Sterilization of skin-piercing equipment and screening of blood and blood products will protect patients who use medical services from both HIV and hepatitis, but appropriate asepsis and the screening of blood products have been beyond the capability of some health services in the developing world. The technology for blood screening is being refined, however, and it may be possible to lower the cost and complexity of testing for HIV seropositivity in blood products in the future. Until then, the best protection for maternal and child health is to insure use of sterile equipment when medical care is given. In addition, the provision of more accessible, better quality obstetric and gynecologic care can reduce the need for blood transfusions. Health workers can be trained – or retrained – to be sure that all transfusions that are administered are necessary, as there is some evidence that transfusions may be overused in certain circumstances.

For hepatitis B, interventions are possible to prevent the transmission of the virus; an effective vaccine has been developed and marketed. Protocols for vaccine plus immune globulin have been developed that can markedly reduce maternal/infant transmission of infection. A dose of immune globulin and of hepatitis vaccine at birth, plus vaccine at three and six months, produces a substantial decline in transmission (on the order of 75%) among infants treated with this regimen.[39]

TETANUS

Neonatal tetanus has been documented to be a major cause of mortality in the first two weeks of life in some areas of the world. It has been calculated that almost one million fatalities are caused by this disease.[40] Rates appear to be highest in South Asia, including Pakistan and Bangladesh. Substantial rates are also found in parts of Africa (including Somalia, Ivory Coast, and Uganda) and Southeast Asia (Indonesia).[2] In addition, in places where the incidence of neonatal tetanus is high, maternal tetanus may also be a reported cause of death after childbirth, although not of the same magnitude as death from infection or hemorrhage.

Retraining of health workers to provide more hygienic services at delivery as well as tetanus toxoid immunization of pregnant women has been known to reduce the incidence of neonatal tetanus. A recent review of both interventions suggests that, although both can reduce the rates of disease substantially, only tetanus immunization has the potential for totally eliminating the problem.[41] It is suggested that future research should be organized to compare tetanus toxoid immunization alone with toxoid and birth attendant training together to know if the combined effort produces a further decrease in neonatal mortality beyond immunization alone.

Most immunization programs focus on pregnant women who have never been immunized. It should be noted that adequate maternal and infant protection can be provided by at least two doses of tetanus toxoid, the second of which must be given at least four weeks after the first and at least three weeks before delivery. Women who appear late for prenatal care will not have enough time to receive all the injections to provide adequate protection for themselves and their children.[42] A wiser course might involve broader outreach for an immunization campaign, including all women of reproductive age and possibly teenage women as well.

MALARIA

A substantial health threat to women and their children is also posed by the worldwide resurgence of malaria. The problems engendered by malaria have become even more serious due to the increasing prevalence of drug-resistant forms of malaria with the potential for serious morbidity and the need to use more toxic drugs for treatment. Malaria during pregnancy appears to increase the risk of severe complication of cerebral malaria and of death.[2] In addition, malaria generally contributes to the problem of anemia, lowering the hemoglobin level by about 1.5 grams per cubic centimeter, and producing lower birth-weight babies, spontaneous abortion, and fetal death.[2] The problem of malaria and the spread of resistant parasites is truly a community-wide problem that has as its severest manifestation the health status of women and children.

IMPLICATIONS FOR RESEARCH AND SERVICES

It is obvious that the health problems of mothers and their children are closely connected in multiple ways. These health problems interact with the environmental detriments to which women and children are subject for cultural, social, and economic reasons.

Many large gaps in knowledge exist, even about the most fundamental issues, such as the prevalence of morbidity in women in different communities. Some knowledge can be gained by a systematic review of existing publications. In particular, national and regional medical journals, especially those not published in English, may contain valuable information not usually accessible in the international literature. For many poorly researched issues, such as the prevalence of various genital tract infections, new studies will have to be designed and carried out.

Some suggestions for community interventions need to be re-examined for efficacy (for example, antibiotics during pregnancy), and, even if proven efficacious, appropriate designs need to be developed for programs. Well established interventions should also be examined to determine whether new program designs might improve long-term successes (for example, prenatal care, iron supplementation). In addition, an important area for research is the efficacy of retraining health personnel. This issue arises in regard to interventions against tetanus, but also in terms of improving the overall safety of medical procedures, including use of blood products, sterile equipment, abortion techniques, and contraceptive service delivery. How much, indeed, can be expected of training lower-level health workers? To what extent is retraining of higher-legal professionals also necessary?

It is clear that a re-examination of the service delivery paradigms that are often taken for granted may help to improve the delivery of both preventive services and primary health care to women and children. To view pregnancy, for example, as the central point of contact between women and health services may appear logical at first. In the long term, it may prove short-sighted because it ignores the potential for effective reduction of morbidity (and mortality) among women and children. If women's lives are seen as a continuum, it is obvious that the morbidity leading to poor outcomes of pregnancy exists for many months before and after pregnancy. Anemia, for example, is very important and widely prevalent precisely because nothing is done to improve the diets of small girls, of growing adolescents, or of married women before the first pregnancy, between pregnancies, and after pregnancies. Similarly, women may suffer the morbidity of genital infection for a long time before pregnancy, yet have no access to medical care for treatment of their problems.

Selecting certain "high-risk" groups as targets of health care interventions has established benefits in terms of directing resources to those at highest risk or most in need. On the other hand, it must be realized that a certain resource expenditure is always involved in the process of finding and serving the target population – that is, in designing services directed at the few rather than the many. Programs need to judge whether this cost is worthwhile. Because of the high incidence of preventable disease which may have serious implications for generations to come, it may be time to look at some less-targeted interventions that are aimed at the female population as a whole. Testing "detargeting" of some interventions might demonstrate pay-offs in greater acceptability and efficiency for the programs themselves.

Re-examining the locus of certain interventions might also prove worthwhile. For example, programs to combat iron deficiency might achieve greater compliance and perhaps better outcomes if supplementation were given to women at times other than, or in addition to, prenatal visits. Postpartum, family planning, or child care visits might be acceptable and effective times to provide preventive care to mothers. This brings up the general need to think about the appropriate points of contact between health services and mothers and the kinds of services that could possibly be provided in a different milieu. It also emphasizes a need for good short- and long-term indicators of program effect. Certainly, it could be the case that some program designs show more immediate results, and others have more sustained or permanent effects. Despite the pressure for short-term or intermediate indicators, there is also a need to verify long-term effects.

Thinking of women as more than simply vehicles for the improved production of the next generation may have dividends in better health for women and also in reorientation of the health services themselves. The importance of such a new perspective, from a human rights orientation, has been emphasized eloquently.[43] Similarly, understanding the close link from mothers to their children and to the next generation of mothers will allow a longer-range perspective to be applied to the design of services. For example, the feeding of young female children may be viewed as a maternal health intervention as well as a pediatric priority. From the point of view of the community, a rethinking of the service delivery packages offered as part of primary health care and of the timing of different interventions in the life cycle may be one way to improve the utilization of resources allocated for health care.

(Note: This chapter has been adapted from "Women's Health: An Alternate Perspective for Choosing Interventions." - Beverly Winikoff, in STUDIES IN FAMILY PLANNING, Volume 19, Number 4, July/Aug 1988, with the prior agreement of the author and Population Council.)

REFERENCES

1. Chen, L., E. Hug, and S. D'Souza. Sex bias in the family allocation of food and health care in rural Bangladesh. Population and Development Review 7, 1;55-70, 1981.

2. Belsey, M. and E. Royston. Overview of the health of women and children. Paper prepared for the International Conference on Better Health for Women and Children Through Family Planning, October, Nairobi, Kenya, 1987.

3. Royston, E. Statistical Enquiry: WHO Programme on the Participation of Women in Health and Development (Item 6). Geneva: WHO, 1977.

4. Winikoff, B., C. Carignan, E. Bernardik, and P. Semeraro. Medical services to save mothers' lives: Feasible approaches to reducing maternal mortality. Background paper for Safe Motherhood International Conference, The World Bank, February, Nairobi, 1987.

5. McFalls, Jr., J.A., and M.H. McFalls. Disease and Fertility. Orlando: Academic Press. pp. 387 - 426, 1984.

6. Fortney, J.A. The use of hospital resources to treat incomplete abortions. Examples from Latin America. Public Health Reports 96,6:574-79, 1981.

7. Corvalan, H. The abortion epidemic. In Birth Control: An International assessment.M. Potts and P. Bhiwandiwala, (eds). Baltimore: University Park Press, pp. 201-214, 1979.

8. Wanjala, S., N. Murugu, and J. Mati. Mortality due to abortion at Kenyatta National Hospital, 1974-1983. In Abortion: Medical Progress and Social Implications. Ruth Porter and Malol O' Connor (eds). London: Pitman (Ciba Foundation), pp. 41-52, 1985.

9 . Chen, L., M. C. Gesche, S. Ahmed, A. I. Chowdury, and W. H. Mosley. Maternal mortality in rural Bangladesh. Studies in Family Planning 5,11: 334-341, 1974.

10. Kramer, M. Forthcoming. Determinants of intrauterine growth and gestational duration: A methodologic assessment and meta-analysis. Bulletin of the WHO (in press).

11. Winikoff, B., and C. Debrovne. Anthropometric determinants of birth weight. Obstetrics and Gynecology 58, 6: 678-684, 1981.

12. _____. The incidence of low birth weight: A Critical review of available information. World Health Stat Quart 33, 3: 197-224, 1980.

13. Trivedi, C., and D. Mavalankar. Epidemiology of low birth weight in Ahmedabad. The Indian J Ped 53, 6: 795-800, 1986.

14. Harrison, K. Child-bearing, health and social priorities: A survey of 22,774 consecutive hospital births in Zaria, Northern Nigeria. British J Ob Gyn, Supplement No. 3, 1985.

15. Brown, S. Can low birth weight be prevented? Family Planning Perspectives 17, 3:112-118, 1985.

16. Crawford, M., W. Doyle, and P. Drury. Relationship between maternal and infant nutrition and the special role of fat in energy transfer. Trop Geo Med 37, 3: 55-516, 1985.

17. Yip, R., N. Binkin, L. Fleshood, and F. Trowbridge. Declining prevalence of anemia among low-income children in the United States. JAM 258, 12 :1645-1647,1987.

18. Stockman, J. Iron deficiency anemia: Have we come far enough? JAM 258, 12:1645-1647, 1987.

19. Murphy, J., R. Newcombe, J.O'Riordan, and E. Coles. Relation of haemoglobin levels in first and second trimesters to outcome of the pregnancy. The Lancet (3 May): 992-994, 1986.

20. Kuizon, M., R. Cheong, L. Ancheta, J. Desnacido, P. Macapinlac, and J. Baens. Effect of anaemia and other maternal characteristics on birth weight. Human Nutrition: Clin Nutrition (5 August): 419-446, 1985.

21. Baynes R., W. Meriwether, T. Bothwell, F. Costa, W. Bezwoda, and A. MacPhail. Iron and folate status of pregnant black women in Gazankulu. SAM/70 (2 August) :148-151, 1986.

22. Mukherjee, M., H. Sandstead, M. Ratnaparkhi, L. Johnson, D. Milne, and H. Stelling. Maternal zinc, iron, folic acid, and protein nutriture and outcome of human pregnancy. Am J of Clin Nutrition 40 (September):496-597, 1984.

23. Jenkinson, D. Single-dose intramuscular iron dextran in pregnancy for anaemia prevention in urban Zambia. J Trop Med and Hygiene 87: 71-73, 1984.

24. Hetzel, B. Iodine deficiency disorders (IDD): A maternal and child health issue. Advances in International Maternal and Child Health. D. B. Jelliffe and E. F. Patrice Jelliffe (eds) Oxford: Clarendon Press, pp. 79-107, 1986.

25. Mtimavalye, L., and M. Belsey. Infertility and sexually transmitted disease: Major problems in maternal and child health and family planning. Prepared for the International Conference on Better Health for Women and Children through Family Planning, October, Nairobi, Kenya, 1984.

26. Rosenbert, M., K. F. Schulz, and N. Burton. Sexually Transmitted Diseases in sub-Sahara Africa: A priority list based on Family Health International's meeting. 19 July: 152-153, 1986.

27. Bishai, D., and M. Bishai. Letter to the Editor. The New Eng J Med 316,24:1549,1987.

28. Berman, S., R. Harrison, T. Boyce, W. Haffner, M. Lewis, and J. Arthur. Low birth weight, prematurity and postpartum endometritis. JAM, 257, 9 :1189-1194, 1987.

29. Schachter, J., M. Gorssman, R. Sweet, J. Holt, C. Jordan, and E. Bishop. Prospective study of perinatal transmission of *Chlamydia trachomatis*. JAM 255,24:3374-3377, 1986.

30. Rosenberg, M., W. Rojanpithayakorn, P. Feldblum, and J. Higgins. Effects of the contraceptive sponge on chlamydia infection, gonorrhea, and candidiasis. JAM 257,17: 2308-2312, 1987.

31. Schulz, K.F., W. Cates, Jr., and P.R. O'Mara. Forthcoming. Pregnancy loss, infant death and suffering; the legacy of syphilis and gonorrhea in Africa. Genitourinary Medicine (in press).

32. Hira, S. Sexually transmitted disease: A menace to mothers and children. World Health Forum 7: 243-247, 1986.

33. McCoremack, W., B. Rosner, Y. Lee, A. Munoz, D. Charles, and E. Kass. Effect on birth weight of erythromycin treatment of pregnant women. Obstetrics and Gynecology 69, 2: 202-207, 1987.

34. Grimes, D. Deaths due to sexually transmitted diseases. JAM 255.13:1727-1729, 1986.

35. Naeye, R. Urinary tract infections and the outcome of pregnancy. Advances In Nephrology 15:95-102, 1986.

36. Wasserheit, J., J. Harris, J. Chakraborty, B. Kay, and K. Mason. Reproductive tract infections in a family planning population. Studies in Family Planning 20, 2:69-80, 1989.

37. Cates, W., T.M. Farley, and P.J. Rowe. Worldwide patterns of infertility: Is Africa different? Lancet 11 (14 September):596–598,1985.

38. World Health Organization. Infections, pregnancies, and infertility: Perspectives on prevention. Fertility and Sterility 47,6:964-968, 1987.

39. Beasely, R., C. Lin, Wang, F. Hsieh, L. Hwang, C. Stevens, T. Sun, and W. Szmuness. Hepatitis B Immune Globulin (HBIG) efficacy in the interruption of perinatal transmission of Hepatitis B virus carrier state. Lancet (22 August): 388-393, 1981.

40. Stanfield, J.P. and A. Galazka. Neonatal tetanus: An underreported scourge. World Health Forum 67,2:127-129, 1985.

41. Ross, D. Does training TBAs prevent neonatal tetanus? Health Policy and Planning I, 2:89-98, 1986.

42. Galazka, A. Control of neonatal tetanus. Indian J Ped 52,417:329-341, 1985.

43. Germain, A. Reproductive health and dignity: Choices by Third World Women. Background Document for the International Conference on Better Health for Women and Children through Family Planning. October. Nairobi, Kenya, 1987.

17

THE STATUS OF FAMILY PLANNING IN DEVELOPING COUNTRIES

Jodi L. Jacobson

Thirty-three-year-old Socorro Cisneros de Rosales, a Central American mother of 13, is neither a demographer nor an economist. But in describing her own plight and that of her country as " an overproduction of children and a lack of food and work," Mrs. Cisneros speaks authoritatively on the conflict between high birth rates and declining economies that faces many in the Third World.

Over the past two decades, steadily declining birth rates have contributed to significant improvements in the health and well-being of millions of people and to the growth of national economies. To date, however, only a handful of countries have reduced fertility rates enough to make these gains universal or to ensure that their populations will stabilize in the foreseeable future. Countries that remain on a high fertility path will find that meeting basic subsistence needs will be increasingly difficult in the years to come.

Despite lower fertility levels for the world as a whole, population increased by 94 million people in 1989. Although birth rates continue to fall in many developing countries, the pace has slowed markedly. And declining death rates have balanced out the modest reductions in fertility of the past few years. Furthermore, slower economic growth in developing countries plagued by debt, dwindling exports, and environmental degradation means that governments can no longer rely on socioeconomic gains to help reduce births. This uncertain economic outlook raises important questions. Can governments successfully encourage fertility reductions in the face of extensive poverty? What mix of policies is likely to promote smaller families, thereby reducing fertility and raising living standards?

Encouraging small families requires a two-pronged strategy of family planning and social change. Few countries, however, have put family planning and reproductive health care at the top of their agendas. In most industrial nations, widely available contraceptive technologies enable couples to choose the number and spacing of their children. But for the majority of women in many developing countries, contraceptive methods remain unavailable, inaccessible, or inappropriate. Surveys confirm that the 463 million married women in developing countries outside of China want no more children. Millions more would like to delay their next pregnancy. Meanwhile, the number of women in their childbearing years is increasing rapidly.

With few exceptions, governments have not changed policies or invested in programs sufficiently to weaken the social conditions underlying high fertility. These conditions include, most significantly, the low status of women and the high illiteracy, low wages, and ill health that customarily accompany it. Until societal attitudes change, national fertility rates are unlikely to decline significantly.

International support for family planning has been considerably weakened in recent years by changes in U.S. policy. By the time the world's population surpassed 5 billion in 1987, the United States had abdicated its role as a leading supporter of reproductive rights worldwide. Political and societal disputes have converged with fiscal constraints to cut funding for contraceptive research and for both domestic and international family planning. This policy change has set worldwide efforts to reduce fertility back by several years, dimming hopes of achieving population stabilization by the end of the next century.

Reducing birth rates to speed the development process is a goal that deserves the immediate attention of the world community. Promoting smaller families throughout the Third World will benefit every segment of society. For women, bearing fewer children means better health for themselves and their offspring. For countries, reducing average family size increases per capita investments and alleviates pressures on the natural resources that underpin national economies. For the world, slower population growth enhances the prospects for widespread security and prosperity.

FERTILITY TRENDS WORLDWIDE

Childbearing trends are most clearly represented by total fertility rates, defined as the average number of children a woman will bear at prevailing levels of fertility. A country that has achieved replacement-level fertility of about 2.1 births per woman is well on the road to a stable population size. Once this level has been reached, births and deaths eventually balance out. A population at or below replacement level may continue to grow for two or three generations, however, if the group reaching childbearing age is larger than that reaching old age and dying.

With few exceptions, total fertility rates in the industrial world are at or below replacement level. In the United States, for example, the rate is 1.9 births per woman; in France and the United Kingdom, 1.8 births per woman; in Italy and West Germany it is below 1.5. As a result of low birth rates and populations distributed about evenly among age-groups, these countries will stop growing in the near future. The United Kingdom, for example, is projected to stabilize at 59 million people, about 5 percent above its current population.

Developing countries can be divided into two groups. In the first, fertility rates declined significantly over the past two decades, although few have reached replacement level. In the second group, mostly countries in sub-Saharan Africa, fertility rates have not declined at all.

Twenty countries for which there are reliable data show fertility declines of more than 20 percent since 1960 (Table 1). The most dramatic change took

Table 1
Fertility Declines in Selected Countries, 1960-89

| Country | Total Fertility rates | | Change |
| | 1960 | 1989 | (percent) |
	(avg. number of children per woman)		
Singapore	6.3	1.6	-75
Taiwan	6.5	1.7	-74
South Korea	6.0	2.1	-65
Cuba	4.7	1.8	-62
Thailand	6.6	2.7	-59
Sri Lanka	5.9	2.5	-58
China	5.5	2.4	-56
Chile	5.3	2.4	-55
Costa Rica	7.4	3.5	-53
Colombia	6.8	3.4	-50
Mexico	7.2	3.8	-47
Turkey	6.8	3.7	-46
Brazil	6.2	3.4	-45
Malaysia	6.9	3.9	-43
Tunisia	7.3	4.3	-41
Indonesia	5.6	3.5	-38
Peru	6.6	4.4	-33
India	6.2	4.3	-31
Philippines	6.6	4.6	-30
Egypt	6.7	5.3	-21

Source: SOURCE: Population Reference Bureau, 1989 World Population Data Sheet (Washington, D.C.: 1989).

place in several East Asian nations and in Cuba, where fertility levels dropped by as much as 75 percent. Only one Middle Eastern country (Turkey) and two African ones (Egypt and Tunisia) have experienced fertility declines of more than a fifth since 1960. China reduced fertility rates by 56 percent since the Sixties; Chile, Colombia, and Costa Rica, by more than 50 percent each. Significant reductions were also achieved in Brazil, Indonesia, Mexico, and Thailand. Nevertheless, fertility rates remain moderately high, above 3.5 children per woman, in several of these countries.

Despite some impressive gains, only 4 of the 20 countries listed in Table 1 achieved replacement-level fertility: Cuba, Singapore, South Korea, and Taiwan. These four have also made tremendous economic strides. In demographic terms, however, they are responsible for only a minuscule fraction of annual increases to the global population.

Trends in the more populous countries are much more important to global population growth. Between 1987 and 2007, five countries in Table 1 – Brazil, China, India, Indonesia, and Mexico – will account for 37 percent of total world population growth. Cumulatively, these five will add nearly 700 million people, slightly fewer than India's current population. By 2020, India, projected to have about 1.3 billion people, will be China's closest rival for the title of the world's largest nation. And Mexicans will then number 138 million, more people than are in all of Central America and the Caribbean today. China, with a current fertility rate of 2.4 births per woman, is the only one of these demographic giants likely to achieve replacement-level fertility in the near future.

Fertility is declining much more slowly now, and in some countries appears to have reached a standstill. A recent report from the Indian National Academy of Science shows that the total fertility rate there declined by about 16 percent between 1972 and 1978, from 5.6 births per woman of reproductive age to 4.7. But the pace has slowed markedly since then. In 1988, Indian women bore on average 4.3 children, only 8 percent below the figure in 1978. Egypt, the Philippines, and Tunisia show similar trends.

Pockets of extremely high fertility – above six children per woman – still exist throughout Africa and the Middle East (Table 2, next page). Sub-Saharan Africa faces the highest fertility rates and population rates in the world. Nigerian women, for instance, bear nearly seven children on average. Most Middle Eastern countries also maintain high fertility levels, as do Bangladesh and Pakistan.

A tradition of large families in countries where young people are predominant means these nations will experience massive population increases over the generation ahead. Pakistan's population will more than double over the next 30 years, from 105 million to well over 240 million; Nigeria's will reach 274 million, up from its current population of 109 million; and Bangladesh's 104 million will grow to 200 million.

Lowering birth rates will help ease the transition from persistent poverty to sustainable development by reducing pressure on national resources. For example, a 1985 analysis by Kenya's National Council for Population and Development projected the country's future population size under two scenarios. It showed that at current fertility rates, Kenyans – now 24 million – would number 57 million in 2010, as opposed to 38 million if total fertility dropped by half, to four children per woman. With the smaller population size, corn requirements would be eased by 3.2 million tons, twice the amount that Kenyan farmers produced in 1980.

Table 2
Countries with High Fertility, 1989

Country	Total Fertility Rate	Population Growth Rate
	(average number of children per woman)	(percent)
Kenya	8.1	4.1
Saudi Arabia	7.2	3.4
Zambia	7.2	3.7
Tanzania	7.1	3.6
Afghanistan	6.9	2.6
Nigeria	6.6	2.9
Pakistan	6.5	2.9
Sudan	6.5	2.8
Zimbabwe	6.5	3.6
Senegal	6.4	2.6
Iran	6.2	3.4
Jordan	6.2	3.5
Ethiopia	6.1	2.1
Zaire	6.1	3.1
Bangladesh	5.8	2.8

SOURCE: Population Reference Bureau, 1989 World Population Data Sheet (Washington, D.C.: 1989).

THE ROLE OF FAMILY PLANNING

Family planning has played an important role in reducing fertility throughout the world. Countries such as China, Mexico, and Thailand have devoted extensive government resources to expanding services and supplying contraceptives. In Brazil, the efforts of private voluntary organizations have been key to declining birth rates. Nevertheless, in a substantial number of high fertility countries, family planning programs are weak or nonexistent, in part because governments have been slow to allocate the necessary resources. But the recent experiences of several nations suggest a close relationship between effective voluntary family planning programs, rising levels of contraceptive use, and declining fertility, even in the absence of broad-based economic gains.

Programs on family planning affect fertility primarily by raising contraceptive prevalence – the share of married women of reproductive age who use modern contraception to prevent pregnancy. Modern birth control methods like the pill and intrauterine device (IUD) are far more effective at preventing pregnancy than their traditional counterparts, such as withdrawal. The cost and availability of birth control dictate the difference between the number of children a couple wants and the number they actually have. Significantly, the demand for contraceptive information and supplies is rising among groups traditionally resistant to family planning, namely the urban and rural poor.

Unmet need, defined as the gap between the number of women who express a desire to limit fertility and the number who actually are able to do so, exists to varying degrees in virtually every developing country. This gap results from inadequate access to or knowledge of family planning methods, even where programs already exist. According to data from the World Fertility Survey (an international reproductive trends survey sponsored by the United Nations between 1974 and 1984), 40-50 percent of women of reproductive age in 18 developing countries desire no more children but have no access to family planning. Fertility rates could be reduced by 30 percent in these countries if unwanted births were prevented.

In India, half the couples contacted in the 1980 All-India Family Planning Survey wished to limit family size, but only 28 percent were using a modern method of birth control. The gap between desired and actual family size spotlights the inadequacy of family planning programs. Two-thirds of the couples surveyed felt three children were ideal, although most couples in India have four or more. Similarly, a 1985 survey showed that while 56 percent of Egyptian women wanted no more children, only 30 percent were using contraceptives. These surveys actually define a minimum level of unmet need: Because a significant share of respondents have never even heard of a family planning method, they are unlikely to identify a need for one even if they desire smaller families.

Not surprisingly, the countries with the strongest commitment to family planning are making the greatest strides in reducing fertility, regardless of their level of development. In Indonesia, a predominantly rural country with a per capita income of $530, a well-organized national family planning program has been in operation since 1969. A 1987 government survey indicates that between 1980 and 1985 contraceptive prevalence increased from 27 to nearly 41 percent of married women of reproductive age. A striking 42 percent decline in the number of births per woman of reproductive age occurred between 1970 and 1985, with the most significant drop after 1980. Due to the government's efforts to make family planning universally available, over 80 percent of Indonesian contraceptive users rely on modern methods.

Examining data from the World Fertility Survey, University of Michigan sociologist Ronald Freedman showed that contraceptive use varies little among Indonesians in different social and economic groups. Couples with low living standards are almost as likely to use contraception as those with the highest standards. Professional and clerical workers are only slightly ahead of farmers with small landholdings. And villages without modern amenities like electricity have contraceptive prevalence levels about as high as those with such facilities.

In Bangladesh, a deteriorating agrarian economy has raised the ante on large families just when a growing family planning program is making birth control cheaper. Agricultural wages today are below those of 150 years ago in constant dollars. Demographer Samuel Preston notes that much of the decline in real wages occurred since the Fifties, a period of rapid population growth. The number of landless families has mushroomed. Parents do not see a very bright future for their children: Land scarcity has undermined traditional inheritance practices, while rising educational costs have foreclosed employment options outside the agricultural sector.

One study based on data from three government surveys found that the adoption of family planning methods in Bangladesh has accelerated gradually in recent years in response to greatly improved services. Between 1969 and 1983, the share of married women who said they did not want additional children increased slightly, from 52 to 57 percent, albeit still a high level. Over the same period, contraceptive use increased steadily among both rural and urban women of all educational levels and all family sizes. In 1969, fully 93 percent of Bangladeshi women who wished to end childbearing were not using contraceptives; by 1983, this unmet need had declined to 71 percent, albeit still a high level. The study concludes that deteriorating economic and environmental conditions "may have influenced couples...to believe that large families are burdensome."

The lowest contraceptive prevalence rates (and the highest fertility rates) are found in sub-Saharan Africa, where the use of modern methods of birth control is rising quite slowly. Until recently, most African governments firmly opposed family planning programs on the grounds that curtailing population growth would limit the region's ability to recognize its economic potential. The low status of women has made childbearing the only rite of passage for girls. And lack of funds and poor service delivery systems hinder the dissemination of information and methods outside major urban areas. Surveys show that fewer than one-fifth of Nigerian women have ever heard of a modern method of birth control. In Kenya, less than 40 percent of women familiar with at least one modern contraceptive method knew of a supply source; fewer than half of these women could reach the source on a 30-minute walk. Despite these constraints, the desire both to space and limit births is increasingly evident in some African countries, particularly among educated women and those living in urban areas. Evidence of fertility decline due to strong family planning programs exists in sub-Saharan Africa. In 1982, a government survey showed that contraceptive prevalence in Zimbabwe stood at 14 percent for both modern and traditional methods. That year, President Robert Mugabe committed his government to a strong family planning effort to slow population growth and promote economic development. The program was immediately incorporated into the Ministry of Health, linking it with training and outreach for maternal and child health care. Zimbabwe made a financial commitment unparalleled among sub-Saharan nations, allocating $24 million to the program. By 1984, total contraceptive prevalence reached 38 percent (27 percent for modern methods), a remarkable increase for any country.

By reducing fertility levels, and hence the total amount of per capita social expenditures necessary just to maintain the economic status quo, family planning programs can help raise living standards. Between 1972 and 1984, for example, every peso spent on family planning by Mexico's urban social security system (IMSS) saved nine pesos that would otherwise have been spent on maternal and infant health care services. During this time, IMSS spent 38 billion pesos ($252 million) to provide nearly 800,000 women with contraceptive supplies, thus averting 3.6 million births and 363,000 abortions. Net savings for IMSS equaled 318 billion pesos ($2 billion), which was rechanneled into pension payments and expansion of general health care services.

Programs to increase the use of birth control are not a substitute for investments in education or efforts to raise per capita incomes. But reducing fertility is integral to any economic development strategy, allowing governments to raise per capita investments in health, education, and other social services. The growing desire for smaller families shows that family planning has a major role to play in virtually every nation. Developing countries that encourage family planning may be the first to experience rapid and widespread social and economic advances.

FAMILY PLANNING AND HEALTH

Family planning is among the most basic of preventive health care strategies, though it is rarely recognized as such. Encouraging fewer and safer births among women in developing countries will reduce unacceptably high rates of maternal mortality from complications of childbirth and abortion. Moreover, by distributing condoms and increasing the public's understanding of reproductive health issues, family planning programs can help control the spread of acquired immunodeficiency syndrome (AIDS), a major threat to Third World health and economic survival.

Each year, at least one-half million women worldwide die from pregnancy-related causes. Fully 99 percent of these deaths occur in the Third World, where complications arising from pregnancy and illegal abortions are the leading killers of women in their twenties and thirties. World Health Organization (WHO) officials caution that maternal deaths – those resulting directly or indirectly from pregnancy within 42 days of childbirth, induced abortion, or miscarriage – may actually be twice the estimated figures. What is more, for every woman who dies, many more suffer serious, often long-term, health problems. That bearing life brings death to so many women is a distressing irony. It is even more distressing given that family planning and preventive medicine could substantially reduce these losses.

In the Third World, maternal mortality accounts for some 25 percent of deaths of women aged 15 to 49. More than 3,000 maternal deaths occur per 100,000 live births annually in parts of Ethiopia and Bangladesh (Table 3, next page). By contrast, the figures in the United States and Norway are only 10 and 2, respectively. Each year, over 20,000 women die from pregnancy or related complications in Bangladesh, compared with about 500 women in the United States, a country with more than twice as many people.

Illegal abortion is one of the major direct causes of maternal death. Rough estimates indicate that only half the estimated 54 million abortions performed annually around the world are legal. Most illegal abortions are carried out under unsanitary conditions by unskilled attendants, leaving women vulnerable to serious complications and infection. By contrast, modern abortion procedures, carried out under proper medical supervision in countries where they are legal, cause fewer maternal deaths than pregnancy or oral contraceptives do.

Forty-four percent of women in the developing world (outside of China) live in countries where abortion is allowed only to save the mother's life. Another 10 percent live in countries where abortion is totally prohibited. Sadly, millions of women unable to obtain a legal abortion on the basis of life-threatening circumstances have subsequently died from the complications of an illegal abortion. Those who advocate abortion policies rarely acknowledge this toll on women's lives.

Estimates of the annual number of deaths due to abortion complications range from 155,000 to 204,000 women worldwide. Abortion-related deaths are especially common among poor and illiterate women living in countries with strict abortion laws. In Latin America, where legal abortion is generally restricted to cases of rape or endangerment of the woman's life, up to half of maternal deaths appear to be due to illegal abortions.

Table 3
Maternal Mortality Ratios, Selected Countries, 1987

Country	Maternal Mortality Ratios	Study Region and Year
	(deaths per 100,000 live births)	
Ethiopia	3,500[1]	Urban, 1984
Bangladesh	3,000[2]	National, 1983
Senegal	700[1]	Rural, 1983
India	400-500[2]	National, 1984
Egypt	190	Rural, 1981-83
Romania	175	National, 1982
Mexico	103	National, 1978
Thailand	81	National, 1981
Chile	73	National, 1980
United States	10[1]	National, 1979
Norway	2	National, 1981

[1]Unknown whether deaths from abortions included.
[2]Deaths from abortions not included.

SOURCE: World Health Organization, Maternal Mortality Rates: A Tabulation of Available Information (Geneva: 1985).

Pregnancy itself takes a greater toll on a woman's body in regions where malnutrition and poor health are the norm. In the Third World, pregnancy is associated with a higher incidence of health-threatening infection, vitamin and mineral deficiencies, and anemia. Due to reduced immunity, common diseases such as pneumonia and influenza cause 50-100 percent more deaths in pregnant than in non-pregnant women.

Three groups of women face the highest risk of pregnancy-related deaths – those at either end of their reproductive cycle, those who bear children in rapid succession, and those who have more than four children. Due to biological factors, women under 19 or over 35 are more susceptible to complications of pregnancy. Women giving birth to children spaced less than a year apart are twice as likely to die from pregnancy-related causes than those who have children two or more years apart. In Matlab Thana, Bangladesh, health workers recorded three times as many deaths among women giving birth to their eighth child as among those giving birth to their third.

At least half of all maternal deaths can be averted through a combined strategy of family planning, legal abortion, and primary health care. According to researchers Beverly Winikoff and Maureen Sullivan of the Population Council, a fertility rate reduction of 25-35 percent resulting from more widely available family planning would also lower maternal mortality by one-fourth. Making abortions legal and safe could reduce the toll an additional 20-25 percent. Making all pregnancies safer through increased investments in prenatal health care and reducing the number of high-risk pregnancies would prevent another 20-25 percent of deaths. Winikoff and Sullivan point out that while, theoretically, this three-pronged strategy could reduce maternal mortality by three-fourths, a 50-percent decrease is a more realistic expectation, given prevailing social and political conditions, such as large desired family size and the opposition to legalizing abortion.

Establishing integrated family planning and health strategies will be well worth the investment. Village-based paramedics and midwives can teach women the benefits of birth spacing, breast-feeding, prenatal care, and contraceptive use. Small-scale maternity centers – on the order of one for every 4,000 people – could promote simple solutions to some of the most pervasive maternal health problems, by providing, for instance, iron supplements to treat anemia. Linked with regional facilities run by doctors, such clinics would constitute a pivotal link between rural populations and the often urban-based medical community. Assuming that maternal deaths run as high as 1 million per year, family planning and health care would save at least 500,000 women's lives annually, and improve the health of millions more.

THE INGREDIENTS OF SUCCESS

Without fertility declines, many governments cannot hope to make the investments necessary to improve human welfare and encourage economic development. But a number of political and social obstacles remain for countries wishing to reduce fertility, improve health, and raise living standards. Attaining these goals will depend on fundamental changes in several areas, including the way governments shape population policies, the degree to which they make contraceptive supplies and information accessible, and the steps they take to improve the status of women and increase their access to education.

Policymakers concerned with population dynamics are faced with two objectives: reducing the unmet need for family planning in medium fertility countries and, in high fertility countries, providing an environment in which small families can become the norm. Helping couples achieve that norm will require a major commitment to family planning from both the international community and the Third World. But uncertain economic prospects, competing investment needs, and international politics have subverted the growing support for family planning in developing countries. Without the resources needed to back that commitment, the trend of declining fertility in developing countries may be reversed.

An increase in international donor assistance can be used to strengthen family planning in several key areas. First, improving the statistics-gathering and analytical capabilities of Third World governments is essential to charting and responding to trends more accurately. Second, priority should be given to the poorest, most rapidly growing countries, such as those in sub-Saharan Africa and parts of Asia, where services are scant, but sorely needed. Third, donors can augment funding for programs in countries where current efforts are inadequate. And new approaches to family planning and social change in these countries deserve more support. India and Mexico, for example, are both using the popular media to spread information and promote the concept of smaller families.

Developing countries themselves need to make a greater commitment to family planning. At the moment, the Third World spends more than four times as much on weaponry and upkeep of military forces as it does on health care – $150 billion in 1986, compared with $38 billion. Increased government funding of family planning and primary health care programs is essential as part of the effort to speed fertility rate declines.

Contraceptive supplies, educational materials, prenatal health care, and information on family health are desperately needed in rural areas throughout the developing world. New approaches to contraceptive marketing and distribution, such as those that rely on local residents and shopkeepers to disseminate information and supplies, are now being tried in a number of countries, and should be considered in others.

The primary goals of a family planning program are to reduce unmet need for fertility control, to improve maternal and child health through birth spacing, and eliminate the need for illegal abortion. But an integrated development strategy that combines family planning with income generation for women, reforestation efforts, small-scale agricultural projects, and improvements in water supply and sanitation will simultaneously reduce births and improve the quality of life.

Although national leadership is needed, encouraging the development of regional, district, and village programs that are responsive to local needs is essential, too. Programs patterned after the Thai loan experiment, relying on village leaders to help develop and introduce new ideas, may be the most successful. The private sector should also be involved. Initiatives in Africa and elsewhere have shown that it is cost-effective for employers to offer primary health care and family planning services, which result in better overall health and higher productivity. In Kenya, a group of 50 companies and plantations is the second largest provider of family planning. Likewise, in Nigeria, Gulf Oil and Lever Brothers Co. are planning to introduce such programs.

Three decades of international family planning experience hold important lessons for designing effective programs and for creating a social environment receptive to smaller families. Countries such as China, India, Mexico, and Thailand can serve as models for different approaches. Sub-Saharan African countries may find that region-wide cooperation on family planning, in the form of training and outreach programs through perhaps a new consortium on population growth, will strengthen the efforts of individual countries.

As the interdependence of nations becomes increasingly clear, so too does the knowledge that the fate of even the richest nations is intertwined with that of the most destitute. Planning families to reduce the number of births, improve health, and raise living standards is a universal responsibility. No nation should exempt itself from this global effort.

18

FAMILY PLANNING: CLINICAL ASPECTS

KULDIP SINGH, M.B.B.S., M.R.C.O.G.,
AND S.S. RATNAM, M.B.B.S., F.R.C.O.G.

INTRODUCTION

Evidence from around the world shows that the risk of maternal and infant illness and death in both the industrialized and developing countries is highest in four specific types of pregnancy: "those too young, too old, too many and too close." In practice, the combination of these four types of high-risk pregnancy is more important than any of the four considered separately. There are both biological and sociocultural reasons for the extra risk in these four types of pregnancies. Age, number of children, and birth spacing affect the mother's ability to carry a pregnancy safely and to provide optimal biological consideration for the developing fetus. After birth, the same factors affect the ability to feed and care for the baby in the increased family.

Family planning addresses the two most common and most serious health problems in developing countries, namely high maternal and child mortality. The demand for family planning is expected to increase in the next 2-3 decades as the number of couples in the reproductive age groups grows. Thus, in this chapter, an update of currently existing methods of family planning prior to conception will be given. In addition, the health rationale for family planning will be discussed.

FAMILY PLANNING METHODS

I. HORMONAL METHODS

1. Combined oral contraceptives (the Pill)

Mode of Action: The pill contains synthetic hormones (estrogen and progestogen) in small quantities. There is suppression of ovulation and since ovulation does not occur, conception cannot occur. There are basically three types of combined pills: monophasic, biphasic and triphasic. The monophasic pill delivers a fixed dose of the hormones during the entire menstrual cycle. The biphasic pill delivers two different dosages of hormones while the triphasic pill delivers three different dosages of hormones during the menstrual cycle (Figure 1, next page).

Frequency of administration: The combined pill needs to be taken daily for 21 days in a cycle.

Effectiveness: The combined pill is highly effective when used regularly. The pregnancy rate per 100 users varies from 0.1-3.0.

Advantages: It is convenient, non-coitus related and relatively easy to use. The combined pill protects against pelvic inflammatory disease, ectopic pregnancy, endometrial cancer, ovarian cancer and common menstrual disorders.

Side effects: Minor side effects include nausea, headache, weight gain, gastrointestinal complaints and intermenstrual bleeding. Thromboembolic phenomenon, increased risk of cardiovascular disease and stroke are the major side effects particularly for women over 35 years and who smoke.[1-5]

Reversibility: Immediate to short delay only.

Recent advances: Reduction in estrogen dosages with the current use of the 'minipill' containing 30 mg of estrogen has brought with it a concomitant reduction of venous thrombosis,[6] that the progestogens may be more important in the etiology of atherosclerosis and myocardial infarction, the trend over the years has been to reduce the overall intake of progestogen per cycle of use without sacrificing efficacy. There also seems to be an affinity between some progestogen and androgen receptors and it is felt that this is what promotes the metabolic side effects of the pill. All synthetic progestogens are derivatives of either 17-hydroxy progesterone or 19-nortestosterone (Table 1, page 207). Since a little androgenic activity is required for better cycle control, the gonanes are the most effective new synthetic progestogens and research therefore is directed at finding a progestogen of strong activity with least androgenic (hence causing least metabolic upset) activity. The important differences between the new progestogens and their influence on lipid metabolism are shown in Table 2.[7] (page 207) Other possible areas of research are in the developing of slow sustained release formulations and the studying of different routes of administration to reduce the first-pass effect on the liver (and thus reduce the metabolic consequences of oral contraceptives).

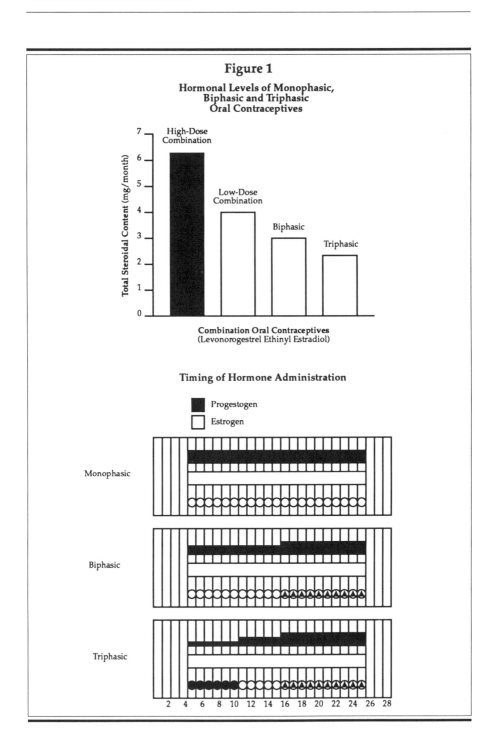

Figure 1

Hormonal Levels of Monophasic, Biphasic and Triphasic Oral Contraceptives

2. Progestin-only pill (minipill)

Mode of action: The minipill contains only a progestin and it acts mainly by thickening the cervical mucous and thus inhibiting the upward migration of sperm. It is also said to cause changes in the endometrium, thus making implantation defective. Ovulation is inhibited in about 50% of cycles.

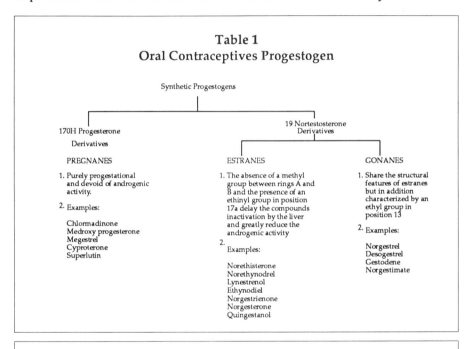

Table 1
Oral Contraceptives Progestogen

Synthetic Progestogens

17OH Progesterone Derivatives

19 Nortestosterone Derivatives

PREGNANES	ESTRANES	GONANES
1. Purely progestational and devoid of androgenic activity. 2. Examples: Chlormadinone Medroxy progesterone Megestrel Cyproterone Superlutin	1. The absence of a methyl group between rings A and B and the presence of an ethinyl group in position 17a delay the compounds inactivation by the liver and greatly reduce the androgenic activity 2. Examples: Norethisterone Norethynodrel Lynestrenol Ethynodiel Norgestrienone Norgesterone Quingestanol	1. Share the structural features of estranes but in addition characterized by an ethyl group in position 13 2. Examples: Norgestrel Desogestrel Gestodene Norgestimate

Table 2
Influence of Monophasic Pills on Lipid Metabolism
(Ref Runnebaum, 1987)

Progestogen	Triglyceride	Total Cholesterol	HDL Cholesterol
Levonorgestrel (30 g EE, 150 g LNG)	0 - 20% increase	Normal range for all preparations	Normal range
Desogestrel (30 g EE, 250 g NG)	0 - 20% increase		Normal to slight ↑
Norgestimate (30 g EE, 250 g NG)	20 - 50% increase		Normal to slight ↓
Gestodene (30 g EE, 75 g GTD)	20 - 30% increase		Normal range

EE = ethinyl oestradiol   LNG = levonorgestrel   DSG = desogestrel

NG = norgestimate   GTD = gestodene

Frequency of administration: To be taken daily throughout the cycle.

Efficacy: It is less effective than the combined pill and pregnancy rates are from 0.5-3.0 per 100 users.

Advantages: The side effects of estrogen associated with the combined pill are eliminated with the progestin-only minipill.

Side effects: Increased menstrual irregularity and increased risk of ectopic pregnancy are the main side effects. Cardiovascular disease risk is now being reduced as a result of indepth studies of progestogens.[7]

Reversibility: Immediate to short delay.

3. Injectable (DMPA, Depo Provera, NET-EN, Novisterat)

Mode of action: Progestin is injected into muscles and, like the minipill, changes in cervical mucous, endometrial changes and inhibition of ovulation are the main modes of action.

Frequency of administration: Once every one, two, or three months.

Efficacy: Pregnancy rate varies from 0.3-0.4 per 100 users. This depends on the woman's compliance to return regularly to the clinic for injections.

Advantages: It is convenient, not related to coitus and does not interfere with lactation.

Side effects: Heavy intermenstrual bleeding and amenorrhoea are the main side effects. The menstrual disturbances are probably related to the fact that the progestins are not released uniformly from the depot side – the drugs are initially released as a burst after injection, reaching high levels, then decline slowly after 4 weeks of injection.[8] Possible effects on carbohydrate and lipid metabolism are the other side effects.[9,10]

Reversibility: Delay of 4-8 months possible.

Recent advances: To reduce menstrual disturbances, research is currently on for the synthesis of newer steroids with better or zero-order release rates profile.[11] Other possibilities are increasing the number of injections using smaller doses of existing progestogens, combining with natural estrogen to achieve a better control of vaginal bleeding[12,13] and using new delivery systems, e.g., norethindrone injectable microspheres to provide better release characteristics.[14]

4. Implants (NorplantR system)

Mode of action: NorplantR consists of 6 silicone rubber capsules filled with levonorgestrel. They are inserted under the skin of the arm and their three modes of action are similar to those of other progestin-only contraception.

Frequency of administration: Once every 5 years.

Efficacy: Pregnancy rates of 0.0 to 0.5 per 100 users.

Advantages: It is a convenient, long acting, reversible method of contraception not related to coitus. The sustained slow release of a low amount of levonorgestrel avoids daily hormonal surges.

Side effects: Menstrual irregularities consisting of either prolonged bleeding, spotting and amenorrhoea are the main side effects. However, the menstrual irregularities are less common than with injectables. Other infrequent minor side effects include headache, dizziness, nervousness, weight gain, skin and hair disorders. Moreover, since insertion and removal involve a minor surgical procedure, infection of the implant site can occur.

Reversibility: Immediate upon removal.

Recent advances: In the face of development and making NorplantR more acceptable, NorplantR-2, consisting of two rods, has been introduced. Results to date have been encouraging.[15,16] However, a recent setback has been that the medical grade elastomer 382 used in the rods has been withdrawn because of its suspected carcinogenic potential in rodents in a dose a thousand times more than that used in the NorplantR2 system. Meanwhile, efforts are being undertaken to find an, alternate elastomer to replace the medical grade elastomer 382.[17] In addition, biodegradable norethindrone (NET) pellet implants, expected to release NET over 12-18 months, are currently undergoing clinical trials.

5. Vaginal Rings

Medical vaginal rings with steroids are being developed. An earlier variety containing both estrogens and progestogens, designed to be worn for 3 weeks and then removed for 1 week to induce withdrawal bleeding, has been terminated because of estrogen-related side effects. A more recent variety contains levonorgestrel only and is worn continuously. A recent setback in its development has been the medical grade elastomer 382 that is used to make the vaginal ring has been implicated with possible carcinogenic effects. Thus, until alternative elastomers are found, further production and evaluation have been discontinued.

II. Intrauterine Contraceptive Devices (IUCDs)

Mode of action: These consist of a plastic or metal device inserted into the uterus. It is not known precisely how the IUCD prevents pregnancy, but it is said to stop the fertilized ovum from implanting in the endometrium. The presence of a metal like copper or silver is said to increase its effectiveness by influencing the fertilizing ability of the spermatozoa in the female genital tract. There are also the progestin-releasing IUCDs which have the additional property of making the cervical mucous impermeable to sperm and often of suppressing ovulation.

Frequency of administration: This varies with the device used. Generally, the metal-containing devices need to be changed once every 4 years while the progestin-releasing IUCDs are effective for only a year.

Efficacy: Varies from 0.3-1.0 pregnancy per 100 users for the metal-containing IUCDs. For the progestin-releasing IUCDs, which are generally less effective, the pregnancy rate varies from 1.9-2.0.

Advantages: It is a convenient, long-term method which is not related to intercourse. Careful patient selection is recommended and the method is best suited for women who have had at least one pregnancy and are in a stable monogamous relationship. In addition, progestin-releasing IUCDs decrease menstrual blood loss.

Side effects: Possible side effects are increased and irregular menstrual bleeding often associated with pain. Perforation and infection are possible. There is the potential risk of pelvic inflammatory disease resulting from ascending infection. There is also an unaccepted high risk of ectopic pregnancy associated with progestin-releasing IUCDs. Hence the use of this device has been discontinued.[21]

Reversibility: Immediate upon removal.

Recent advances: The increased bleeding and pain experienced by some IUCD users is said to be associated with the size of the plastic skeleton which supports the metallic wire. Currently, new IUCDs have been designed to combat this. The Cu-fix, which is to be tested soon, consists simply of a chain of copper cylinders hanging on a nylon thread from the fundus of the uterus. In order to place the thread, it is necessary to deliberately push the insertion needle into the myometrium and it has not been established how safe this procedure would be.[22] The Multiload Mark 2 is yet another new device with a radically new insertion system. The device itself has barium in the frame and is easier to remove than the earlier version.[23]

III. CHEMICAL BARRIERS — SPERMICIDE

Mode of action: Foams, cream, jelly or a suppository is inserted into the vagina before intercourse to kill sperm on contact, thus preventing them from entering the uterus.

Frequency of administration: Prior to sexual intercourse.

Efficacy: Pregnancy rate of 3-28 per 100 users.

Advantages: No obvious health risks.

Side effects: It is messy and chemicals in preparations may cause irritation.

Reversibility: Immediate.

IV. PHYSICAL BARRIER METHODS

1. Condoms

Mode of action: This consists of a thin rubber sheath put on the man's penis before intercourse. It collects the semen during ejaculation and thus prevents sperm from entering the vagina.

Frequency of administration: Required prior to every act of sexual intercourse.

Efficacy: Effectiveness of this method is somewhat variable and increases with the use of spermicide. The pregnancy rate is about 3-15 per 100 users.

Advantages: No apparent health risks. Added advantage of providing protection against sexually transmitted diseases, including AIDS.

Side effects: Condom use may disrupt sexual pleasure for some.

Reversibility: Immediate.

Recent advances: Besides the development of the female condom, which is being tested, it seems unlikely that any novel improvement is going to emerge as far as barrier methods and spermicide are concerned.

2. Diaphragm/Cervical Cap

Mode of action: A soft rubber dome or thimble-shaped cap coated with contraceptive cream or jelly is inserted into the vagina to cover the cervix to prevent sperm from entering. The contraceptive cream or jelly kills the sperms on contact. The diaphragm or cap comes in different sizes and requires individual fitting by a health care professional. In addition, a woman should be refitted following any situation they may change the size and/or shape of her vagina, e.g., childbirth, a weight change of 10 or more pounds, or pelvic surgery.

Frequency of administration: Must be used prior to sexual intercourse. Diaphragm must be left in place 6 hours after intercourse, whereas cervical caps can be in place for 2 days with additional application of spermicide.

Efficacy: Pregnancy rates vary from 3-19 per 100 users.

Advantages: No apparent health risks.

Side effects: Some women have pelvic conditions that rule out use. Diaphragm may be dislodged during intercourse or may interfere with spontaneity. Some find it messy. It may increase chances of bladder infections.

3. Sponge

Mode of action: A soft synthetic sponge containing spermicide is moistened and inserted into the vagina up to 24 hours before intercourse. The sponge continuously releases a spermicide and also acts as a physical barrier to block and absorb sperm to prevent them from entry into the uterus.

Frequency of administration: Prior to sexual intercourse. The sponge must be kept in place 6 hours after intercourse and should be removed within 24 hours.

Efficacy: Pregnancy rate is 3-28 per 100 users.

Advantages: Chemicals in the sponge may cause irritation.

Reversibility: Immediate.

V. NATURAL METHODS

1. Withdrawal or coitus interruptus

Mode of action: The man withdraws his penis from the vagina just before ejaculation, to keep sperm away from the uterine opening.

Frequency of administration: Applicable at each coital act.

Efficacy: 20-25 pregnancies per 100 users.

Advantages: Does not involve use of any physical, hormonal or chemical methods.

Side effects: May interrupt spontaneity of sexual intercourse.

Reversibility: Immediate.

2. Periodic abstinence or rhythm method

Mode of action: The couple refrains from intercourse when the woman is ovulating. The woman has to keep track of her menstrual cycles to predict when ovulation is likely to occur each month. She takes her temperature daily so that she knows when ovulation occurs. She may also monitor cervical mucous, which changes during ovulation.

Frequency of administration: Abstinence for one-third to one-half of cycle.

Efficacy: 2-40 pregnancies per 100 users.

Advantages: No obvious health risks.

Side effects: Has a high failure rate, particularly if the woman's cycle is irregular or she is ill. It is not used during lactation.

VI. STERILIZATION

1. Vasectomy (male)

Mode of action: Through a minor surgical procedure, the vas deferens is cut so sperm cannot enter the seminal fluid.

Frequency of administration: Once.

Efficacy: 0.10-0.15 pregnancies per 100 users.

Advantages: A permanent method which should be selected only if no more children are desired. It is not coitus-related and there is no impairment of sexual function.

Side effects: Potential risk of operative and post-operative complications. Temporary pain and swelling are common.

Reversibility: Irreversible, for all purposes.

2. Tubectomy (female)

Mode of action: Fallopian tubes are cut or occluded so ovum cannot be transferred to be fertilized.

Frequency of Administration: Once.

Efficacy: 0.1-0.3 pregnancies per 100 users.

Advantages: Permanent method with no long-term health or safety risks.

Side effects: Has risk of operative and post-operative complications requiring medical care.

Reversibility: Generally irreversible, for all purposes.

HEALTH RATIONALE FOR FAMILY PLANNING

1. EFFECTIVE PREVENTION FOR HIGH MORTALITY AND MORBIDITY

Family planning offers high effective technology that can reduce maternal and child mortality by preventing high-risk pregnancies. Besides the intrinsic properties of a method,[24] the effectiveness of a contraceptive method also depends on why it is used. With most methods, couples who have all the children they want and so intend to prevent any more births experience fewer unplanned pregnancies than couples who want more children eventually but intend to delay births. This personal motivation and valid health reasons often reinforce one another to encourage the use of family planning.

2. RISKS OF CHILDBEARING VERSUS FAMILY PLANNING

The risks of family planning methods are very slight in the majority of cases. Estimates based on the most recent data conclude that childbearing is generally far more dangerous than using oral contraceptives, IUCDs or condoms.[25,26] Oral contraceptives raise the risk of certain potentially fatal cardiovascular problems, which are almost limited to older women who smoke. Primary health care workers can identify these women and urge them to use other methods. Still, where the risks of childbearing are great, oral contraceptives are safer than childbearing for women of any age.[27]

3. SAFETY OF FAMILY PLANNING METHODS

Compared with other drugs, surgical procedures and childbearing, family planning methods are safe and free from substantial risk of major complication. They are also not toxic and have a wide margin of safety. Use of contraception, again, does not build up psychological resistance in the population. Serious problems with some contraceptive methods can be largely avoided by following simple rules; for example, about who should use oral contraceptives or about sterile techniques for performing IUCD insertions or voluntary sterilization. Other problems that develop can often be solved by switching to another contraceptive method. As with most other primary health care measures, the rare special problems that may arise with certain family planning methods can be handled through a referral system that takes clients to sources of more sophisticated diagnosis and care.

4. HEALTH BENEFITS OF FAMILY PLANNING

Some family planning methods offer substantial health benefits (as mentioned above) besides preventing pregnancy. To re-emphasize briefly, condoms, spermicide and diaphragm, when properly used, protect against sexually transmitted diseases and pelvic inflammatory disease. Oral contraceptives also furnish protection against pelvic inflammatory disease, ectopic pregnancy, endometrial carcinoma, ovarian cysts and relieve a variety of common menstrual disorders.[28,29]

5. REDUCE THE NUMBER OF ABORTIONS AND ABORTION-RELATED COMPLICATIONS

Family planning reduces the number of abortions by offering women an alternative way to control their fertility. For example, increased contraceptive use and liberalization of abortion legislation have led to a remarkable decrease in the number of abortion deaths and complication.[30,31]

6. UNMEASURED COST SAVING

By monitoring and preventing high-risk, often unwanted, pregnancy, family planning saves health expenditures that would be necessary later in treating mothers and infants in higher risk. Other savings due to family planning in terms of education, social service and health care are also substantial. These long term saving costs are, however, more difficult to calculate.

CONCLUSION

Knowing the health rationale for family planning, it is essential that all family planning methods be made available to the population at large in so far as their use is legal and in accordance with prevailing social values. Moreover, in order to ensure the individual's free choice and strengthen the acceptability and practice of family planning, all available methods should not merely be provided for inservice programs but also be dealt within information and educational activities. There is also the need for continued clinical and psychosocial research into making the various contraceptive methods more safe, effective and acceptable. By these ways, we can hope to promote and sustain high levels of contraceptive practice among couples and thus help to bring the goal of "Health for All by the Year 2000" closer to realization.

REFERENCES

1. Inman, W.H., and M.P. Vessey. Investigation of deaths from pulmonary, coronary and cerebral thrombosis in women of childbearing age. British Med J 11: 193-199, 1968.

2 Royal College of General Practitioners' Oral Contraception Study. Effect on hypertension and benign breast disease of progestogen component in combined oral contraceptives. Lancet 1:624, 1977.

3. Prasad, R.N.V., and S.S. Ratnam. The cardiovascular and thromboembolic risks of oral contraception - A review. Sing J Obstet Gynecol 11:1-19, 1980.

4. Ratnam, S.S., and R.N.V. Prasad. Oral Contraceptives, Practice of Fertility Control - A Comprehensive Textbook. S.K.Chaudhuri (ed). Calcutta: Current Book Publishers, 1983, pp. 79-107.

5. Fotherby, K. Oral contraceptives, lipids and cardiovascular disease. Contraception 31: 367-338, 1985.

6. Vankeep, P.A. The birth and development of the pill: A short history of oral contraception. Sing J Obstet Gynecol 15;1-5, 1980.

7. Runnebaum, B. and T. Rabe. New progestogens in oral contraceptives. Am J Obstet Gynecol 157: 1059-1063, 1987.

8. Crabbe, P., S. Arcjer, and G. Benangiano, et al. Long-acting contraceptive agents: Design of the WHO chemical synthesis programme steroids, (in press).

9. Benangiano, G., E. Diczfaluzy, and J.W. Goldzieher, et al. Multinational comparative clinical evaluation of two long-acting injectable contraceptive steroids: Norethisterone enanthate and medroxy progesterone acetate 1. Use effectiveness. Contraception 15: 153-533, 1977.

10. World Health Organization. Special Programme of Research, Development and Research Training in Human reproduction. Tenth Annual Report. Geneva: WHO, 1981, p. 167.

11. Weiner, E., and E.D.B. Johansson. Plasma levels of norethindrone after intramuscular injection of 200 mg norethindrone enanthate. Contraception 11: 419-423, 1975.

12. Prasad, K.V.S., K.M. Nair,and B. Sivakumar et al. Plasma levels of norethindrone in Indian women receiving norethindrone enanthate (20mg) injectable. Contraception 23: 497-506, l981.

13. Hall, P.E. Long-acting injectable formulation, fertility regulation today and tomorrow. E. Diczfaluzy and M Bygdemen (eds). USA: Raven Press, 1987, pp. 119-141.

14. World Health Organization. Task force on long-acting systemic agents for fertility regulation. A multicentered pharmacokinetic, pharmacodynamic study of once-a-month injectable contraceptives I: Different doses of HRP112 and of Depoprovera. Contraception 36: 441457, 1987.

15. Singh, K., O. Viegtas, and S.S. Ratnam. Norplant contraceptive subdermal implant: One year experience in Singapore. Contraception 37: 457-469, 1988.

16. Singh, K., O.Viegas, and S.S. Ratnam. Norplant-2 rods: A one year experience in Singapore. Contraception 38: 429-440, 1988.

17. Population Council Recommendation on the Conduct of Clinical and Introductory Trials of Norplant II. New York: The Population Council, 1987.

18. World Health Organization. Task force on long-lasting systemic agents for fertility regulation. Pharmacokinetic profiles and pharmacodynamic effects of capronor contraceptive implants in the human. Contraception (In Press).

19. Rowe, P.J. Steroid-releasing vaginal rings – A review, fertility and sterility. R.F. Harrison, J. Bonnar, and W. Thompson (eds). Lancaster, UK: MTP Press Ltd., 1984, pp. 301-309.

20. Landgren, B.M. Vaginal delivery system, fertility regulation today and tomorrow. E. Diczfaluzy and M. Bygdeman (eds). New York: Raven Press,1987, pp. 165-180.

21. World Health Organization. Special programme of research development and research training in human reproduction task force on intrauterine levonorgestrel for contraception. Contraception 35: 363-379, 1987.

22. Sivin, I., and F. Schmnidt. Effectiveness of IUDs – A review. Contraception 37: 55-84, 1987.

23. Population Reports. IUDs - A New Look. Population Reports B(5) 1-31, 1988.

24. Population Council. Comparing family planning methods. NORPLANT Fact Sheet, No. 5. New York: Population Council, 1988.

25. Kols, A., and P.T. Piotrow, et al. Oral contraceptives in the 1980s. Population Reports A(6), 1982.

26. Ory, H.W., J.D. Forrest, and R. Lincoln (ed). Making Choices: Evaluating the Health Risks and Benefits of Birth Control Methods. New York: Alan Guttmacher Institute, 1982.

27. Henderson, B.E., S. Preston-Martin, and H.A. Edmondson, et al. Hepatocellular carcinoma and oral contraceptives. Br J Cancer 48: 437-440, 1983.

28. Lincoln, R. No support for pill – breast cancer link, but cervical connection more ambiguous. Int Fam Plan Perspect 10: 27-31, 1984.

29. Vessey, M.P., M. Lawless, and K. MacPherson, et al. Neoplasia of the cervix uteri and contraception – a possible adverse effect of the pill. Lancet 2: 930-934, 1983.

30. International Planned Parenthood Federation (IPPF). Family Planning in Child - A Profile of the Development of policies and Programmes. London: IPPF, 1980.

31. Lim, L.S., M.C.E. Cheng, and M. Rauff, et al. Abortion deaths in Singapore 1968-1976. Singapore Med J 20: 391-394, 1979.

19

THE CHALLENGES OF SAFE MOTHERHOOD

MAHMOUD F. FATHALLA, M.D., PH.D., F.A.C.O.G.

Maternal mortality in developing countries is a neglected tragedy. It is a tragedy in terms of magnitude of the problem. The World Health Organization (WHO) estimates that at least one-half million women die from causes related to pregnancy and childbirth each year.[1] This amounts to one death every minute. Women who die are in the prime period of their life, and they sacrifice their lives in the course of fulfilling a physiological reproductive duty. As mothers, their death has a major health and social impact on their families. Moreover, maternal mortality should be viewed as only the top of an iceberg of maternal morbidity and acute or chronic suffering. It has been estimated that for every maternal death, 16 women suffered from illness during pregnancy, childbirth or within six weeks after delivery.[2]

Maternal mortality in developing countries is also a tragedy in terms of equity and social justice. The WHO estimated (about 1983) that the maternal mortality rate (MMR) is 150 times more in developing countries (450 per 1000,000 live births) than in developed countries (30).[1] Even this large discrepancy is a gross underestimate of the degree of inequity. It does not reflect the fact that national maternal mortality rates range from 2 in certain European countries to 1100 in certain African countries.[3] It also does not reflect the great differences within countries, particularly in rural areas. A recent community study in a rural area of Gambia found a maternal mortality rate of 2200, or about one woman dying for every 50 births.[4] The discrepancy in MMR also underestimates the discrepancy in numbers. When the number of live births is considered, the WHO estimates that all but 6000 of the annual half million deaths take place in developing countries.[1] This amounts to 99% of all maternal deaths. It should also be noted that maternal mortality is a recurrent risk. The overall risk to women dying from pregnancy-related causes, expressed as the lifetime chance of maternal death, is estimated to be 1 in 21 for a woman in Africa, and only 1 in 9850 for a woman in Europe.[5]

The tragedy of maternal mortality in developing countries has been neglected. One reason is that the magnitude of the problem is often not appreciated. Although maternal mortality accounts for the greatest proportion of deaths among women of reproductive age in most of the developing world, its importance is not always evident from official statistics. In areas where the problem is most severe, the majority of maternal deaths simply go unrecorded, or the cause of death is not specified; hence the tendency to underestimate the gravity of the situation. Only 75 of WHO's Member States were able to provide information on maternal mortality.[3] Of the 117 developing countries, 73 were unable to give a rate; and a number of the figures that were provided were grossly underestimated. It was only recently that systematic efforts have been made to collect valid data from different sources on the prevalence of maternal mortality.[3] Another reason why maternal mortality has been neglected is that it is a woman's problem in regions where women do not enjoy a high social status. It could also be that people have lived with the problem of maternal death for so long, that a sense of fatalism has developed. The health service also shares some of the guilt for this neglect. The traditional MCH services have tended to be oriented towards the child. Even the care extended to the pregnant and parturient woman often had its implicit justification in the benefit that goes to the child. This has provoked the recent outcry: Where is the M in MCH?[7]

There are now signs of hope that the tragedy of maternal deaths will receive more global and national attention. A major international conference on safe motherhood was held in Nairobi, Kenya, in February 1987, under the sponsorship of the World Bank, WHO, and the United Nations Population Fund. The WHO established the Safe Motherhood Initiative in 1987 to fund short-term operations research projects on maternal health interventions. A large number of regional and national conferences on safe motherhood have been held or are being planned.

CAUSES OF MATERNAL MORTALITY

A maternal death is defined as the death of a woman while pregnant or within 42 days of termination of pregnancy, irrespective of the duration and the site of the pregnancy, from any cause related to or aggravated by the pregnancy or its management but not from accidental or incidental causes.[8] According to the International Classification of Diseases, maternal deaths are divided into two groups: direct and indirect obstetric deaths. Direct obstetric deaths are those resulting from obstetric complications of the pregnant state (pregnancy, labor and puerperium), from interventions, omissions, incorrect treatment, or from a chain of events resulting from any of the above. Indirect obstetric deaths, on the other hand, are those resulting from previously existing disease or disease that developed during pregnancy and which was not due to direct obstetric causes, but which was aggravated by physiologic effects of pregnancy.

Although regional variations exist, the following five major complications account for most of the direct obstetric deaths: hemorrhage, infection, toxemia, obstructed labor (and rupture of the uterus), and unsafe abortion. A study in Bangladesh, for example, has estimated that out of the 600 women who died per 100,000 live births, 132 died from hemorrhage, 18 from infection, 114 from toxemia, 186 from abortion, 54 from obstructed labor and 96 from other causes.[9] Most of these deaths should be avoidable. Certain diseases are particularly important in the causation of indirect obstetric deaths in developing countries. These include viral hepatitis, malaria, anemia, and rheumatic heart disease.[10]

This medical perspective, however, provides only a partial answer to the causes of the tragedy of maternal mortality. The question still remains as to why women die in large numbers from these complications, when women in developed countries do not. To illustrate the point, let us consider, as an example, the case of one maternal death. The medical cause of the death of Mrs. X was hemorrhage caused by placenta praevia. Death from this life-threatening complication, however, should be avoidable. Inquiry reveals that it took her four hours to reach the hospital, during which she was bleeding severely. This was because of the lack of facilities for emergency transport. Moreover, the district hospital to which she was referred was not well prepared with the essential obstetric functions to save her life. Blood transfusion was not readily available, and she had to wait for three hours before Caesarean section could be performed. Further questioning shows that Mrs. X should have been considered a case of high-risk pregnancy even before the development of the fatal complication. This attack of bleeding was not the first. She had had two minor episodes of bleeding in the last month of pregnancy, the serious significance of which could have been heeded, and she could have been referred earlier for appropriate management. However, Mrs. X did not have access to the services of a trained birth attendant who could have alerted her. Moreover, she was also suffering from chronic iron deficiency anemia because of parasitic infestation and malnutrition Her reserves were so low that she could not stand the severe attack of bleeding. But she never had the benefit of any community-based prenatal services, where her anemia could have been corrected by simple treatment. Further probing in the circumstances of Mrs. X shows that she had more than her desired number of children, and had not wanted to become pregnant. She did not, however, have access to information and services for birth planning. We have to add to these circumstances her low social status as a woman. She was an illiterate housewife, with no gainful employment. Finally, we need to put this picture within the frame of the poor socio-economic development of the community in which she was born and in which she lived.* This case illustrates the concept that maternal deaths in developing countries should not be looked upon from a narrow medical perspective, as the result of isolated disease episodes. Maternal mortality is commonly the last stop in what we may metaphorically call "THE ROAD TO MATERNAL DEATH."[11] Understanding of this concept is essential for developing an effective strategy for safe motherhood.

A STRATEGY FOR SAFE MOTHERHOOD

An integrated strategy for safe motherhood should have the following basic elements to address the reproductive health needs of women in general, and those at risk, in particular:

Advancement of the status of women: for all females.
Birth planning: for all women in the reproductive age period.
Community-based prenatal services: for all pregnant women.
Delivery by a trained birth attendant: for all women in labor.
Essential obstetric functions: for women with high-risk pregnancy.
Facilities for emergency transport: for women with obstetric life-threatening complications.

ADVANCEMENT OF THE STATUS OF WOMEN

The social status of women around the world, particularly in developing countries, leaves much to be desired. A recent global survey has labeled the status of women as POOR, POWERLESS, and PREGNANT.[12] The study has indicated that over 50% of all women and girls in the world live under conditions which threaten their health, deny them choice about childbearing, limit educational attainment, restrict economic participation, and fail to guarantee them equal rights and freedom with men. Women need to be healthy in order to fulfill their reproductive duty safely and efficiently, and health is not merely the absence of disease or infirmity, it is a positive state of physical, mental, and social wellbeing. Where the social status of women is low, sex

---

* A video-tape with the title of "Why did Mrs. X die?" is available in English, French, Spanish and Arabic from the World Health Organization.

discrimination begins from the time of birth (and thanks to new technologic advances in prenatal diagnosis, even before birth). The girl child may not receive the same care as her brother when she gets sick. She does not get her full nutritional share of the family pot. Her family does not make the same investment in her education. She may be subjected to certain harmful practices as female circumcision.

Moreover, women will not be able to take full advantage of the other essential elements of the strategy of safe motherhood, without advancement of their status. The ability of women to plan their births is directly proportional to their educational attainment.[13] A study in India has confirmed that the available rural health services were utilized more by men, even when the services were manned by women.[14] Another recent study in Jordan reported that the utilization of prenatal services was much less by illiterate women and women with only a few years of education.[15]

BIRTH PLANNING

The importance of sound birth planning for a successful and safe outcome for the mother and child is now well documented. Birth planning will reduce the prevalence of high-risk pregnancy and of unwanted pregnancy.

Prevention of high-risk pregnancy

In addition to medical conditions that may necessitate the postponement of pregnancy, there are health indications related to the mother's age, the spacing between pregnancies, and the number of pregnancies. Pregnancy carries a higher risk if it is too early (adolescent pregnancy), too close (short spacing), too many (grand multiparity), or too late (elderly gravida). These unfavorable patterns of childbearing account for about half of all pregnancies in many developing areas.[16] Some studies have attempted to provide an answer to what extent birth planning would contribute to safer motherhood by prevention of high-risk pregnancy. In one study in the rural areas of Bangladesh, it was estimated that the maternal mortality will be reduced by one-third, if births were limited to women between 20 to 39 years of age, and for a number of times from 1 to 5.[17]

Prevention of unwanted pregnancy

The prevention of unwanted pregnancy protects the mother from being exposed to the unnecessary risks of pregnancy and childbirth, and to the risks of induced unsafe abortion. Some studies have tried to evaluate the potential impact of the prevention of unwanted pregnancy on maternal mortality. One study based on data from the World Fertility Survey in 26 developing countries, estimated the proportion of deaths that would be prevented if all future births were avoided by women who want no more children and are not using selective contraceptives.[18] The percentage ranged from 5% in the Ivory Coast to 62% in Bangladesh, with a regional median of 17% for 8 countries in Africa, 35% for 10 Asian countries, 33% for 8 Latin American countries, and an overall median of 29%. The World Health Organization estimates that unsafe induced abortion accounts for almost one-half of all maternal deaths in several Latin American countries.[3]

The objective of the strategy for safe motherhood would be to ensure universal access to family planning information and services to all women in the reproductive age group. A recent global survey of 95 developing countries has scored the access to birth control as very poor in 31 countries, poor in 33 countries, fair in 16 countries, good in 10 countries, and excellent in only 5 countries.[19]

COMMUNITY-BASED PRENATAL SERVICES

Prenatal services have as objectives: The screening of pregnant women to detect those at high risk and to direct them to appropriate higher service levels; monitoring the progress of pregnancy for the early detection of complications; and health promotion, including health education.

Community-based prenatal services by trained health workers are by no means readily accessible to pregnant women in developing countries. Country data reported to the World Health Organization show that there are large sectors of the population in developing countries with poor coverage of services. Eight countries reported a coverage of less than 20%, and 9 countries with a coverage of 20 to less than 40%.[3]

DELIVERY BY A TRAINED BIRTH ATTENDANT

The presence of a trained birth attendant is essential at every delivery. The attendant should have the basic training to suspect that labor be abnormal or of high risk, to monitor the progress of labor to detect at an early stage deviations from the normal course, and to take adequate safeguards in the management of labor, including the prevention of puerperal infection.

The World Health Organization estimated that only 55% of a world total of 128.3 million births were attended by trained personnel. The percentage for developed countries was 98 and for developing countries, 48. This does not reflect the regional and country variations, and the variations within countries particularly between urban and rural areas.

Community health workers and traditional birth attendants (TBAs) are often the only potential source for birth planning, prenatal care and delivery. Improving the skills of community health workers and TBAs, providing them with basic equipment and supplies, and integrating them in the health care system are critical steps to improving health care at the community level. Success will also depend on the active participation of the communities and the mobilization of community resources.

ESSENTIAL OBSTETRIC FUNCTIONS AT THE FIRST REFERRAL LEVEL

The availability of community-based prenatal services and trained birth attendants will not be enough to ensure safe motherhood. There will always be a certain percentage of cases in which assistance at birth will be needed, of a type that can only be provided by trained professionals in equipped centers. There are also cases of high-risk pregnancy which need special care. Moreover, life-threatening complications cannot always be prevented, and in many cases cannot be predicted.

The World Health Organization has prepared a technical report detailing the essential obstetric functions that should be available at the first referral level, as well as their requirements in terms of health manpower, training and facilities.[21] These seven functions include:

1) Surgical functions such as Caesarean section, surgical treatment of sepsis, repair of high vaginal and cervical tears, laparotomy for ruptured uterus, removal of ectopic pregnancy and evacuation of the uterus in cases of abortion;
2) anaesthetic functions;
3) blood replacement, which includes blood transfusion and plasma expanders;
4) manual and/or assessment functions, which include manual removal of the placenta, delivery by vacuum extraction or forceps and use of the partograph;
5) medical treatment functions, which include treatment of shock, medical treatment of sepsis, control of hypertensive disorders of pregnancy and eclamptic seizures;
6) family planning functions, which include surgical contraception, IUDs, Norplant, and other contraceptives; and
7) management of women at high risk.

FACILITIES FOR EMERGENCY TRANSPORT

The occurrence of a life-threatening complication will necessitate immediate transport to a facility where the complication can be adequately managed. The median time period between the onset of the complication and death has been estimated at two hours for postpartum hemorrhage, twelve hours for antepartum hemorrhage, one day for rupture of the uterus, two days for eclampsia, three days for obstructed labor, six days for puerperal sepsis, and seven days for complicated abortion.

Facilities for emergency transport are not readily available in developing countries, particularly in rural areas. The shortage is compounded by a poor communication system and the bad condition of the roads. Innovative approaches have to be explored. Some health care systems have established the feasibility of providing maternity waiting homes for women with high-risk pregnancies, where they can wait for the onset of labor close to a health care facility well prepared to handle obstetric problems, without occupying the limited number of hospital beds.[22]

The six basic elements of the strategy for safe motherhood should be considered a package of interrelated elements, and not as different options. The potential impact of each element is in fact partly dependent on the presence of the other elements. Advancement of the status of women and birth planning have a two-way relationship. Without birth planning, maternity services will be over-burdened by the large numbers of unwanted pregnancy, induced abortions, and high-risk pregnancies. Without community-based prenatal services and delivery by trained birth attendants, cases at high-risk and life-threatening complications will not be detected at an early stage to allow their successful management at the first referral level. Without the back-up of essential obstetric functions at the first referral level and the facilities for emergency transport, community-based services by trained personnel will not be effective in ensuring safe motherhood.

REQUIREMENTS FOR A SUCCESSFUL STRATEGY FOR SAFE MOTHERHOOD

The 40th World Health Assembly passed a resolution on Maternal Health and Safe Motherhood in 1987, urging Member States to give high priority to improving the health of women and reducing maternal mortality and morbidity.

A lowering of maternal mortality by one-half in developing countries by the year 2000 is a feasible target. It needs, however, a strong political commitment: The mobilization, rational allocation and effective utilization of the necessary resources; adaptation of the already available know-how to the cultural environment, socio-economic situation and health services organization; and the active participation of the communities and particularly of women.

REFERENCES

1. World Health Organization. Maternal mortality rates. A tabulation of available information, 2d ed. Geneva: WHO, 1986, pp. 1-3.

2. Datta, K,K., R.S. Sharma, P.M.A. Razack, et al. Morbidity pattern among rural pregnant women in Alwar, Rajasthan – a cohort study. Health and Population Perspectives and Issues 3:282-292, 1980.

3. World Health Organization. Evaluation of the strategy for health for all by the year 2000. Seventh report on the world health situation. Vol 1: Global overview. Geneva: WHO, 1987, pp. 74-75, 41.

4. Greenwood, A.M., B.M. Greenwood, and A. K. Bradley, et al. A prospective survey of the outcome of pregnancy in a rural area of the Gambia. Bulletin of the World Health Organization 65:635-643, 1987.

5. Herz, B., and A.R. Measham. Safe motherhood initiative. Proposals for action. Washington, DC: The World Bank, 1987, p. 7.

6. World Health Organization. Studying maternal mortality in developing countries. Rates and causes. A guidebook. Division of Family Health. Geneva: WHO, 1987.

7. Rosenfield, A., and D. Maine. Maternal mortality – a neglected tragedy. Where is the M in MCH? Lancet 2:83ff, 1985.

8. World Health Organization. International classification of diseases. Vol 1. Geneva: WHO, 1977, p. 764.

9. Rochat, R.W. The magnitude of maternal mortality: Definitions and methods of measurement. Background paper for Meeting on Prevention of Maternal Mortality. Geneva: WHO, 1985.

10. Lettenmaier, C., L. Liskin, and C.A. Church, et al. Mothers' lives matter: Maternal health in the community. Population Reports 16:1-31, 1988.

11. Fathalla, M.F. The long road to maternal death. People 14:8-9, 1987.

12. Population Crisis Committee. Country rankings of the status of women: Poor, Powerless and Pregnant. Population Briefing Paper no. 20. Washington, DC: Population Crisis Committee, 1988.

13. London, K.A., J. Cushing, and S.O. Rutstein, et al. Fertility and family planning surveys: An update. Population Reports 13:289-348, 1985.

14. Murthy, N. Reluctant patients – the women of India. World Health Forum 3:315-316, 1982.

15. Abbas, A.A., and G.J.A. Walker. Determinants of the utilization of maternal and child health services in Jordan. Int J Epi 14:404-406, 1986.

16. Rinehart, W., A. Kols, and S.H. Moore. Healthier mothers and children through family planning. Population Reports 12:658-696, 1984.

17. Trussel, J., and A. R. Pebley. The potential impact of changes in fertility on infant, child and maternal mortality. Studies in Family Planning 15:267-280, 1984.

18. Maine, D., A. Rosenfield, and M. Wallace, et al. Prevention of maternal mortality in developing countries. Program options and practical considerations. Background paper for Safe Motherhood International Conference, Nairobi, 1987.

19. Population Crisis Committee. Access to birth control: a world assessment. Population Briefing paper no. 19. Population Crisis Committee, Washington DC, 1987.

20. World Health Organization. Coverage of maternity care. A tabulation of available information. Geneva: WHO, Division of Family Health, 1985, p. 4.

21. World Health Organization. Essential obstetric functions at the first referral level. Report of a technical working group. Geneva:WHO, 1986.

22. Cardoso, U.F. Giving birth is safer now. World Health Forum 7:348-352, 1986.

20

TRADITIONAL BIRTH ATTENDANTS

A. MANGAY-MAGLACAS, R.N.,DR.P.H.

INTRODUCTION

The traditional birth attendant (TBA) has been defined as "a person (usually a woman) who assists the mother at childbirth and who acquired her skills delivering babies by herself or by working with other traditional birth attendants."[1] Traditional birth attendants are found in most villages of Africa, Asia, and Latin America. They serve in many rural communities as the main source of assistance for maternal and child care. Just how many TBAs there are in the world is not known, since only a few countries have made national surveys and introduced the registration of TBAs. However, it is estimated that in the developing world, about 50% of all births are still attended by TBAs.

In many societies, traditional birth attendants do much more than this name suggests. Some would be better described as "traditional healers," since they are the only ones available to care for the health needs of women and children. For example, in Niger, the ratio of traditional birth attendants to 10,000 population is 11.9; for physicians it is 0.3; and for midwives, 0.3.[2] Given the number of TBAs, the broad range of health-related activities in which they engage, and the general lack of other available health services in communities where they practice, training and articulating them into the formal health care system appear to be the best alternative approach for improving not only maternal and child health, but primary health care services in many countries.

Formal global attention to the TBAs was encouraged by the World Health Organization when it launched a worldwide survey of TBAs in 1972.[3] This review underlined the importance of the role played by the TBA. Since then, the World Health Organization assiduously gathered and analyzed a mass of information; from this certain, basic truths have emerged.[4,5,6]

Among them are the following: That large numbers of TBAs exist in many countries and, for the time being, they are the major source of assistance to millions of pregnant women, mothers, and infants; and that in many countries several decades will pass before national health resources will be sufficient to allow the development of an adequate number of staff qualified to provide the type of "excellent" care that may be desired by or for society, but which is currently unavailable to most of its population.

It becomes apparent that efforts will need to be focused on enhancing the vast potential that lies in communities themselves for providing basic health care, thus making it possible for such communities to improve their capacity for serving themselves. TBAs constitute a large segment of that potential.

THE ROLE OF TBAs

In all countries where the TBAs exist, the TBA is accepted by local communities, a very important fact indeed. The functions of TBAs vary considerably from country to country, and in most countries they reach beyond the major functions of attendance at, and assistance with, birth. In fact, the term "traditional birth attendant" reflects a gross understatement of the actual function of the category of midwife. A review of several reports from many countries of Asia and Africa shows that these health workers carry out a varied range of activities, and these are as follows:

- basic care to mothers before, during, and after delivery
- care of the newborn
- undertaking referrals to health facilities
- participating in promotion of family planning
- helping in notification of communicable diseases
- helping in organizing mothers' classes and community immunization campaigns
- participating in primary health care services

In some countries of the Middle East, in addition to delivering babies, treating female infertility and gynecological disorders, TBAs give sex education, induce abortions, perform female circumcision, and give nutrition education.[9]

The role of the TBA frequently extends to more than just the range of activities enumerated above. They provide housekeeping services to the family, look after children when ill, perform rituals at weddings, deaths, and when girls reach menarche. Their <u>accessibility</u> and <u>acceptability</u> are two key factors that demonstrate the immense potential of their services to mothers and children.

The acceptance and use of TBAs since the early 1970s can be attributed to two factors: First, the countries' adoption of primary health care as the key to the attainment of the social goal of "Health for All"; and second, the countries' commitment to the increased coverage of their underserved populations, especially in rural areas. The accelerating movement towards the wide acceptance of the value of the trained TBA has encouraged countries to design more effective TBA training programs.

While TBA training programs have gained a lot of support, not only nationally but internationally, it is the <u>sustained</u> support for utilizing TBAs that presents a formidable problem. Of import is the lack of an organized system to supervise trained TBAs, provide continuing training for them, and make available to them basic supplies, such as cord care kits. Supervision continues to be a problem. Walt has identified the constraints on supervision as falling into five major categories:

- weak technical, organizational, and administrative support
- dispersed and isolated communities
- lack of rapport between health system personnel and TBAs
- low involvement of community in TBA programs
- limited financial support for training and supervision.[10]

Supervision of TBAs constitutes the major link between them and the formal health care system. A shortage of supervisory health personnel, inadequate transportation systems, and insufficient financial resources – problems cited in the WHO survey of 1972 remain the primary obstacles to the development of good supervision. Many countries are exploring alternative approaches to resolve the problem of supervising TBAs and are focusing greater attention on involving people in their own health. The constraints to supervision identified above have been expanded and a matrix lay-out has been proposed by the World Health Organization.[11] Because of the practicality and relevance of the identified support mechanisms, they are reproduced on the next three pages.

THE TRAINING OF TBAs

During the past decade and a half, there has been a great deal of interest in training TBAs. Many United Nations agencies, notably WHO, UNICEF,

SUPERVISION MATRIX[7]

CONSTRAINTS ON SUPERVISION	MECHANICS TO IMPROVE SUPERVISION
Weak technical, organizational, and administrative support	
Poor transport system	- Thorough initial TBA training. - Arrange 2-3 day annual or bi-annual meetings as refresher courses.
Shortage of health personnel; little time for supervision	- Schedule supervision into the normal work routine, with guidelines on what is expected of supervisors. - Appoint health staff with knowledge about childbirth to provide supervision. - Establish a system of community intermediaries to support trained TBAs. They may be teachers, religious leaders, other traditional practitioners, perhaps with specialist skills, a women's committee, and so on.
Lack of support for health personnel	- Provide regular supervision for health workers at all levels of the health infrastructure. - Set up refresher courses, or workshops, or meetings for supervisors (and trainers) at least once a year.
Response to referral poor because of technical incompetence of health staff	- Improve the practical training in childbirth in education programmes for health centre staff. - Consider pairing health staff to work with TBAs as part of professional training.
Supplies and salaries arrive irregularly	- Establish a regular, realistic routine to re-supply; do not widen TBA's functions unless supplies can be guaranteed; do not supply kits with material that cannot be locally replaced. Do not rely on material incentives.
Lack of integration between health units in the referral network	- Set up clear structure for referral and ensure that feedback occurs.

SUPERVISION MATRIX (continued)

Dispersed and isolated communities	TBAs do some deliveries, but many are done by relatives of pregnant women	- Consider health education for all older women in community on specific aspects of birth, such as cord care, rather than training TBAs only, using mobile teams, and specially-trained health educators.
	Health units inaccessible	- Identify intermediaries in community who can support TBAs. Health committees may be useful, or village leaders, religious leaders, other traditional practitioners. They could keep records of births, etc. - Use technical aids like radio to keep in touch. - Health staff arrange to visit a cluster of villages at specific time of year, if only once annually.
Lack of rapport between health systems personnel and TBAs	Health systems personnel not sympathetic to TBAs	- Try to change attitudes in training. Ensure contact with TBAs during training and that trainers have positive attitudes about TBAs. - Leave trained TBAs accountable to community and not to health staff.
	TBAs fear or have reservations about health system personnel	- Bring TBAs into health units. Provide regular meetings with health staff. Ensure they are treated with respect.
	TBAs view health personnel as young and incompetent	- Pair health professionals with TBAs so they learn from their experience and build up mutual trust.
	TBAs and clients have a complex set of beliefs and customs not shared by health system personnel	- Support understanding of harmless traditional rituals and promote safe, technical procedures. - Identify any harmful practices, and explain why they are harmful within the context of the TBAs understanding and the local situation.

SUPERVISION MATRIX (continued)

Low involvement of community in TBA programme	Communities indifferent to or un- aware of TBA training programme	- Ensure that community and TBAs want training. - Involve community in selection of TBAs for training. - Hold graduation ceremony. - Encourage community to support trained TBAs by: providing a place for deliveries; setting up a health committee to sup- port TBAs' material needs; keep records; help provide trans- port for at-risk women.
	Communities suspicious of trained TBAs	- Hold meetings between the community (and especially the men, in some cases) and health centre personnel (in some cases male health professionals) explaining the advantages of training TBAs. - Meet all the women, discuss the problems relating to preg- nancy and labour; set up women's committee to support and also heighten expectations of trained TBA. - Hold joint meetings of men and women to reinforce the value of trained TBAs' work.
Limited financial support for training and supervision	Limited funds available from government or external sources	- Use funds as incentives to TBAs to come into health units or for health staff to visit TBAs in field, taking into account atti- tudes, distances involved, and so on. - Use for occasional workshops, refresher courses for TBAs. - Provide health education, including guidelines for community health development to women's groups or health committees.
	No extra funds available	- Build training TBAs into routine work of health units. - Establish community mechanisms of material support, e.g., village insurance schemes, village cooperatives for drugs and supplies.

and UNFPA, and such other agencies as USAID, IPPF, and Save the Children Fund are supporting and providing assistance to TBA training programs. Although a few countries started training TBAs as early as 1922, as in the case of the Sudan, which has perhaps the longest history of experience in the formal training of TBAs, other countries, such as India, Philippines, and Thailand, started formal training of TBAs only in the early 1950s.[12]

More training is now being made available to TBAs. The increase in training programs is especially marked in the African region; whereas, only one training program was reported in 1972, now all countries with TBAs operate some kind of training. While no recent survey has been undertaken, it is safe to deduce that in all countries where TBAs exist, training programs have been instituted – whereas, in 1972 only 37% of countries with TBAs had some form of TBA training. The greatest increase in the number of countries with TBA training programs, and in the number of countries where TBAs are registered or certified, has occurred in the African region.

The emphasis of most training programs is placed on:

- increased safety in the TBAs' practice, such as cleanliness, especially washing of the hands, and clean or sterile cord-cutting procedures
- non-interference during labor
- care of mothers before, during, and after delivery
- identification and referral of mothers at risk
- doing away with traditional harmful practices and leaving alone or supporting those that contribute to psychosocial support.

Because most TBAs cannot read or write, the teaching/learning sessions must be oral and based on pictures, role-playing, and demonstrations. In most training programs the use of clean or boiled cord-cutting instruments and clean hands are stressed very much because tetanus is an important cause of neonatal death.

Many countries have developed their own training programs using or adapting the WHO/BLAT TBA Trainer's Kit.[13] This kit focuses special attention on planning relevant course content, ensuring that current safe and beneficial practices of TBAs (either physically or psychologically) are reinforced, and abandoning those practices that are harmful, while ignoring those that are harmless. In cases where harmful practices reflect the cultural and religious beliefs and demands of the community, rather than solely the idiosyncracies of the TBA, the latter may find it difficult to abandon such practices, and TBA trainers will need to provide appropriate health education to the community, particularly the women.

Experience has shown that successful TBA training programs are those that are planned and linked with the organized health care system of the countries. Perhaps most important, in some if not all countries, are the changes that are made in support of the new role of the TBAs and their articulation with the health system. The attitudes of health personnel should reflect their acceptance of the TBA as a legitimate health worker. Aspects of the training program that are usually considered are: TBA tasks on which the training will focus; the specification of learning objectives; preparation of trainers; selection of trainees; course content and methods; the place and duration of the training; and teaching/learning materials.

Most countries with TBAs have organized formal training programs. After successful completion of the course, a certificate of attendance, equivalent to permission to practice, is often granted. Although not given a legal status, the TBA is entitled to practice. Moreover, TBAs, whether recognized or not, trained or untrained, are not restricted to practice in the majority of countries where they exist. Because of the recognized need to fill the gap, health authorities have benignly tolerated their activities without interference and have not objected to their training and utilization. In Latin America, Africa, and Asia, where trained TBAs have been upgraded, and also trained in family planning and health promotion, there is an indication that TBAs are the indigenous practitioners most easily incorporated into the formal health care system. Case studies from Bangladesh, Guatemala, Liberia, and Tanzania also report successful incorporation of TBAs into the health system.

In a large number of countries, the responsibility for developing and conducting TBA training courses and for TBA supervision has been assigned to midwives or nurse-midwives. There is still a dearth of trainers who are prepared to teach and who are familiar with the sociocultural background and practices of the TBAs and their communities.

Numerous problems still underlie the effectiveness of TBA training programs. Of the utmost importance is the selection of appropriately prepared trainers of TBAs – trainers who are not only proficient in midwifery, but who are knowledgeable in teaching illiterate or semi-literate groups, and who are familiar with the TBAs' practices, influence, and status in the community, including the role they play in providing psychological support to families. There is still a dearth of training materials for trainers, and of programs for the training of trainers. Trainers need to focus on the knowledge TBAs already have in order to <u>adapt</u> content and training or learning strategies to TBAs who are different in terms of age, literacy, and cultural background.

EVALUATION

What are the effects of training TBAs? A review of the literature reveals that there has been a lot of work on evaluating training programs per se, but very little has been done in evaluating the trained TBAs and assessing their impact on factors influencing maternal and child health. This is understandable because the decrease in mortality rates is due to a number of factors, not simply to the performance of a trained TBA. Besides, TBAs are powerless to deal with many of the causes of poor health among mothers. However, specific indicators of training programs can be designed and monitored. When this is done, some yield of effectiveness can be shown as a direct result of the trained TBA's performance.

In the Philippines, the impact of TBA training on neonatal tetanus was investigated by studying the decline in deaths from this disease in relation to the extent of TBA training.[14] In the provinces, where the training of TBAs was nominal (i.e., where 25% or less of TBAs had been trained) the average annual incidence of death from neonatal tetanus declined from 49 in 1973-75 to 41 in 1976-77, and to 29 in 1978 – an overall decline of 41%. On the other hand, in those provinces where 50% or more of the TBAs had been trained, the incidence declined from 41 in 1973-75 to 28 in 1976-77 and to 6 in 1978 – an overall decline of 85%.

In Bangladesh, Rahman studied birth outcomes by a two-fold approach, i.e., giving tetanus toxoid vaccine to pregnant mothers, and training TBAs in hygienic delivery techniques.[15] Three areas for the study were established: one with trained TBAs, the second where tetanus toxoid was given, and the third as a control area.

Neonatal Death Rates at Beginning of Study	
Area	No. of deaths/1000 live births
Control	85
Tetanus Toxoid	39
Trained TBAs	24

The study showed the following results:

Neonatal Deaths Due to Tetanus	
Area	No. of deaths by percent
Control	24%
Tetanus Toxoid	1%
Trained TBAs	6%

The preceeding results augur well for high effectiveness when a dual intervention of tetanus toxoid immunization and TBA training is undertaken.

Very few countries determine the effects of training on TBA practice, but some countries have attempted to evaluate the efficiency of their training programs. Mangay-Maglacas and Simons collected a few experiences of countries in assessing the effectiveness of their TBA training programs.[16] The results briefly described below illustrate some of the effects of such programs.

Sierra Leone undertook a survey in 1981 involving about 50% of all trained TBAs. The majority of the TBAs were seen to be giving regular antenatal care to pregnant mothers and tackled normal deliveries quite satisfactorily. Furthermore, an interview of community leaders (N=102) showed that 96% felt that TBA training had led to a recognizable improvement in the TBAs' work after training. The acceptance of the TBA by the community and the evidence that the TBA's work has changed for the better have been firmly acknowledged.

The results of an evaluation of the DANFA Comprehensive Rural Health and Family Planning Project in Ghana showed that the project was "favorable on the midwifery care given to women in the study area...the vast majority of women seen by the trained TBAs were referred to the local health center for at least one prenatal visit, and the use of sterile cord packs by TBAs increased considerably."

Most of the evaluation carried out does reveal very encouraging results about the TBAs' practice. However, many of these studies are restricted to defined local areas and are not always the results of rigorous field research, nor do they always stand up to detailed methodological scrutiny. Given that, one could ask if it is really necessary to undertake vigorously designed research to establish valid results when the cost of such research can easily be more expensive than most TBA training programs? Certainly, more will be gained if a TBA is trained rather than not trained; the investment in training is very small compared with the gains that have been so far observed and evaluated.

The need for further research is not negated. This is especially true in the areas of traditional practice that should form part of the content of training programs, and the need to search for better teaching/learning methods for a group such as the TBAs. The expanded role of TBAs in primary health care is another area that has to be studied for a better understanding of the potential in community health programs.

FUTURE OF TBAs

In 1978, at Alma-Ata, USSR, where primary health care was endorsed as the key to the attainment of the social goal of health for all, the following statements were also endorsed:

"Traditional medical practitioners and birth attendants are found in most societies. They are often part of the local community, culture and traditions, and continue to have high social standing in many places, exerting considerable influence on local health practices. With the support of the formal health system, these indigenous practitioners can become important allies in organizing efforts to improve the health of the community. Some communities may select them as community health workers. It is therefore well worth while exploring the possibilities of engaging them in primary health care and of training them accordingly."[17]

The acceptance and use of TBAs have come a long way since the Declaration of Alma-Ata. Many countries have undertaken seriously the training and utilization of TBAs. For many of the developing countries, there is no choice, given the worsening economic conditions, but to use all available potential manpower to extend wider health care coverage, especially in underserved communities where the TBAs live and work. It can be assumed with a fair degree of confidence that trained TBAs can contribute to the health of mothers and children, and a considerable proportion of infant deaths can be averted by clean hands and the use of clean instruments.

Each country has to decide for itself whether or not TBA training should be intensified in terms of numbers, amplified in terms of numbers, amplified in terms of content, and/or extended to include expanded primary health care functions. The latter seems to be gaining ground and should be discussed more intensively; TBAs are now more involved in oral rehydration, immunization programs, and other primary health activities, and not just those related to midwifery. The many problems surrounding supervision, the lack of continuing training, and the lack of adequate referral systems could dilute the effectiveness of the TBAs' role in midwifery practices, which is their "expertise," so to speak. Considering that many are semi-literate or illiterate, expanding their tasks or roles without adequate supervision may be counterproductive and may even become unsafe. A little knowledge could be potentially dangerous. This extended role needs to be studied and analyzed, and safeguards should be established. Efforts would be focused on making the very best use of the greater numbers of TBAs and more work should be undertaken to ensure their effective and full participation in health care in their communities.[8]

Although there is considerable literature on the training and utilization of TBAs in primary health care, little research has been undertaken to discover the nature and efficacy of their practices. There is also a paucity of policies developed to articulating TBAs to the formal health system. In many instances they work as appendages to formal health care workers and mainly out of the stream of organized health care services. The absence of comprehensive, clear, and positive policies on TBAs has left them as a "fringe" issue, and for the most part TBA training programs have become a means to an end.

What is the future of TBAs? TBAs should be phased out gradually; that is, if countries would make relevant health manpower plans that would include a gradual replacement of TBAs. Timing for a gradual phase-out will depend on the capability of countries to support a sustainable plan for manpower development. TBAs should be replaced by village midwives, drawn from females or males who have had some primary education, and then trained accordingly and progressively to reach higher and higher levels, becoming literate trainees. Where health manpower plans are developed, the staged development of midwives could very well become part of it. This plan could in the long run be directed at developing a career ladder leading to professional midwifery. If there continues to be an absence of clear and well-defined policies and plans on TBAs, and a laissez-faire attitude towards them, then the training and utilization of TBAs will continue to be merely tolerated and the present problems will continue unabated. The future would, at best, be exemplified as is the present state.

REFERENCES

1. Verderese, M. de L., and L. M. Turnbull. The traditional birth attendant in maternal and child health and family planning: A guide to her training and utilization. Geneva: World Health Organization, (WHO offset publication no. 18).

2. World Health Statistics Annual. Geneva: World Health Organization, 1988, p.46.

3. Verderese, M.L. Report of review and analysis of information and data on traditional birth attendants. Geneva: World Health Organization, 1973 (Document HMD/NUR/73.3).

4. Traditional birth attendants: A field guide to their training, evaluation, and articulation with the health services. Geneva: World Health Organization, 1979 (WHO offset publication no. 44).

5. Mangay-Maglacas, A., and H. Pizurki, (eds). The traditional birth attendant in seven countries: Case studies in utilization and training. Geneva: World Health Organization, 1981 (Public Health Papers no. 75).

6. The extension of health service coverage with traditional birth attendants: A decade of progress. WHO Chronicle, 36(3):92-96, 1982.

7. The supervision of traditional birth attendants (TBAs). Geneva: World Health Organization, Division of Health Manpower Development, 1984 (Document HMD/NUR/84.1).

8. Mangay-Maglacas, A., and J. Simons, (eds). The potential of the traditional birth attendant. Geneva: World Health Organization, 1986 (WHO offset publication no. 95).

9. Kamal, I.T. A survey of the training and utilization of the traditional birth attendants in the eastern Mediterranean Region of WHO. Alexandria, Egypt: World Health Organization regional office for the eastern Mediterranean, 1984, p.13.

10. The supervision of traditional birth attendants (TBAs), op cit., pp. 23-25.

11. Ibid.

12. Mangay-Maglacas, A., and H. Pizurki, op cit.

13. Lovedee, I.M., W.D. Clarke, A. Mangay-Maglacas, and K.P. Shah. A TBA trainer's kit. Joint production of the World Health Organization, Geneva, and the BLAT Center for Health and Medical Education, London, 1982.

14. Mangay-Angara, A. Philippines: The development and use of the national registry of traditional birth attendants. In: Mangay-Maglacas, A. and H. Pizurki. The traditional birth attendant in seven countries, op.cit., pp. 37-70.

15. Rahman, S. The effect of TBAs and tetanus toxoid in reduction of neonatal mortality. Dhaka, NIPORT, 1981 (Unpublished paper).

16. Mangay-Maglacas, A., and J. Simons. The potential of the traditional birth attendant, op.cit.

17. Alma-Ata, 1978: Primary health care. Geneva: World Health Organization, 1978 ("Health for All" series, no. 1), p.63.

21

IMPLEMENTATION OF RISK APPROACH IN MATERNAL HEALTH

W. Phuapradit, M.D., M.P.H.; S. Pongthai, M.D., M.P.H.;
S. Sudhutoravut, M.D.;
K. Chaturachinda, M.B., Ch.B., F.R.C.OG.;
V. Benchakan, M.D.

CONCEPT OF HIGH RISK

Pregnancy and parturition, a natural process, still carry a risk, often fatal to both the mother and infant – a major problem in developing countries where health care and services are severely limited.

The concept of high risk originates from the fact that the vulnerability to death and disability is not equally distributed among all pregnant women and their babies. Only a certain proportion of women and infants face the tragedy while the majority have uneventful pregnancies and deliveries. Unfortunately it is this "high-risk" group of women who at present receive the least adequate health care. (Figure 1, next page.) With hindsight most of those who die or are disabled could be identified before the events occur because they usually share some common features or characteristics which are related to their biological make-up or their environments or both. These characteristics are usually called "risk factors." If these risk factors as well as their effects are identified, diseases and death could be prevented by providing appropriate health care and services. Thus the risk approach is a method for measuring the need of individuals and groups for care (and thus for assisting them to determine their priorities), and a tool for the reappraisal and reorganization of health and other services to meet that need. Its aim is to improve care for all, but to pay special attention to those in greater need.

242

CRITERIA OF HIGH-RISK WOMEN

Criteria used to identify high-risk women can be based on 2 classifications.[1-5]

1. Relationships between risk factors and adverse outcomes; these are of three kinds:

    a. causative, triggering of pathological process; for example, maternal malnutrition and low birthweight, placenta previa, and fetal death from anoxia, or first trimester rubella infection and congenital malformations.

    b. contributory, such as grand-multiparity predisposing transverse lie, and prolapse of the umbilical cord.

    c. predictive, or associative in the statistical sense; for example, a woman with previous fetal loss is at greater risk of losing her next pregnancy.

2. Biological, medical and social conditions: These include biological risk factors (age, birth order, birth interval); nutritional factors (height, weight, weight gain); health care utilization (antenatal care); pregnancy complications (anemia, hypertension, diabetes mellitus, antepartum bleeding, twins, abnormal presentation); and social conditions (work load, birth attendance).

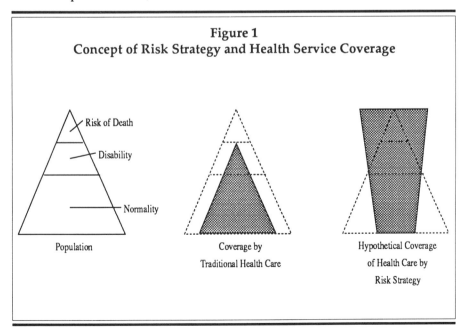

Figure 1
Concept of Risk Strategy and Health Service Coverage

Risk of Death

Disability

Normality

Population

Coverage by
Traditional Health Care

Hypothetical Coverage
of Health Care by
Risk Strategy

The following are examples of maternal risk factors and expected adverse outcome, based on 1977-1978 perinatal study at Bang Pa-In, Ayuthaya Province, Thailand, under collaboration of World Health Organization.[4,5] (Table 1.)

Table 1
Maternal Risk Factors and Their Adverse Outcomes

Risk Factors	Adverse Outcome	
	Perinatal	Maternal
1. Biological		
1.1 Age ≤ 17 yrs	perinatal	–
1.2 Age ≥ 30 yrs, first birth order	death & low	–
1.3 Age ≥ 35 yrs	birthweight	–
1.4 Birth order ≥ 4		APH, PPH retained
1.5 Birth interval < 18 months		placenta
2. Nutritional Status		
2.1 Height ≤ 144 cms.	perinatal death	prolonged labour
2.2 Weight at delivery ≤ 44 kgs.	& low	–
2.3 Weight gain < 7 kgs.	birthweight	–
2.4 Weight delivery ≥ 70 kgs.	perinatal death & high birthweight	hypertension
2.5 Hemoglobin ≤ 8 gm.	–	APH, PPH
3. Medical Complication		
3.1 DM	perinatal death & low	–
3.2 Chronic hypertension	birthweight	–
4. Obstetric Complication		
4.1 Pre-eclampsia	perinatal death & low birthweight	
4.2 History of difficult labour	birth asphyxia	–
5. Health Care Utilization		
5.1 No ANC	perinatal death & low birthweight	

RISK-SCORING SYSTEM

A risk-scoring system is a simple method for detecting and classifying pregnant women at risk. Steps used to develop risk-scoring system are as follows:[2,7]

1. Collect risk factors that influence health of mother and fetus during pregnancy from previous studies, journals and theoretical papers.

2. Categorize the risk factors according to the criteria based on biological, medical and social conditions.

3. Scoring marks are given to each risk factor according to its severity and its effect on pregnancy and labor on the basis of measurements of the actual risks in the same population. Those with the highest score are at greatest risk for the defined adverse outcome. In case of multiple risk factors the score for each factor is added and the "cut-off" point above which the mother is referred is arbitrarily given. However, this point must always be lower than the score given to a single risk factor which is known to be associated with a major adverse outcome.

4. Test for validly of the scores and the scoring criteria.

The following conditions should be considered in risk scoring:

1. Due to different health problems and different level of health personnel, the development of risk-scoring system should be individually tailored in different communities, and simple to be used by the primary health care workers.

2. Pregnancy is a dynamic process. Complications may occur anytime during pregnancy, labor and puerperium. Health care providers should screen expectant mother at proper time setting.

3. The "cut-off" point of the risk factors must be appropriately chosen, taking into account the balance between the serious outcome of the false negative readings and the inconvenience and waste of resources on false positives.

APPLICATION TO PLANNING AND DELIVERY OF SERVICES

Having made the decision to proceed with the concept of risk approach strategy in maternal health, one has to collect data regarding the health information for the implemented area as follows:[1,4,5]

- The age and sex distribution of the population and its geographical distribution by community and household
- area maps, communication facilities and local climate
- perinatal and maternal mortality according to age and sex and by cause
- local cultural patterns, education level and facilities, occupation, religious customs and attitudes toward health, disease and death in particular related to family planning and child rearing
- health services such as accessibility, quantity, quality, distribution, availability, technology, utilization, organization, and referral system, including health education services
- environmental risk factors, such as inadequate sanitation, water supplies, and sewage disposal
- role of health volunteers, birth attendants, traditional healers and their training.

In order to obtain the above information, it may be necessary to undertake surveys or make estimates from the existing reports. The next step is to set up the objectives of the project including plan of action and evaluation based on the problems to be tackled. Planning should concern the method to be used, including descriptions of population sampling, instruments of survey, data coding, data processing and constraint analysis. The alternative sampling method of the study population is to include either all newly pregnant women or only women in confinement or after delivery. The latter strategy has an advantage of lower utilization of manpower and expenses for data collection. However, it is not very informative if the study is carried out in a place where antenatal care coverage is poor and information in the record of risk factor identification is inadequate. For such a place the former sampling method is more suitable. Where the sampling method includes all currently pregnant women, more time, workload and expenses are required.

Two types of study designs are available: the case-control trial and the study without control area with evaluation of the result before and after the study against the expected outcome. The advantage of the case-control trial is having pairs of areas for evaluation. During the study period, factors affecting the paired areas should be comparable. The disadvantage is "contamination" of the risk approach strategy in the control area, psychologically and practically, with both the control and the implemented area competing "to be better." There would also be difficulty in getting paired areas with comparable social, economic, educational, health care and geographic aspects. The disadvantage of the study design without control area is the difficulty in evaluation of morbidity, mortality, health care utilization and coverage against expected outcome, which are affected by time elapsed; but this can be overcome by the study of the trends of rates of health indicators before and after project implementation or by comparing with the trend of national data.

Evaluation of service innovation is a process which should be going on in all health care systems based on primary health care, if progress toward the idea of health for all is to be achieved. To see whether the risk approach project is successful, one should evaluate the impact the study has in antenatal care coverage, knowledge and use of risk data by the community, referral pattern, relevant training program, risk factor intervention and maternal, perinatal morbidity and mortality.

EXAMPLE OF APPLICATION

Our experience in the application of risk approach in maternal and child care was carried out during the years 1981-1983 at Bang Pa-In district, Ayuthaya province, which is approximately 60 kilometers north of Bangkok, the capital city of Thailand. In this district there already existed a WHO collaborative study on perinatal mortality. The population is approximately 42,000 and during the study period there were 1800 deliveries. The infrahealth structure of Bang Pa-In district consists of regional, provincial, district, subdistrict, village and primary health care level. (Figure 2,3, next page.) The overall objective was to see if application of risk approach could reduce maternal, perinatal mortality and morbidity in the rural area within the national health infrastructure.

The specific aim and plan of action in each objective were as follows:

Objective 1. To identify mothers, newborns and infants at risk by the existing health personnel.

Plan of Action

- Develop subsystem for report of pregnant women, newborns, and deaths by community volunteers to peripheral health team.

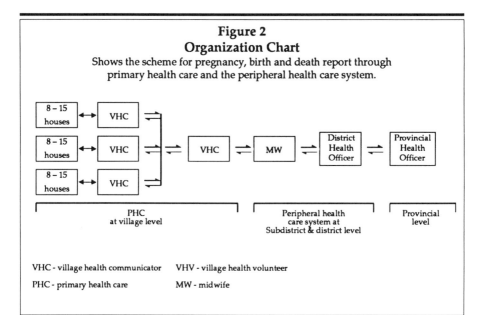

Figure 2
Organization Chart
Shows the scheme for pregnancy, birth and death report through
primary health care and the peripheral health care system.

VHC - village health communicator   VHV - village health volunteer

PHC - primary health care   MW - midwife

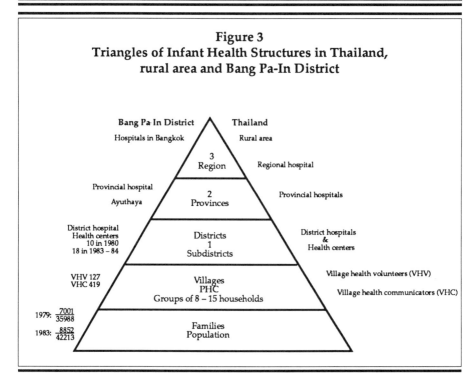

Figure 3
Triangles of Infant Health Structures in Thailand,
rural area and Bang Pa-In District

- Screen for high-risk group by community volunteers, and village health volunteer (primary screener); and by auxiliaries of the health station and community hospital (secondary screener).
- Support the reporting subsystem by setting up village clinics as data collecting points. Auxiliaries can perform risk screening and provide care for the needs.
- Develop simple forms for reporting pregnancy, birth and death, risk screening by health volunteers.
- Train existing health workers and volunteers on risk-screening technology.

Objective 2. To provide health care for identified risk group according to risk strategy.

Objective 3. To provide wider coverage through the package of integrated primary health care elements for mothers, newborns, and infants by peripheral health workers in the existing health delivery system.

Plan of Action for Objectives 2 and 3 included:

- Identify focal point persons including auxiliaries, community leaders and volunteers.
- Obtain permission and co-operation from the Ministry of Health at policy and operational level.
- Orient and train auxiliaries and volunteers on the use of manuals.

The evaluation design of this project employed the study without control area with evaluation of the result before and after the project comparing with the trend of national data. Sampling method was the total target population approached in a defined area and included the antenatal period in order to investigate risk factors accurately.

The maternal and child health indicators are presented in Table 2, (next page) compared before the project was implemented (1979-1980) and during the project (1981-1983). The coverage of health care during antenatal period increased approximately 14 percent. Attendance in early pregnancy had increased, as was the number of total visits. Delivery was increased in district and provincial hospitals, while there was a noticeable reduction in traditional birth attendant role. The perinatal mortality rate had declined especially in the early neonatal period but the late fetal mortality rate had not changed significantly. Maternal mortality had also reduced appreciably. The growth of newborns showed marked improvement with decrease in low birthweight incidence, and approximately 60 percent of all newborns weighed 3,000 grams or over at birth.

The improvement in maternal and child health indicators in this project was clearly demonstrated as was the reduction in rates of adverse conditions which compared favorably with the trend of national data. This must be due to the outcome of the project on risk approach strategy in MCH care as the facility for special care for mother and newborns remains the same. Better utilization of existing health care is approaching to acceptable coverage and also more booking in the first half of pregnancy which indicated better quality of health care utilization. The role of health volunteers in this project is not as yet optimal; there are still some high-risk mothers who were not properly managed or referred. There is still a need for further education of the health team with emphasis on more practical points. It is a long-term approach in order to reach the goal and needs determination and commitment.

Table 2
Maternal and Child Health Indicators
Comparing Before and During the Project

Indicators	Before Project 1979 - 1980	During Project 1981 - 1983
Antenatal care		
- coverage	73.0	87.9
- first visit before 24 wks.	18.6	34.5
- no. ≥ 3 visits	25.0	55.8
Perinatal mortality rate	22.0	15.1
Late fetal mortality rate	8.0	7.6
Early neonatal mortality rate	12.0	7.6
Maternal mortality rate	2.0	0.5
Low birthweight	8.0	7.2
Birth weight ≥ 3 kg.	55.9	59.8

REFERENCES

1. World Health Organization. Risk approach for maternal and child health care. Geneva:WHO offset publication no. 39, 1978.

2. Sirivongs, B., and S. Parisunyakul. Risk pregnancy screening: A simple method for non-physicians to screen the high-risk pregnancy. J Med Assoc Thailand 67(Supp 2):15-21, 1984.

3. A workbook on how to plan and carry out research on the risk approach in maternal and child health including family planning. WHO document FHE/MCH/RA 84.1.

4. Khanjanasthiti, P., S. Watthanakasatr, and V. Benchakarn. Report on risk approach strategy in MCH service research, Thailand. May 1981 - Jan 1984. Ramathibodi Faculty of Medicine, Mahidol University.

5. Backett, E.M., A.M. Davies and A. Petros-Barvazian. The risk approach in health care. With special reference to maternal and child health, including family planning. Public Health Papers No. 76. Geneva: World Health Organization, 1984.

6. Risk approach for maternal and child care. World Health Forum 2(3):413-422, 1981.

7. Coopland, A.T., L.J. Peddle, and T.F. Baskett. A simplified antepartum high-risk pregnancy screening form: Statistical analysis of 5459 cases. Can Med Assoc J. 116:999-1001, 1977.

22

WOMEN AND NUTRITION IN DEVELOPING COUNTRIES: PRACTICAL CONSIDERATIONS

C. Gopalan, M.D., Ph.D., D.Sc., F.R.C.P.

In recent years there has been a remarkable upsurge of interest in the health and nutrition problems of women, thanks to the vigorous "women's movement," which has served to highlight current disabilities of our women. In order that this new awakening is channeled into truly constructive directions, it is important that the scientific foundations of our present concern with respect to women's health and nutrition are clearly articulated and understood. This presentation is based largely on observations made on poor communities in India. It appears likely that these observations may be applicable to a wide range of developing countries.

To be sure, during the last forty years, there have been some impressive gains with respect to women's health. For example, life expectancy at birth for the female in India, which stood at 31.7 in 1950, rose to 54.7 in 1980.[3,4] Female-infant mortality had declined to 97 (1986) and female-child mortality (0-4 years) to 38.6 (1986).[6] But while more women are thus "surviving" in many developing countries, there is unfortunately not much evidence of substantial improvement in the health and nutritional status of the survivors. Two illustrative observations from the Indian experience will serve to highlight this point.

1. The hallmark of poor maternal nutrition and poor antenatal care in a community is the high proportion of babies born with low birth weights – less than 2.5 kg (small gestational age). This proportion was reported to be nearly 38% in poor rural communities in South India in 1955.[13] Studies carried out nearly 30 years later indicate that the situation today is not much better. Indeed, a recent study in Calcutta[2] has actually revealed a shocking propor-

tion of 56% of low birth weights among deliveries in its urban slums. This figure of 56% is probably much higher than what generally pertains in India and in other developing countries; however, available evidence would suggest that it is still the case that nearly one-third of babies born in most poor countries are of low birth weights. Low birth weight of offspring is not only an evidence of poor maternal nutritional status but is also an indicator of possible poor future development of the baby.[7] Maternal nutritional status thus determines not only the state of the offspring at birth, but also, to some extent, the future course of its development. We have, therefore, reason to feel concerned over the persistent high proportion of deliveries of low birth-weight infants in most developing countries.

2. The Indian Council of Medical Research (ICMR) had carried out a countrywide study of growth and development of children in 1955.[9] Almost 20 years later, the National Nutrition Monitoring Bureau (NNMB) of the ICMR had also published its findings of heights and weights of children of different ages covering a large part of the country.[5] It will be seen from Figures 1 and 2 (next page) that the ICMR data of 1955 and the NNMB data of 20 years later, both of them for rural girls, are almost identical. There is no evidence of secular trend indicating improved growth performance in the succeeding generation – a feature expected of all successful developing societies.

It can be computed, on the basis of available growth data, that today nearly 24% of adult women in the reproductive period in India, and possibly in other developing countries as well, have body weights less than 38 kg and 16% have heights less than 145 cm.[5] These women, according to the generally accepted criteria proposed by WHO, fall into the high-risk category; i.e., they are likely to suffer obstetric complications and give birth to offspring of low birth weight, especially in situations where antenatal care and obstetric services are below par. These observations broadly indicate the magnitude of the unfinished tasks with respect to improvement of health and nutritional status of women in developing countries. The current picture regarding the prevalence of anemia, maternal mortality, sex ratio and the state of health care, serve to reinforce this broad conclusion.

THE WASTED YEARS OF ADOLESCENCE

Even with the existing levels of poverty, a significant impact of maternal nutritional status and birth weights of offspring can be achieved through just

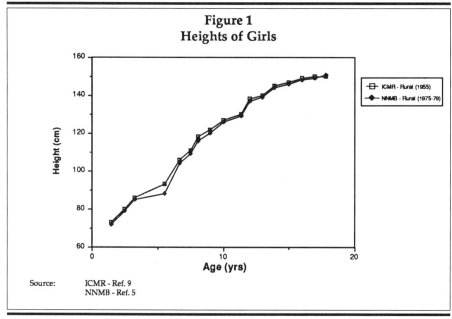

Figure 1
Heights of Girls

Source: ICMR - Ref. 9
         NNMB - Ref. 5

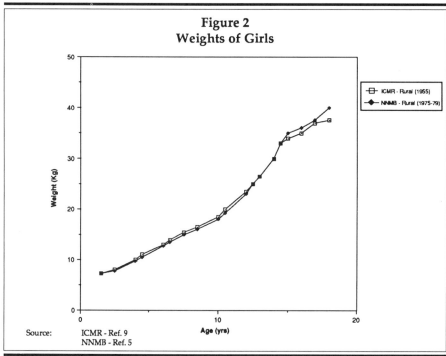

Figure 2
Weights of Girls

Source: ICMR - Ref. 9
         NNMB - Ref. 5

bringing about a rise in the age at marriage of our rural girls. It will be seen from Table 1 (based on NNMB data) that between their 14th and 18th years, girls in poor rural communities gain on an average 6.8 kg in their body weights and 5 cm in their heights. The period 14-18 years is a period of active growth for rural girls of developing countries. The mean age at menarche in the rural girls in India at present is about 14 years.[9] A very large percentage of these girls are pushed into marriage very early, the marriage being consummated almost immediately after menarche; a large proportion thus embark on their arduous reproductive journeys almost from their 14th year, and teenage pregnancies are the rule.

The proportion of girls of poor communities who can be estimated to be at obstetric risk (as per the WHO criteria) at 14, 15 and 18 years of age is indicated in Table 2 (next page). The data in the table will show the remarkable impact that raising the age at marriage could have on maternal, fetal and infant nutrition even in the current context of poverty in poor rural communities. Indeed, the data in Table 2 could probably underestimate the order of this impact. It must be remembered that in addition to the increased risk posed by their current immature body stature, there is also a crucial difference with respect to pregnancy between a 15-year-old girl and an 18-year-old girl. In the latter case, there are two competing nutrient demands on the mother during pregnancy – the demand for repair and maintenance of her own tissues and

Table 1
Heights and Weights of Poor* and Affluent** Girls at 14 Years and 18 Years

Age	Height (cms)		Weight (kg)	
(years)	Poor	Affluent	Poor	Affluent
14	145.9	156.6	35.1	47.5
18	150.9	158.9	41.9	52.5

* NNMB (Rural) [5]
** NFI study (SR. 10) [8]

the demand for fetal growth and development. In the case of the former, however, in addition to the above two demands, there is also the added competing nutrient demand of the mother for her own further growth which could be quite exacting and significant. It is not surprising for this reason that the incidence of low birth-weight deliveries is significantly greater in young primipara.

Between 14 and 18 years, according to the NNMB data, girls of poor rural communities in India gain over 5 cm in height and nearly 6.8 kg[5] in body weight as against only 2.3 cm in height and 3.5 kg in body weight by girls of the affluent sections of the population[8] (Table 1). This is because menarche and consequently the adolescent growth spurt is delayed by almost one year in the case of poor rural girls. Between 14 and 18 years, there is a significant degree of catch-up of the growth levels of poor rural girls with those of the affluent girls. Thus the growth process continues for a longer time in the poorer group than in the well-to-do. For this reason, it is even more important that conception be delayed until about the 18th year in the case of the poor rural girls than in the case of the affluent. Actually, however, it is the poor rural girls who are married off at a much younger age and have to start their reproductive career much earlier than the well-to-do.

In the developmental programs in most developing countries as they stand today, there are no special efforts specifically beamed to adolescent girls. These girls, having generally dropped out of school before their 8th or 9th year, are not reached by the school system; antenatal services start only after the onset of pregnancy. The intervening crucial years of adolescence between their dropping out from school and the onset of pregnancy, during

Table 2
Percentage of Rural Women* at Obstetric Risk at Different Ages

Ages	% below 38 kg	% below 145 cms
14	68	45
18	47	39
18	24	16

* NNMB, 1980 [5]

which period much can be done by way of equipping the girls for better and more productive citizenship, and safer and more competent motherhood, are truly wasted years – years of wasted opportunities. This is the basic deficiency in the present developmental system which needs to be addressed if significant improvement in the health and nutritional status of the women and children of the Third World is to be achieved within the next 20 years.

ANTENATAL CARE

Antenatal services in many underprivileged populations around the world have not made the desired impact for the reason that the system of antenatal care in developing countries is patterned on lines which may be appropriate and adequate for the affluent and not for the poor. At present a pregnant woman is contacted by the health services for antenatal care (if at all) only half-way through her pregnancy. Even this contact takes place in only a small proportion of cases because of the poor outreach of health services in most developing societies; and the contact may be no more than one or two visits to the health center throughout pregnancy. It must be remembered that the woman is already anemic (in a high proportion of cases) and stunted and of low body weight even at the start of her pregnancy. In the interval of barely 12 weeks between the time of contact by the health system and the delivery of her baby, even with an efficient antenatal service, it will be extremely difficult to correct, to any significant degree, the fairly large prepregnancy deficits that she is already suffering from and, in addition, provide for her added demands of pregnancy. Thus, a stunted woman, who starts on her pregnancy with a body weight of 38 kg or less and a hemoglobin level below 8 g% is unlikely to achieve a body weight increase of more than 5-6kg, and a hemoglobin level of 11 g%, by the end of her pregnancy with the type of inputs which our health system is now able to provide. Clearly, therefore, the answer lies in ensuring that the opportunities provided by the precious years of adolescence are not wasted by our health system. Programs of improving the health and nutritional status of girls during their adolescence and programmes such as regularly supplying iron and folate tablets right through adolescence are necessary so that the girls can enter into their pregnancy with no serious initial handicaps. In such a situation, even the type of antenatal care which alone is now possible in our health system, may still prove adequate.

SUPPORT TO NURSING MOTHERS

While adolescent girls are totally out of focus in the present health systems, a great deal of lip-service is being paid to nursing women with, however, no concrete action plans. While we extol the value of breast milk and laud women of poor communities for breast-feeding their babies for prolonged periods, no special attention is being bestowed toward improvement of the health and nutritional status of nursing mothers even during the first six months of their lactation. One of the great physiological marvels, which is still not fully explained, is the fact that poor women in developing countries, despite meals which generally provide no more than 2000 Kcal per day with about 45 gms of vegetable protein daily, are able to produce 450 ml to 600 ml of breast milk; and are able to do so for several months together. It is going to be expected that they are able to achieve this feat only at considerable cost to themselves through depletion of their own tissues. The marginal loss of body weights in the course of lactation does not fully reflect the extent of tissue depletion. A study on body composition among poor nursing women in India has shown that the mean figure for the percentage of total body water in a group of poor nursing women was 59.2 against 51 reported for normal European women;[14] indeed, in one-third of the subjects studied, body water accounted for over 60% of the body weight. It seems possible, therefore, that the true extent of depletion of lean body mass in nursing women is being masked by concurrent absolute increase in total body weight.

An important finding indicative of serious tissue depletion in these women is the evidence of markedly increased avidity for protein, as reflected by their capacity to retain high levels of nitrogen. A study carried out at the National Institute of Nutrition, Hyderabad,[17] showed that at an intake of 61 g of protein daily, lactating women of poor undernourished communities were in marginal nitrogen balance; when, however, the protein intake was raised to 99 g daily, there was substantial several-fold increase in nitrogen retention. A further increase of protein intake to 114 g daily was not accompanied by a further increase in nitrogen retention, showing thereby, that a level of at least 99 g of protein daily was needed in these undernourished women in order to achieve the maximal possible nitrogen retention. Apparently, undernourished nursing women, severely depleted of tissues, need increased levels of protein for correcting their tissue deficit. They are more able to successfully retain the needed additional levels of nitrogen if these are forthcoming in their diets. Unfortunately, supplementary feeding programs in most developing countries, wherever they exists, hardly cover nursing women to any significant extent.

The facile assumption that no matter how poorly fed the mother is, she will still be able to deliver the milk her baby needs, may be wholly erroneous. Indeed, it would appear that a significant proportion of poor women in India are currently not able to achieve a level of lactation performance which they could have achieved if their nutrition were adequate. This inadequacy in lactation is being reflected currently in the poor growth performance of their infants. Two studies carried out under the auspices of the Nutrition Foundation of India,[11] had indicated that a good proportion of poor women in urban slums and peri-urban areas of Calcutta and its rural environs were unable to breast-feed their infants for even up to two months despite their strong desire to do so. Excessive use of commercial baby foods (in a highly unhygienic manner) by the poor in the Calcutta area and the consequent diarrheal diseases and severe growth retardation observed in a large proportion of children even in early infancy in this region should be directly attributed to this fact.[12] The NNMB survey data[5] also show that hemoglobin levels, body weights and heights of poor women in Calcutta are poorer than those of the women of the Bombay region who are apparently able to breast-feed their infants fairly well for at least four months.

We depend highly on breast-feeding for up to 4-6 months, as being the sheet-anchor of infant nutrition. It follows that we must also ensure that women in our poor communities are in fact not only able to breast-feed their infants adequately for at least this period but also that they do so without detriment to their own health and nutritional status. This apparently is not the case at present in a considerable proportion of poor women in many parts of the world.

FAMILY PLANNING

According to the Indian Registrar General's Report (1984),[1] 43.1% of all births in India were accounted for by births in women less than 24 years of age, and 69.5% in women less than 29 years old. Family planning programs which are directed largely to women over 30 years of age, thus, in effect, address barely less than one-third of the problem – very much like bolting the door after the horse has escaped! It is not surprising that flattering official claims regarding "couple protection" rates do not tally with the actual observed impact on birth rates. Obviously many couples who do not stand in need of "protection" are now being "protected" and serve to inflate official records. Claims that several million births have been "averted," again based on the numbers of sterilizations or vasectomies suffer from obvious fallacies for the same reason.

These considerations underscore the imperative need for sex education to teenage girls and the extension of a family planning program – not terminal methods, but "a family-planning education program" designed to promote and propagate methods for spacing of births, including particularly contraceptive procedures not dependent on drugs or gadgets, such as "periodic abstinence method" (safe period). Such a family-planning education program beamed to adolescent girls cannot be carried out in isolation. It can be undertaken only as part of a comprehensive program of "education for better living" and vocational training, for our rural girls, of the type which the Nutrition Foundation of India has repeatedly advocated.[11]

ANEMIA

Among nutritional deficiency states currently afflicting women, anemia is the most widespread. Its clinical manifestations are not spectacular and for this reason the disease is often ignored. Recent studies have indicated that in states of iron deficiency apart from anemia there are impairments of physical stamina, of learning ability, of immunocompetence, and of behavior in general. Severe anemia also adds to obstetrical risks. Because of its high phytate content, bioavailability of iron present in habitual high-cereal diets (which are the staple of poor populations in developing countries) is expected to be poor. It will be necessary to provide the additional iron needed either through a programme of fortification of some commonly used food item (i.e., common salt) with iron, or through a regular and intensive program of distribution of iron-folate tablets to women and children of poor communities. Although the technique for fortification of common salt with iron has been developed successfully at the National Institute of Nutrition, it would seem unrealistic to expect that an effective program of fortification of common salt could be undertaken in many countries on a scale sufficient to make a substantial impact on the problem of anemia before the turn of the century. Therefore, we will have to rely heavily on distribution of iron-folate tablets. Unfortunately, this program, though it exists on paper, is being implemented very tardily on most poor countries. Anemia is at least one nutrient deficiency disease which can be controlled even under current conditions of poverty. Every effort must be made to intensify the distribution of iron tablets and to increase the availability of these tablets for the poor. This must go hand-in-hand with a program of nutrition education. Apart from health centers, rural schools, post offices and a number of public institutions could be used as outlets for distribution of iron-folate tablets.

ENDEMIC GOITRE

Millions of people in South East Asia live in the goitre-endemic regions and many are actually suffering from goitre.[10] Recent studies[15,16] have revealed new disturbing dimensions of the problems. The incidence of neonatal hypothyroidism, as reflected in cord-blood thyroxin and thyrotrophin levels, is highly disturbing. In populations with high incidence of neonatal hypothyroidism, an increased prevalence of nerve deafness and a shift of IQ of children towards lower scores were demonstrated. Thus iodine deficiency is of great public health significance and of far-reaching implications. Adolescent girls and pregnant women and their offspring need to be protected. The answer lies in the vigorous implementation of the salt iodation program. Kochupillai[15] has warned against resorting to iodine injections in pregnancy. There are no doubts whatsoever about the efficacy and safety of the well-tried salt iodation procedure and this is what developing countries should pursue without allowing ourselves to be defected by powerful vested interest.

HEALTH CARE OF THE PEOPLE BY THE PEOPLE

The major reason for the poor quality and outreach of rural health care and especially for the relatively poor utilization of health services by women, is that health services in many developing countries are now being perceived by the rural communities largely as a bureaucratic governmental operation which must be availed of only when absolutely necessary and that, too, rather guardedly. The psychological distance that now seems to divide the provider and the beneficiary can be bridged only through bringing about a radical qualitative change in the basic orientation of health systems in developing countries, whereby health/nutrition/welfare operations at the village level become largely people's movements operated by the people for their own betterment with the government providing such logistic, technical and financial support as may be necessary. In such a qualitative shift in the health strategy, it is the women of the rural communities who must be enabled to play the central role. There are some heartening examples of this approach in some developing countries – such as Indonesia and Thailand.

Voluntary health brigades composed of young girls (and boys) in the village – somewhat like the Scout movement – could be encouraged. The recruits could be provided a general broad-based training; and from among these candidates, all recruitment to village level operations could be made with such further special training as may be necessary for the jobs to which they are being recruited.

The Nutrition Foundation of India had advocated a program of "Education for better living and vocational training of rural adolescent girls."[11] A program of this nature can help to generate the health brigade referred to above. It can also help to train candidates for specific jobs which are available in the villages.

The problems which beset women in developing countries are formidable, but these problems are now getting increasing attention. Specific programs and proposals for combating the current disabilities of men, especially with respect to their health and nutrition, are being discussed more intensively today than ever before. It is to be hoped that the enthusiasm that is now being generated will lead to tangible results within the next two or three decades.

REFERENCES

1. Office of the Registrar General. Birth order differentials in India 1984. New Delhi: Ministry of Home Affairs, 1989.

2. Birth weight: A major determinant of child survival. Report of the project completed by the Indian Council of Medical Research. Future 17, Winter, UNICEF, 1985-1986.

3. Office of the Registrar General. Census of India 1981. Occasional paper no. 4 of 1988. Report of the Expert Committee on the Population Projections. New Delhi, 1988.

4. Office of the Registrar General. Census of India 1981 (ser. 1 India; paper 2 of 1983). Part II: Key population statistics, based on 5% sample data. New Delhi: Ministry of Home affairs, 1983.

5. National Nutrition Monitoring Bureau. Report for the year 1974-79. Hyderabad: National Institute of Nutrition, 1980.

6. Office of the Registrar General. Sample Registration System 1986, Vital Statistics Div. New Delhi: Ministry of Home Affairs, 1988.

7. Scientific Report 9: Maternal nutrition, lactation and growth of infants in urban slums. New Delhi: Nutrition Foundation of India, 1988.

8. Scientific Report 10: Growth of affluent Indian girls during adolescence. New Delhi: Nutrition Foundation of India, 1989.

9. Technical Report Series No. 18: Growth and physical development of Indian infants and children. New Delhi: Indian Council of Medical Research, 1984.

10. Gopalan, C. The National Goitre Control Program – A sad story. NFI Bulletin. July, 1981.

11. Gopalan, C. Home science and vocational training for rural girls - A proposal. NFI Bulletin, 5 (1), 1984.

12. Gopalan, C. et al. Infant feeding practices: With special reference to use of commercial infant foods. Scientific Report 4. New Delhi: Nutrition Foundation of India, 1984–5.

13. Gopalan, C., C. Varkki, P.S. Venkatachalam, and S.G. Srikantia. Study of birth weights of infants in relation to the incidence of nutritional oedema syndrome (kwashiorkor). Indian J Med Research 43:291, 1955.

14. Gopalan, C., and P.S. Venkatachalam. Basal metabolism and total body water in nursing women. Indian J Med Research 48:507, 1960.

15. Kochupillai, N., and M.M. Godbole. Iodized oil injections in goitre prophylaxis – Possible impact on the newborn. NFI Bulletin 7 (4), 1986.

16. Kochupillai, N., et al. Iodine deficiency and neonatal hypothyroidism. Bulletin of World Health Organization, 64 (4), 547-551, 1986.

17. Ra, B.S.N., S. Pasricha, and C. Gopalan.. Nitrogen balance studies in poor Indian women during lactation. Indian J Med Research 46:325, 1958.

Section III
Infant and Child Health

23

PERINATAL MORTALITY

BHASKER RAO, M.D.

Pregnancy and childbirth, though mostly physiological, carry certain risks to both the mother and child. These may vary in different countries. With marked reduction in the maternal mortality rates in some of the developed countries during the last four decades, the focus has shifted to perinatal outcome. The deaths in the neonatal period form about 50 percent of all deaths in infancy.

If the maternal mortality rate is an index of socio-economic status of a country, the perinatal mortality indicates the standard of perinatal care available there. In countries where the perinatal mortality is very low, steps are now being taken to reduce perinatal morbidity and prevent neurological, mental and physical handicaps in children.

Definition: Perinatal mortality is defined as the number of late fetal deaths (also called stillbirths) and early neonatal deaths (or deaths in the first week of life) per 1000 total births. Until 1977, the lower limit of the definition was 28 weeks of gestation. But as babies less than 28 weeks do survive, due to advances in neonatology, WHO[1] recommends that all fetuses and newborns with a birth weight of 500 gm (gestational age of 22 weeks or crown-heel length of 25 cm, when birth weight is not known), whether alive or dead, should be included in the national perinatal statistics. For international purposes, however, the WHO recommendation is that all newborn infants with 1000 gm (or when weight is unknown, gestational age of 28 weeks and crown-heel length of 35 cm) be used for both the numerator and denominator of these rates. Thus birth weight, rather than gestational age, is used to obtain accurate data.

Global Picture: In most developed countries, the perinatal mortality rates (PMR) have been reduced to one-third to one-fourth of those prevalent three decades ago.[2,3,4] (Table 1) However, in the developing world where 80 percent of global births occur, too many lives are lost around birth. The PMR is about 70 per 1000 births in these countries and is comparable to those prevalent in the developed countries four decades ago. In India alone, out of about 23 million births, over 1.2 million perinatal deaths take place annually.

Perinatal Mortality Rates: In most developed countries, the PMR is about 10 per 1000 births but in Third World countries it varies from 25 to 60 per 1000 births (Table 1). Its accuracy depends on the extent of under-registration of vital events like births and infant deaths. When national statistics are not available, the information obtained from careful epidemiological surveys[5,6,7] is more dependable than the hospital figures [8,9] which are high due to a large number of referrals of high-risk cases and unbooked obstetric emergencies (Table 2, next page). Even in these countries, the perinatal death rates are higher in urban slums and in rural areas. In a recent field study conducted by the Indian Council of Medical Research[10] the PMR was 52 per 1000 in urban slums and 61.8 for rural areas; it was as high as 85.6 per 1000 births in rural Varanasi.

Table 1
Perinatal Mortality Rates For Selected Countries
(per 1000 births)

Country	Perinatal Mortality Rates 1956	1982
Sweden	28.8	6.6
Netherlands	28.7	10.0
England & Wales	37.6	10.4
France	33.8	13.0
Hungary	38.1	20.2
Japan	–	13.0
Singapore	–	13.0
Chile	–	16.4
Kuwait	–	23.2
Mauritius	–	34.5
India	–	53.2

Causes: Stembera[11] believes that the cause-effect relationship in perinatal outcome has passed through four phases. In the early period of classical obstetrics, mechanical causes as cephalo-pelvic disproportion, malpresentations and anoxia due to antepartum hemorrhages were considered important. Later on, the maternal diseases like anemia, diabetes, infections and toxemia were blamed. In the third phase, it was the functional derangement of the materno-placental-fetal unit like placental insufficiency. The more recent studies, however, point to socio-economic and cultural factors as leading causes of perinatal deaths.

To determine the causes of perinatal deaths, several studies have been conducted in the past few decades (Table 3, next page), but these were limited to certain institutions, areas or short periods of time. Important among these are the British Perinatal Mortality Survey[12] and the multicentric Perinatal Mortality Survey sponsored by the Federation of Obstetric and Gynecological Societies of India (FOGSI).[9] For obtaining national data and for international comparisons a standard protocol or classification is necessary. For this purpose, classification of perinatal deaths according to the WHO[1] is recommended by the FIGO Standing Committee on Perinatal Mortality and Morbidity. The WHO recommends a separate certificate of the cause of perinatal death based on the minimum of information on the mother, baby, birth attendant and autopsy, if any. It includes the most important factor, maternal as well as

Table 2
Perinatal Mortality Rates For Selected Developing Countries
(from epidemiological surveys)

Author(s) and Year	Country	PMR per 1000 births
Barrows et al (1987)	Brazil	33.7
Perera and Lwin (1984)	Burma	51.2
	India	48.6
	Indonesia	45.0
	Thailand	28.3
Voorhoeve et all (1979)	Kenya	46.7

fetal/neonatal, responsible for the perinatal loss in addition to listing secondary contributory factors (Table 4). Three other classifications based on obstetric factors,[13] fetal and neonatal causes,[14] and according to different groups of birth weight are also known.

Table 3
Perinatal Mortality Rates in Developing Countries
(data from selected hospitals)

Author(s) and Year	Country	PMR per 1000 births
Harrison (1985)	Nigeria	103.0
Mehta	India	66.3
Perera & Lwin (1984)	Burma	47.6
	Indonesia	120.0
	Thailand	13.2

Table 4
Classification of Perinatal Deaths
(ICD 9th Revision, WHO, 1977)
(Figures in brackets are 3-digit codes)

Maternal Causes	Fetal & Neonatal Causes
Maternal Conditions	Congenital anomalies (740-759)
Unrelated to present pregnancy (760)	IUGR (764) Prematurity (765)
Maternal complication of pregnancy (761)	Postterm (760)
Complications of placenta, cord and membranes (762)	Birth trauma (767)
	Asphyxia (768)
	RDS (769)
(APH, placental dysfunction, cord prolapse etc.)	Perinatal infections (771)
	Fetal & neonatal hemorrhage (772)
Other complications (Malpresentations, operative delivery, rupture uterus, etc.)	Isoimmunisation (773)
	Others (774-779)

In the FOGSI study[7] of 10,285 deaths, the leading causes were prolonged and difficult labor (24%), maternal diseases (21.2%), antepartum hemorrhages (13.5%) and congenital malformations (6.7%); in one-third of these, no obvious cause was noted. When analyzed according to fetal/neonatal factors, asphyxia/birth trauma was the most important (seen in 42.8%), followed by prematurity (17.9%), congenital anomalies (6.7%), infections and respiratory distress syndrome in 2.2% each. In a 10-year British Study,[15] anoxia and birth trauma were responsible for 43% of perinatal deaths, followed by congenital malformations in 22.3%, prematurity (14.9%) and others. In 15 percent no cause could be found. In most published series[5,6,16] trauma/anoxia, congenital malformations and prematurity were the important etiological factors. It is particularly so in the hospital experience of developing countries where obstructed labor, prematurity and antepartum hemorrhages were predominant.[8,9]

FACTORS INFLUENCING PERINATAL MORTALITY

A. Birth Weight: It is the most important single factor influencing perinatal mortality rates. The more the low birth weight (LBW) rate in a country, the higher its PMR.[17] India has the highest LBW rates in the world,[18] contributing to a high perinatal loss. Only few babies less than 1000 gm survive in well-equipped specialized neonatal units. Between 1000-1500 gm, the PMR is about 400 per 1000. In Cuba, babies less than 2.5 kg formed 10% of all births but 57 percent of all perinatal deaths.[3] In the south-east Asian studies, the PMR was 7-10 times higher in babies weighing less than 2.5 kg compared to those with 2.5 kg and over.[6] It is lowest between 2.5 to 3.5 kg; but after 4.5 kg the PMR rises. In prematurity, it is the physiological immaturity, particularly of the lungs; and in intrauterine growth retardation (IUGR) it is the poor storage in the liver that contributes to the perinatal death.

B. Time of Death: In the Indian Study,[9] 25.5% of perinatal deaths were macerated, 39.5% fresh stillbirths and 35% neonatal deaths. In a comparative 10-year study of 8 developed countries, Foster[2] found that though the PMR was declining, the decrease in neonatal mortality rate was more rapid than of late fetal deaths due to the improved neonatal services. As a result, the ratio of early neonatal deaths to late fetal deaths tended to approach 1.0. In Scotland in 1984, the antepartum, intrapartum and early neonatal period (7 days) were 4.37, 1.03 and 4.36 per 1000, respectively.[19] However, in the developing countries, the fetal loss is higher in the intrapartum period due to delayed labor and its sequelae (trauma, anoxia and infections). The neonatal deaths were due mainly to prematurity, congenital malformations, hypothermia, infections and rarely pulmonary hyaline membrane.

C. Age and Parity: The PMR is higher at extremes of age and parity. Though it is high with maternal age of 35 years and parity of 7 or more, the comparison of relative risks shows that the age of 35 years and over is more significant than high parity.[3]

D. Multiple Pregnancies and Malpresentations: In malpresentations like breech, the risks are 3-5 times more due to complications during delivery resulting in anoxia and trauma. It is worst in shoulder presentations.

E. Maternal Health Status: The complications like hypertensive disorders of pregnancy or diseases associated with pregnancy like anemia, malaria, syphilis, heart disease and diabetes are responsible for higher perinatal mortality rates. Anemia is widely prevalent in developing countries, often resulting in premature labor. In one study,[20] the perinatal loss was found to be three times higher when the hemoglobin levels were between 5-8 g/dl and nine times more so when it was below 5 g/dl compared to the healthy pregnant women.

F. Social Factors: The social environment in which the mother grows up influences the PMR. In unexplained perinatal deaths, the mothers are smaller, underweight, cigarette smokers and from large families in lower socio-economic groups like their own mothers.[21] Babies belonging to the poorest families were three times more likely to die in the perinatal period than those with highest income.[5]

G. Prenatal Care: The more the number of antenatal visits starting early in pregnancy and the better the quality of such care, the less is the PMR. In Korea,[22] the PMR was eleven times higher in emergency admissions than in those with good prenatal care. The PMR was 16.2 per 1000 in those attending the antenatal clinic in Brazil compared to 56.2 per 1000 for the non-attenders.[5] In Indonesian hospitals the unbooked and late referrals had three times higher PMR than those with prenatal care.[6] With vigilant and skilled intranatal attention and good neonatal services, the PMR could be reduced.

PREVENTION OF PERINATAL MORTALITY

This can be brought about mainly by removing the factors contributing to the perinatal mortality.

A. Female literacy is closely related to crude birth rates and reproductive mortality rates in developing countries.[23] (Table 5) The better the education of girls, the later the age of marriage, the fewer and well-spaced are the births with increased chances of child survival. In India, Kerala state with the highest female literacy has the lowest birth rate and infant mortality though it is economically worse off than most other states in the country.

B. Health Education: The need for prenatal care and early booking for delivery has to be encouraged, as the course of pregnancy and delivery is not always smooth. Avoidance of drugs and infections in early pregnancy to prevent fetal malformations, routine testing of blood for Rh and VDRL and campaigning against smoking in pregnancy are beneficial.

C. Immunization of pregnant women: About 1 million deaths due to neonatal tetanus take place annually in developing countries.[24] The incidence of neonatal tetanus varies from 5-60 per 1000 in India, Indonesia, Pakistan and Bangladesh. These deaths could be

Table 5
Female Literacy and Reproductive Mortality Rates
In Selected Developing Countries (1985)

Country	Female Literacy (%)	CBR	PMR	IMR	MMR
Nepal	5	41.6	—	144	850
Bangladesh	16	45.2	—	132	3000
India	29	33.3	48.6	114	460
Burma	40	37.1	51.2	94.3	170
Indonesia	61	30.8	45.0	86.7	300
Sri Lanka	82	27.7	—	40.6	80
Thailand	83	29.6	28.3	50.6	80

CBR – Crude birth rate (per 1000)

IMR – Infant mortality rate (per 1000 live births)

MMR – Maternal mortality rate (per 100,000 births)

prevented by routine immunization of all pregnant women and care of the cord during delivery. If customs and tradition contribute to increased risk of tetanus, health education about cord care is imperative.

D. Nutritional supplements in pregnancy: Protein/energy supplements for a few weeks do not materially alter the fetal outcome though it is claimed that it increases the birth weight, especially when the weight gain during pregnancy is not satisfactory.[25] The nutrition during adolescence and prior to pregnancy is more important.

E. Prevention of Low Birth-Weight Babies: Important causes of LBW in developing countries are anemia and toxemia. These can be detected and treated early. Routine oral iron and folates prevent nutritional anemias in the tropics.[26] Those with hemoglobin of 8 g/dl and below need hospitalization for investigation and appropriate therapy. Similarly, toxemias have to be carefully monitored and pregnancy terminated in selected cases to save the fetus. Judicious induction of labor in pregnancy associated with diabetes, Rh, IUGR, postmaturity, etc., contributes to reduction of PMR.[27] Where very low birth weight is anticipated, it is better to transport the baby in utero to an institution where specialized care is available.

F. Better Intranatal Care: In most developing countries, the majority of births take place in rural areas where few trained birth attendants are available. Currently, only about 25% of the parturients receive any skilled attention at delivery in rural India.[28] There is a need for training thousands of additional health workers to provide coverage during pregnancy and labor. Obstetric ultrasound is a useful diagnostic tool during pregnancy. But cardiotocograpy helps only in reduction of perinatal morbidity and not perinatal mortality.[29,30] It is necessary for high-risk pregnant women. Clean hands, sterilized instruments and cord ligatures, avoidance of delayed or difficult vaginal deliveries contribute to lowered perinatal death rates.

G. Family Planning: Reproductive efficiency is optimum in the third decade of life. Pregnancy is better avoided in early adolescence and after 35 years. Similarly, too many or too close births increase maternal and infant deaths. If the birth interval is less than 18 months, the risk of PMR was 97.8 compared to overall rate of 40.9 per 1000 in Thailand.[6] An interval of at least 36 months is desirable.

PERINATAL CARE IN THE COMMUNITY

There is a need for supervision of all mothers during pregnancy, labor and following delivery.

A. Risk approach to MCH care has to be adopted in all developing countries where the health manpower and resources are limited. The mothers with high risk factors (universal or social factors like illiteracy, elderly primiparae, grand multiparae, or those due to previous bad obstetric history or associated complications) have to be screened or identified by the health workers in the field and referred to appropriate institutions early.[31] Provision of transport and feedback facilities yield better results. Community education and involvement is essential if one has to prevent these cases being brought in late as emergencies to the referral centers.

B. Organized Intranatal and Neonatal Services: The city/state of Singapore has reduced PMR sharply by having over 80% of deliveries in institutions and strengthening the domiciliary care following early discharge from the hospital.[32] But this is not possible in most developing countries where most low-risk cases could be delivered in their homes or health centers by the midwives and those needing further assistance sent to the nearest hospitals. Regionalization of perinatal care at primary, intermediate and tertiary care centers with appropriate grades of specialization and technology is useful. Well-trained and equipped neonatal centers are required at all tertiary care levels.

C. Continuing Education: Refresher training of TBAs, nurses and general practitioner has to be organized periodically to improve the quality of perinatal care. They should be exposed to the newer trends in the diagnosis and management of prenatal and neonatal complications, clinical monitoring during labor, importance of breastfeeding and postpartum contraception.

D. Liberalization of maternity benefits and social support during pregnancy, exemption from strenuous work in the second half of pregnancy,[33] nutritional supplementation, free or subsidized perinatal care nearer their homes contribute to lowered perinatal mortality.

E. Genetic counseling should be available to those with family/ previous history of fetal malformations.

F. Perinatal audit: Field studies and institutional perinatal audit meetings could help in determining the leading causes of perinatal deaths and help physicians, paramedics, health administrators and the public in reducing the PMR.

It is possible to reduce the present high levels of PMR in developing countries by analyzing their causes and remedying them. In addition to better health education, the commitment by the community and the health personnel is necessary to provide health care to all pregnant and parturient women and the newborn. With improvement in socio-economic conditions and reduction in the LBW rates, the perinatal mortality could be reduced to an "irreducible" minimum – perhaps to less than 5 per 1000 (as gross congenital malformations incompatible with survival and very low birth weights may not be completely eliminated). In the meanwhile, health administrators in all developing countries should aim to bring down the PMR to at least 15 per 1000 births by the year 2000.

REFERENCES

1. World Health Organization. Manual of International Statistical Classification of Diseases, Injuries and Causes of Death, 9th rev. Geneva: WHO, 1977.

2. Foster, F.H. Trends in perinatal mortality. World Health Statistical Quarterly 34:138-1446, 1981.

3. Edouard,L. Epidemiology of perinatal mortality. World Health Statistical Quarterly 38:289-301, 1985.

4. Health Information of India 1986. New Delhi: Ministry of Health, 1986, p. 47.

5. Barros, F.C., C.G. Victoria, and J.P. Vaughan, et al. Perinatal mortality in S. Brazil. Bulletin WHO 65:95-104, 1987.

6. Perera, T., and K.M. Lwin. Perinatal mortality including low-birth weight. A South East Asia Regional profile. SEARO Regional Health Papers no. 3. Geneva: WHO.

7. Voorhoeve, A.M. et al. Agents affecting health of mother and child in a rural area of Kenya. Trop Geo Med 31:607-627, 1979.

8. Harrison, R., U.G. Lister, and C.E. Rossiter, et al. Perinatal mortality in Zaria. Brit J. Obstet Gynecol 92: Suppl 5, 86-99, 1985.

9. Mehta, A.C. Perinatal mortality in India. J. Obstet Gynec India 33:721, 1983.

10. Indian Council of Medical Research. National Collaborative Study on High Risk Families. New Delhi: ICMR. Provisional report. Unpublished data, 1988.

11. Stembera, Z. Environmental and social factors influencing perinatal outcome. IPA/WHO Precongress Workshop on Perinatology. Honolulu, July 1986.

12. Butler, N.R., and D.G. Bonham. Perinatal Mortality. Edinburgh: E&S Livingstone, 1963, p. 833.

13. Cole, S.K., E.N. Hey, and A.N. Thomson. Classification of perinatal deaths – An obstetric approach. Brit J Obstet Gynecol 93:1204, 1985.

14. Hey, E.N., D.J. Lloyd, and J.S. Wigglesworth. Classification of perinatal deaths, fetal and neonatal factors. Brit J. Obstet Gynecol 93:1213, 1986.

15. Edouard, L., and E. Alberman. National trends in certified causes of perinatal mortality 1968-1978. Brit J Obstet Gynecol 87:833, 1980.

16. Tamby, Raja R.L. Trends in Perinatal Mortality in Developing World, Recent Advances in Obstetrics and Gynecology. J. Bonnar (ed). London: Churchill-Livingstone, 1982, pp. 201-212.

17. Alberman, E. Prospects for better perinatal health. Lancet 1:189, 1980.

18. Kramer, M.S. Determinants of low birth weight, methodological assessment and analysis. Bulletin WHO 65:663-737, 1987.

19. MacFarlane, A., S. Cole, and E. Hey. Comparison of data from regional perinatal mortality surveys. Brit J Obstet Gynecol 93:1224-1232, 1986.

20. Annual Report for 1979. National Institute of Nutrition, Hyderabad. 1980, p. 70.

21. Baird, D. Changing problems and priorities in obstetrics. Brit J Obstet Gynecol 92:115, 1985.

22. Martin, B.H., and Y.S. Kim. Progress through antenatal care in Korea. Proc of 6th Asian Congress Obst & Gynecology. Kuala Lumpur, 1974, p. 139.

23. World Health Organization. Regional Health Papers no. 3. SEARO. New Delhi: WHO, 1985.

24. Cook, R. Neonatal Tetanus – A Global Review. The Control of Neonatal Tetanus in India. Bhargava, I., and J. Sokhey (eds). New Delhi: Ministry of Health, 1983, pp. 16-25.

25. Raman, L. Nutrition in pregnancy and lactation. Postgraduate Ob and Gyn. Rao, K.B. (ed). 4th ed. Madras: Orient Longman, 1989, p. 40.

26. World Health Organization. Nutritional Anaemias. Technical Report Series no. 503. Geneva: WHO, 1972.

27. McNay, M.B., G.M. McIlwaine, and P.N. Hawie, et al. Perinatal deaths – analysis of clinical causes to assess value of induction of labor. Brit Med J 1:347,1977.

28. Rao, K.B. Vital statistics for the obstetrician. Postgraduate Ob and Gyn, p. 210.

29. Kubli, F. Perinatal Mortality. Proc. of 27th All India Obst & Gynecologic Congress. Part II. Madras, 1983, p. 57.

30. MacDonald, D., A. Grant, and P.M. Sheridan, et al. The Dublin randomised controlled trial of intrapartum fetal heart monitoring. Amer J Obstet Gyn 152:524-39, 1985.

31. Gupta, A.N. High risk pregnancy. Postgraduate Ob and Gyn, p. 150.

32. Lean, T.H. Influence of obstetric service on perinatal health – The Singapore experience. Proc of 6th Asian Congress of Ob and Gyn. Kuala Lumpur, 1974, p. 162.

33. Manshande, J.P., R. Eickels, and D.V. Manshande, et al. Rest versus work during last weeks of pregnancy; influence on fetal growth. Brit J Obstet & Gynecol 97:1059-67, 1987.

24

CHILD MORTALITY IN DEVELOPING COUNTRIES

BIRGITTA BUCHT, FIL. KAND (MA)*

WORLDWIDE PICTURE

Considerable progress has been made in reducing infant and child mortality in recent decades. For the world as a whole, it is estimated that mortality under age five has declined by more than half in the last 30 years.[1] Mortality has declined in most countries, but the pace of change and the magnitude of improvement have varied considerably between countries. Among developed countries there has been a general convergence of the levels of infant and child mortality so that the differences between the countries with the highest and the lowest mortality are now smaller than in the early 1950s. In the developing regions, the situation has become increasingly diverse. Some countries have experienced very rapid mortality declines and have reached mortality levels as low, or nearly as low, as those in developed countries. In others, the progress has been slow and mortality remains high. The disparity between more and less developed regions also remains large and the relative difference between the two groups of countries has widened.

It is estimated that about 14 million children under the age of 5 will die each year during 1985-1990. Most of these deaths, 99 percent, occur in developing countries. Africa and South Asia together account for 12 million deaths, or 85 percent of the world total. The annual number of deaths has declined significantly since the early 1950s when it was estimated at nearly 24 million. The most dramatic change has occurred in East Asia, where the yearly number of deaths under age 5 declined from an estimated 7 million in 1950-1955 to 1 million in 1980-1990. This decline is the result of very rapid declines in both

---

*The views and opinions expressed in this paper are those of the author and do not necessarily reflect those of the United Nations.

279

fertility and mortality. The number of deaths has declined in most regions, except in Africa where, despite declining infant and child mortality, the annual number of deaths of young children has been increasing and is expected to continue to increase. The reason for the increase is that the young age structure and high fertility cause the number of births to increase at such a rate as to offset the decline in mortality.

In developed countries, deaths under age 5 now constitute only a very small proportion of all deaths, while in many developing countries deaths of young children constitute a large share of total deaths. On average, nearly 40 percent of all deaths in developing countries are deaths of children under age 5 and nearly 30 percent of all deaths in the world are deaths of young children in developing countries. Figure 1 (next page) illustrates the contrasting distributions of deaths by age in a developing country, Egypt, and a developed one, Sweden. In Egypt, despite a high under-registration of deaths in infancy and early childhood than of deaths at older ages, deaths of children under age 5 made up 45 percent of all registered deaths in 1979.[2] In contrast, in Sweden, less than one percent of all deaths are deaths of young children.

LEVELS AND TRENDS OF CHILD MORTALITY IN DEVELOPING REGIONS

United Nations estimates and projections of probabilities of dying by age 5, by region, 1950-2000, are presented in Table 1 (pages 282-283). Measures of under-five mortality are presented instead of the conventionally used infant mortality since in developing countries these measures tend to be more reliable than those of infant mortality. The majority of developing countries lack satisfactory vital registration data and consequently, the estimates are based mainly on retrospective data gathered by censuses and surveys. Given the inaccuracies in the data available and the known limitations of existing estimation techniques, estimates of the probability of dying by age 5 are more reliable than those of infant mortality. It is only in countries where vital registration is complete – the developed countries and a few low-mortality developing countries – that reliable estimates of infant mortality can be derived directly from registration data.

Estimates based on census and survey data are generally less current than those derived from vital registration. Censuses and surveys are usually taken at infrequent intervals, and since the estimates they yield are based on retrospective data, they refer to a period of a few years prior to the census or survey date. Therefore, in Table 1, the values for the 1980s have been obtained mostly by projection.

Figure 1
Distribution of Registered Deaths by Age in Egypt, 1979 and Sweden, 1983

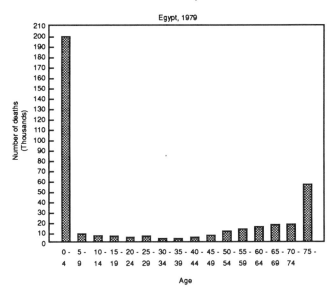

Egypt, 1979

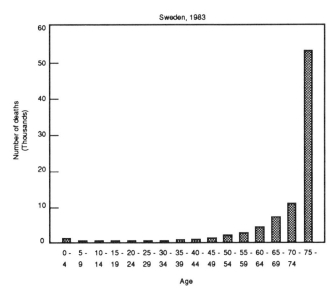

Sweden, 1983

Source: Based on United Nations: *Demographic Yearbook*, 1984

Table 1
Estimates and Projections of Child Mortality, by Region, 1950-2000

Probability of dying between birth and age 5, $_5a_0$ (per 1,000 births)

Region	1950-1955	1955-1960	1960-1965	1965-1970	1970-1975	1975-1980	1980-1985	1985-1990	1990-1995	1995-2000
World	240	215	182	161	144	131	118	105	94	83
More developed regions (1)	73	51	39	32	26	24	19	17	14	13
Less developed regions (2)	281	255	213	184	164	149	134	119	106	94
Africa	322	300	280	261	233	203	182	163	147	132
Eastern Africa	286	266	249	234	222	214	204	188	170	153
Middle Africa	307	289	271	251	229	212	195	178	161	144
Northern Africa	326	295	271	250	219	183	152	129	107	89
Southern Africa	220	202	188	173	158	136	119	103	87	73
Western Africa	347	329	310	289	258	225	206	188	170	154
Latin America	189	166	146	131	115	99	88	78	69	61
Caribbean	186	164	138	123	109	100	91	82	76	71
Central America	205	169	143	126	110	96	84	73	64	56
Temperate S. America	107	101	93	81	64	49	34	34	31	28
Tropical S. America	196	176	157	142	126	109	97	87	77	68

Table 1 (continued)

East Asia (3)	261	235	158	111	81	57	53	43	35	30
China	266	242	162	113	83	58	55	44	36	30
Other East Asia	163	137	97	75	60	47	38	31	26	21
South Asia	305	273	243	219	199	180	157	139	122	106
Southeastern Asia	244	216	193	170	148	129	111	96	81	67
Southern Asia	327	294	263	238	220	203	177	160	142	125
Western Asia	307	271	235	198	170	142	115	95	78	65
Oceania (4)	238	213	187	155	119	96	81	66	54	35
Melanesia	255	233	205	171	131	105	88	72	58	47
Micronesia-Polynesia	156	123	97	76	62	49	39	33	28	24

Source United Nations: Mortality of Children under Age 5: World Estimates and Projections, 1950-2025.
(1) More developed regions include Northern America, Japan, all regions of Europe, Australia-New Zealand and Union of Soviet Socialist Republic.
(2) Less developed regions include all regions of Africa, all regions of Latin America, China, other East Asia, all regions of South Asia, Melanesia and Micronesia-Polynesia.
(3) Excluding Japan.
(4) Excluding Australia-New Zealand.

The highest mortality levels and the slowest rates of improvement are estimated for Africa, followed by South Asia. Mortality is high throughout most of Africa, with the only exception of two small islands in the Indian Ocean, Mauritius and Reunion, where registered infant mortality rates were 25 and 11 per thousand, respectively, in 1986. With the exception of these two tropical islands, the probability of dying by age 5 was estimated to be above 100 deaths per thousand births in all countries in 1980-1985, ranging from just above 100 per thousand in Cape Verde to over 300 per thousand in Gambia, Mali and Sierra Leone. The countries of Northern and Southern Africa have somewhat lower mortality than those of the other African regions. In the early 1950s, Western Africa had the highest child mortality of any region in the world, but the decline in Western Africa has been faster than in Eastern Africa, so that the two regions now have similar mortality levels. Sierra Leone, a country in Western Africa, exhibits the highest mortality ever measured in a contemporary country: Over 390 deaths of children under age 5 per thousand births according to the 1974 census.

The situation in South Asia is considerably more varied than in Africa. The highest mortality levels and the slowest rates of decline are estimated for Southern Asia, although one country in that region, Sri Lanka, has attained relatively low mortality (an estimated probability of dying by age 5 of 52 per thousand in 1980-1985). In Western Asia, several countries have experienced very rapid declines in their probabilities of dying by age 5 – in particular, the smaller oil-producing countries of the region. In Bahrain, for instance, the probability of dying by age 5 is estimated to have declined from 303 per thousand in 1950-1955 to 38 per thousand in 1980-1985, a decline of 87 percent. Rapid declines have also been observed in some of the non-oil-producing countries, such as Jordan and the Syrian Arab Republic. The estimates for Southeastern Asia are more uncertain than those for other regions. The region includes Singapore, the country with the lowest mortality among all developing countries (a registered infant mortality rate of 8 per thousand in 1986-1987), but it also includes countries such as Democratic Kampuchea, Lao People's Democratic Republic and Viet Nam for which no data on mortality are available.

Remarkable progress in reducing mortality has been made in the countries of East Asia, most notably in China where the probability of dying by age 5 is estimated to have declined from 266 to 55 per thousand between 1950-1955 and 1980-1985.

In Latin America, mortality levels and trends vary substantially between countries. In Haiti and Bolivia mortality is as high as in parts of Africa. Low mortality is found in most of the Caribbean (excluding the Dominican Republic and Haiti), temperate South America and in two countries in Central America, namely, Costa Rica and Panama. Most of the countries where the mortality levels are currently low have experienced very rapid declines. In Barbados, the probability of dying by age 5 declined from 165 to 17 per thousand between 1950-1955 and 1980-1985, that is, by 90 percent. Other countries with rapid rates of reduction in under-five mortality levels (over 80 percent) include Chile, Costa Rica and Cuba. Several of the small Caribbean islands with complete vital registration had registered infant mortality rates below 15 per thousand in the mid 1980s.

The developing countries of Oceania have all experienced steady mortality declines and, with the exception of Papua New Guinea (included in Melanesia), all have achieved relatively low levels of infant and child mortality.

The rate of mortality decline has varied considerably among developing countries, but few have enough data to permit the estimation of a change in the pace of decline. However, countries with sufficient data often display a somewhat faster decline in the 1970s compared to earlier periods. Data that have become available after the United Nations' study was completed indicate a continuing decline during the 1980s, some times at an accelerating pace. Thus, it is possible that the actual mortality levels during the 1980s may be somewhat lower than those projected by the United Nations (Table 1).

MAJOR CAUSES OF DEATH

In general, the higher the level of infant and child mortality, the greater the contribution of infectious, parasitic, respiratory and diarrheal diseases to overall mortality. Diarrhea is the most common illness among children in developing countries and mortality caused by dehydration from diarrhea is the largest single contributor to the mortality of young children in those countries. Diarrhea is also a major cause of childhood malnutrition. Other major causes of death in childhood include acute respiratory infections, measles, malaria and tetanus. WHO and UNICEF have estimated that in 1987 approximately 5 million children died before reaching age five years of diarrheal diseases, 2.9 million of acute respiratory infections, 1.9 million of measles, 1 million of malaria, and 0.8 million of tetanus.[3] It should be emphasized, however, that there is much uncertainty attached to these estimates since accurate and comprehensive data on causes of death are scarce in high-mortality populations.

Malnutrition is important both as an underlying and a contributing cause of child mortality in developing countries. WHO and UNICEF have estimated that malnutrition is a contributing cause in approximately one-third of all child deaths.[4] It is estimated that, in developing countries, 12 percent of children under age 5 suffer from acute malnutrition and that almost 40 percent suffer from chronic malnutrition.[5] The nutritional status of a child is influenced not only by diet and feeding practices but also by the frequency of infectious disease. Repeated episodes of diarrhea and infections lower the child's resistance to further disease and increase the risk of a fatal outcome. Measles, for example, is a relatively innocuous disease with a low case fatality ratio among well-nourished children in developed countries, but it is one of the leading causes of child death in developing countries.

Malnutrition can affect a child's chances for survival even before its birth. Maternal malnutrition before and during pregnancy is one of the main causes of fetal growth retardation and low birth weight which are associated with significantly higher mortality in childhood. An estimated 17 percent of infants born in developing countries during 1985 (25 percent in South Asia) had low birth weight, compared to 7 percent in the industrialized countries.[6]

Another factor contributing to increased mortality risks is poor timing of births. Children born to teenage mothers and children born at short intervals suffer higher mortality risks. One of the most important findings from the World Fertility Surveys concerns the exceptionally high mortality risks among children born after a short birth interval.[7]

PREVENTION

A large proportion of the child deaths in developing countries is believed to be preventable through relatively low-cost actions. It has been shown that it is possible to reduce mortality significantly even in societies where levels of economic development are low, if there is strong political will and commitment to implement effective health policies. The cases of the state of Kerala in India, Sri Lanka, China, Costa Rica and Cuba are well known examples.

Access to health services during pregnancy and childbirth, which includes provision of prenatal care, nutritional supplements to pregnant women and vaccination of pregnant women against tetanus can reduce infant and child mortality. Family planning programs aimed at altering birth spacing patterns and avoiding high-risk pregnancies can help reduce infant, child and also maternal mortality. Family planning may also have indirect positive effects on the survival chances of a child, since fewer children will permit more household resources to be allocated to each child.

Other steps to prevent excess child mortality include promotion of breast-feeding and growth monitoring. Breast-feeding has been shown to have an important effect upon the survival chances of children.[8] In addition to the nutritional value of mothers' milk, it imparts a degree of immunity to infectious diseases. One of the simplest indications of a child's overall health status is given by his or her pattern of growth. Growth monitoring of children by periodic weighing and measuring provide parents and health workers with an early warning if growth begins to falter. Appropriate and timely care provided to such children can significantly reduce their mortality.

Diarrheal dehydration, which is responsible for the largest number of child deaths, can now be prevented by the use of oral rehydration therapy (ORT), a treatment that is inexpensive, safe and so simple that it can be learned by any parent. The treatment consists of giving orally a solution to replace the water and salts lost by the body during diarrhea. ORT, which has only recently become well known and widely used, has the potential for preventing more child deaths than any other medical treatment.

Deaths from many of the most common childhood diseases are preventable through immunization or by the use of low-cost drugs. Immunization against a disease may also reduce mortality from other causes. By preventing specific diseases which can precipitate malnutrition, immunization can help break the cycle of malnutrition and infection and contribute more broadly to the reduction in childhood mortality. In addition, when immunization coverage reaches 80 percent or more, disease transmission patterns are affected and a degree of protection is conferred even on unimmunized children.[9]

There is now overwhelming evidence that maternal education reduces infant and child mortality. Research in many countries has consistently shown a strong inverse relationship between female education and child mortality.[10] Thus, an effective way to prevent future child deaths is by educating female children now.

OBJECTIVES FOR THE YEAR 2000

The reduction of mortality, in particular infant and child mortality, is regarded as a universally desirable goal. Specific targets for reducing mortality have been set during recent years by governments and international organizations. In 1974, the United Nations World Population Conference held in Bucharest recommended that countries with the highest mortality levels should aim at reducing their infant mortality to fewer than 120 deaths per thousand live births by 1985.[11] This target was later updated in connection with the Global Strategy for Health for All by the Year 2000, adopted by the World Health Assembly in 1981,[12] and at the International Conference on Population in Mexico City, 1984.[13] According to the updated targets, countries with high mortality levels should strive to reach an infant mortality of fewer than 50 deaths per thousand live births by the year 2000. The Mexico City Conference also recommended that countries with intermediate levels of mortality should aim at lowering their infant mortality to fewer than 35 deaths per thousand births by the year 2000.

While the earlier targets were expressed only in terms of infant mortality, the most recent are also expressed in terms of under-five mortality, the probability of dying between birth and exact age 5, a measure that is becoming more frequently used as an indicator of mortality in childhood. The most recent targets were adopted at a conference on child survival held in Talloires, France, in 1988.[14] At this conference, which was sponsored by WHO, UNICEF, the World Bank, UNDP and the Rockefeller Foundation, it was recommended that the 1980 levels of infant and under-five mortality should be reduced by at least half by the year 2000, or that they should be reduced to 50 and 70 per thousand live births, respectively, whichever achieves the greater reduction.

Many developing countries have already attained or are expected to attain those targets. However, if the mortality trends assumed in the United Nations projections prove accurate, the goals would not be met by all countries. In Africa, only seven out of 51 countries are expected to have mortality levels below the targets set for the year 2000. In South Asia, the most populous countries – Bangladesh, India, Indonesia and Pakistan – are also projected to have mortality rates above those targets. As a result, average child mortality levels for Africa and South Asia, as well as the average levels for all developing regions are expected to remain above the targets. As was mentioned earlier, recent data for many developing countries indicate that child mortality may have declined somewhat faster than expected according to the United Nations' projections. However, even with an accelerating decline, it is unlikely that all countries will reach the goals set for the year 2000.

RECENT EFFORTS IN DEVELOPING COUNTRIES

In the last few years, governments and international organizations have intensified efforts to improve child health and survival. These efforts have consisted mainly in making a few simple and low-cost but effective health technologies widely available, in particular immunization and oral rehydration therapy (ORT). Favorable results from programs to disseminate these technologies have already been reported in a number of countries, but because many of the programs have only recently gained momentum, and the data collection systems in developing countries are often inadequate, a comprehensive assessment of their impact on child survival has not as yet been possible.

In 1974, the World Health Organization launched its Expanded Programme on Immunization (EPI), a collaborative effort by WHO, UNICEF, other organizations and governments. The goal of EPI is to provide immunization against six target diseases – measles, pertussis (whooping cough), neonatal tetanus, poliomyelitis, diphtheria and tuberculosis – for every child in the world by 1990 (in the case of neonatal tetanus, to provide protection to all pregnant women).[15] When EPI was initiated, fewer than 5 percent of children in the developing world were estimated to be immunized.[16] Since then, many countries have sharply increased their coverage, and it is now estimated that almost 50 percent of children born each year are vaccinated against measles, and over 55 percent against the other five diseases. Immunization of women against tetanus still lags behind at just under 25 percent.

The EPI goal of universal coverage by 1990 now appears unlikely to be achieved. If recent trends should continue, 70 percent or more of the world's children are expected to be immunized in 1990, nevertheless an impressive achievement.[17] The main difficulty in improving coverage has been the organization of resources within countries. The programs require political commitment, mobilization of health professionals and the means for wide dissemination of the relevant information.

ORT, which was largely unknown outside the scientific community in the early 1980s, is now being used by approximately one-quarter of the world's families.[18] The majority of governments of developing countries are committed to the use of ORT, but many of the programs are still in their early stages. Although the last few years have seen an acceleration in its use, the spread of ORT has been less rapid than that of immunization. The most well-documented case of a successful program is that of Egypt, where dehydration from diarrhea has been the leading cause of death among children. After some small-scale test projects in Alexandria and Menoufia, Egypt launched a nation-wide campaign in February 1984 through an extensive use of the mass media, in particular television, and the mobilization of health professionals. Less than two years after the campaign began, 98 percent of mothers with young children reported in a survey that they had heard of ORT, and 70 percent said that they had used it in their child's most recent bout of diarrhea.[19] Such high levels of knowledge and use should have an important impact on child mortality. Registered infant mortality showed a fairly sharp drop in 1985, but because vital registration is incomplete and because there have been large fluctuations in the registered rates in the past, it is not possible to tell how much of this decline is attributable to the ORT program.

REFERENCES

1. United Nations. Mortality of Children Under Age 5: World Estimates and Projections, 1950-2025. United Nations publications, Sales no. E.88.XIII, 1988.

2. United Nations. Demographic Yearbook 1984, United Nations publication, Sales no. E/F.85.XIII.l, 1986, table 19, pp. 374-375 and 390-391.

3. Grant, J.P. The State of the World's Children 1988. New York: Oxford University Press for UNICEF, 1988, p. 3.

4. Ibid.

5. World Health Organization. Evaluation of the Strategy for Health for All by the Year 2000, Seventh Report on the World Health Situation, vol 1, Global Review. Geneva:WHO, 1987, p. 90.

6. Ibid, p. 89.

7. Hobcraft, J., J. McDonald, and S. Rutstein. Child-spacing effects on infant and early child mortality. Population Index 49:4, 1983.

8. Palloni, A., and S. Millman. Effects of inter-birth intervals and breastfeeding on infant and early childhood. Population Studies 40:2, 1986; DaVanzo, J., W.P. Butz, and J.P. Habicht. How biological and behavioural influences on mortality in Malaysia vary during the first year of life. Population Studies 37:3, 1983.

9. Grant, J.P. The State of the World's Children 1988. New York: Oxford University Press for UNICEF, 1988, p. 13.

10. Caldwell, J.C., and P.F. McDonald. Influence of maternal education on infant and child mortality: levels and causes. International Population Conference, Manila, 1981: Solicited Papers. Liege: International Union for the Scientific Study of Population, 1983, vol 2, pp. 79-96; Hobcraft, J., J. McDonald, and S. Rutstein. Socio-economic factors in infant and child mortality: A cross-national comparison. Population Studies 38:2, 1984.

11. United Nations. Report of the United Nations World Population Conference, 1974, Bucharest, 19-30 August 1974. United Nations publication, Sales no. E.75.XIII.3, 1975, p. 10.

12. World Health Organization. Formulating Strategies for Health for All by the Year 2000. Geneva:WHO, 1979, para. 63, World Health Organization. Taking off into health for all by the year 2000. World Health Statistics Quarterly 35:1, 1982, pp. 2-3.

13. United Nations. Report of the International Conference on Population, 1984, Mexico City, 6-14 August 1984. United Nations publication, Sales no. E.84.XIII.8, 1984, p. 19.

14. Grant, J.P. The State of the World's Children 1989. New York: Oxford University Press for UNICEF, 1989, p. 64.

15. World Health Organization. The WHO's Expanded Programme on Immunization: A global overview. World Health Statistics Quarterly 38:2, 1985, pp. 232-252.

16. Grant, J.P. The State of the World's Children 1989, New York: Oxford University Press for UNICEF, 1989, p. 4.

17. Ibid, p. 8.

18. Ibid.

19. Williams, G. A simple solution: How oral redydration is averting child death from dehydration. New York: A UNICEF special report, 1987, pp. 55-56.

25

LOW BIRTH WEIGHT

S. Olu Oduntan, M.D., M.P.H., F.F.C.M.

INTRODUCTION

The birthweight has long been recognized not only as a sensitive index of the viability of newborn infants and a determinant of infantile and childhood survival,[1] but also as a powerful indicator of the economic and social development of communities.[2,3]

Birthweights vary between and within communities depending on fetal, maternal and environmental factors.[4] The use of birthweight measurement as a predictive tool in the overall management of babies has necessitated the development of objective criteria and terminologies which are based on scientific, clinical and biological considerations, such as gestational age, and the observed clinical performance of the categorized low birthweight, but gestationally mature babies. The terminologies that have been used include low birth weight (LBW), preterm, small-for-date or small for gestational age (SGA). Detailed descriptions and definitions of these terminologies are fully discussed by Davidson,[5] and could also be obtained from WHO, Geneva.

DEFINITIONS

Low birth weight (LBW) infants are infants with birthweight of less than 2500 gram (up to, and including 2499 gm).[6] This definition does not take account of the etiology or the period of gestation. It does not represent a homogeneous group, and it consists of two broad categories of infants: the preterm infants and the small-for-gestational age (SGA) infants.

The preterm infants are those infants born before 37 completed weeks of gestation, from the first day of the last menstrual period.

The small-for-gestational age (SGA) or light-for-dates are those infants whose birth weights fall below the tenth percentile of the standard for the gestational age.[5]

MAGNITUDE OF THE PROBLEM

Information on birthweight is easily obtained from many developed countries, but correct figures on the global problem of low birth weights are, however, not available, as accurate and comprehensive data on birth weights in many developing countries of the world are scarce and even nonexistent.[3] Most data obtained from these countries are only estimates. Information on gestational ages is also lacking in most data, thus making it impossible to estimate correctly the proportion of LBW infants who are pre-term or full term.

LBW is a worldwide public health problem. Lechtig and his colleagues[7] estimated that in 1975, 22.2 million LBW infants (or 18% of all live births) were born all over the world. Petros-Barvazian and Behar[8] on the other hand, recorded 17% LBW rate (or 23.4 million LBW births) for the same year. The WHO also estimated that 17% of all 122 million global live births in 1979 were low birthweight infants. On a global level, only about 5-10% of all LBW infants were estimated to be born in the developed countries of the world.[8] The summary of the findings of the comprehensive WHO global review of studies on LBW in 90 counties which accounted for 90% of all world births for 1979 is presented in Table 1 (next page). According to that study, there was a wide geographical variation in the incidence of LBW, with rates ranging from 7% in North America, 8% in Europe, 11% Latin America, 15% in Africa to 20% in the whole of Asia and 31% in Middle South Asia.[3] The LBW rates recently reported by Grant[9] for the period 1982-1987 did not differ significantly from those of 1979, considering the inaccuracies of data from most developing countries (Table 2, page 295).

Significant differences and variations in LBW rates were recorded within countries and regions, and this rightly reflected the prevailing heterogeneity of genetic, biological and other environmental factors. For example, China and Japan in Asia had LBW rates which compared favorably with the lowest rates in Europe; rates as high as 17% and 20% were reported for countries in Africa, while the lowest rate of 4% was reported for the Scandinavian countries.[3,9]

In the 1979 WHO study, an estimate of the proportion of SGA full-term infants was possible for a few countries in which the gestational ages were recorded. The proportion of full-term SGA infants ranged from 24% in Finland, 45% in Sweden and the United States of America, to 57% in England and Wales. Similar figures recorded for the developing countries were 34% in Kenya, 38% in Cuba, 56% in Tanzania, 83% in rural Guatemala, about 75% in India, Malaysia and Indonesia and Sri Lanka.[3] The higher proportion of LBW infants who were full term that had been reported in some developing countries had been attributed to unfavorable environmental factors, and which exercised adverse influence before and during pregnancy and had given rise to intrauterine growth retardation.[8]

ETIOLOGY OF LOW BIRTH WEIGHT

The two main determinants of birth weight are the gestational age and the rate of intrauterine fetal growth. Any factor that will exert negative influence on these two determinants will invariably give rise to LBW. Many factors have been associated with the occurrence of low birth weight, and they can be categorized into fetal, maternal and environmental factors. Fetal factors in-

Table 1
Estimated Proportion of Low Birthweight Infants by Region in 1979

Region	Low Birthweight Infants %
Africa	15
Northern America	7
Latin America	11
Asia	20
Europe	8
Oceania	12
U.S.S.R.	8
World	17
Developed Countries	7
Developing Countries	18

Source: WHO, World Health Statistics Quarterly, 33, 1980, 197-224.

Table 2
Estimated Proportion of Low Birthweight Infants
by Selected Countries 1979 and 1982-1987

Countries	Low Birthweight Infants %	
	1979*	1982 – 1987
Bangladesh	50.0	31
India	30.0	30
Pakistan	27.0	25
Papua New Guinea	25.0	25
Sri Lanka	21.0	28
Philippines	19.5	18
Nigeria	18.0	25
Guatemala	17.9	10
Kenya	17.5	13
Zimbabwe	15.0	15
Zambia	14.0	14
Egypt	13.5	7
Thailand	13.0	12
Chile	13.0	7
Italy	11.0	7
Jamaica	10.2	8
Cuba	10.1	8
Colombia	10.0	8
U.S.S.R.	8.0	6
U.S.A.	7.4	7
Tunisia	7.3	7
United Kingdom	7.0	7
France	6.5	5
Canada	6.4	6
China	6.0	6
Australia	5.8	6
Japan	5.1	5
Finland	3.9	4
Sweden	3.6	4

Source: WHO. The incidence of low birth weight. A critical review of available information. World Health Statistics Quarterly, 33, 197-224, 1979.

Grant, J.P. The State of the World's Children. UNICEF Oxford University Press, 1989, pp. 96–97.

* Note: Countries are listed in descending order for 1979 LBW rates.

clude the sex of the fetus, multiple births and congenital malformations.[5] The maternal factors are numerous and have been shown to be interrelated; they are the maternal age, parity, height, educational and socio-economic status.[8,10] The illiterate women, women of short stature, women of 16 and below, women of ages 35 and above, women in the low socioeconomic status tend to have more LBW infants than the more privileged women.[11] Diseases in pregnant women such as anemia, hypertension, toxemia in pregnancy, placenta praevia, sickle cell disease, undernutrition and maternal infections such as rubella, syphilis and malaria also contribute to the occurrence of LBW infants.[5,12] Women who smoke cigarettes and drink alcohol heavily, and those who perform hard physical work or are undergoing severe psychosocial stress, are similarly affected.[10,13] The previous reproductive history of the woman is a well known risk factor as women who have had LBW babies in previous pregnancies or have had repeated abortions are more likely to be similarly affected in future pregnancies. The environmental factors that have been positively associated with LBW infants are high altitude, short intergestational intervals,[8,14] and the non-utilization of antenatal care.[12]

THE PUBLIC HEALTH SIGNIFICANCE OF LBW

LBW is a major contributory factor in perinatal, neonatal and infant mortality and morbidity.[3,15] LBW can have long-term adverse effects on the physical growth of children and their intellectual performance.[7] The development of cerebral palsy and other kinds of brain damage of varying degrees is recognized sequelae of LBW.[3] Some longitudinal twin studies have also shown that there may be differential and abnormal physical and mental development in LBW infants particularly those with intrauterine growth retardation, which are most frequently seen in the developing countries. A small weight difference of about a hundred grams at birth in these LBW infants may result in statistically significant differences in school performance of the children at least up to the age of 11 years.[10,16] It had also been postulated that the long-term effects of LBW on the physical and the intellectual growth of children, especially in the developing countries, might eventually lead to suboptimal learning in childhood and adolescence; and this coupled with other prevailing adverse environmental factors might give rise to inequity in employment opportunities, lower productivity, lower income and a general poor quality of life, including chronic malnutrition, short statured women and low socio-economic status.[17] All these are capable of creating a vicious cycle which will perpetuate the problem of LBW in these countries.[16] The high incidence of LBW and its resulting high-cost care, coupled with its long-term debilitating economic and social effects will also impose a severe economic burden which can further deplete the already overtaxed resources of most impoverished developing countries.

PREVENTION OF LOW BIRTH WEIGHT

The prevention of LBW is of great importance to the overall development of any country as it will promote the health of the children, it will reduce human suffering and wastage, and will also avoid the high costs associated with the immediate and long-term care of LBW infants. Any program for the control of LBW must be multidisciplinary and intersectoral and must entail promotive, preventive, curative and rehabilitative care. The approach to be adopted will, however, depend on the social and cultural characteristics of the communities to be served.

In most developing parts of the world, where the problem is most paramount, about 60-80% of deliveries take place outside the conventional health institutions, and are carried out by traditional birth attendants;[18] a great proportion of the population also dwell in rural areas where health facilities are either not available, or are inadequate. It is therefore obvious that for many programs of intervention to succeed and have a lasting effect, the primary health care approach which will involve community motivation and participation, and which will attack the problem from the grass root level must be adopted. The control and prevention of LBW should be based on interventions that will be short term and long term, and will be carried out at the primary, secondary and tertiary levels of care.

SHORT–TERM MEASURES

These will include the following:

1. The collection of comprehensive data on LBW in the communities to assess the magnitude of the problem.
2. The distribution of nutritional supplements to all identified high-risk pregnant mothers to improve the birth weights of the infants.
3. The provision of medical facilities at primary, secondary and tertiary levels of care for the management of the LBW infants.
4. The provision of rehabilitation facilities for the management of handicapped children and their families.

LONG–TERM MEASURES

These will include the following:

1. The compulsory registration of all births and the compulsory recording of birth weights on all birth certificates.
2. The development of primary health care programs in all communities which will include comprehensive Maternal and Child Health programs.
3. The training of traditional birth attendants and other primary health workers in (i) the identification of high-risk pregnant women and their prompt referral to higher centers; (ii) the art of safe and hygienic delivery, and (iii) the taking of accurate birthweight measurements using appropriate techniques and instruments.
4. The development of appropriate instruments for the measuring of birth weights by primary health workers and traditional birth attendants. These instruments must be cheap, sturdy, accurate, portable and easy to operate and interpreted by illiterate health workers.
5. The adoption of a "risk" approach in the care of mothers and children. The adverse risk factors must be identified, scored and interpreted in such a way that the illiterate primary health workers will be able to utilize them to screen pregnant mothers.
6. The development of a workable referral system for smooth and easy referrals of high-risk infants from the grass root level to the specialized units, and the organization of specialized neonatal units at the secondary and tertiary levels of care for the proper management of LBW infants.
7. The mobilization for and education of all members of the communities to appreciate the problem of LBW as a health priority, and their mobilization for positive action. Special attention should be paid to community and religious leaders, womens' groups, school teachers and other identified non-governmental voluntary organizations.
8. The development of adequate food production to provide much needed nutritious food especially to women and children. This will involve active cooperation, and participation of nutritionists, agriculturists and agricultural extension workers.
9. The control of all infections and the intestinal parasitic infections that might have synergistic or antagonistic effects on the nutrition of the people.

10. The development of acceptable standards of environmental sanitation including the provision of potable water, the hygienic disposal of refuse, provision of adequate housing, ensuring food hygiene as well as the control of all other physical factors which may exert negative effects on the health of mothers and children.

11. The organization of an acceptable fertility control program which will help to reduce parity, to prolong intergestational intervals and thereby improve the quality of life generally.

12. The abolition of traditional practices such as early marriages and excessive physical exertion by pregnant women through appropriate health education activities and governmental legislative measures.

13. The promotion of the socio-economic development of the communities through initiation of special welfare programs, the creation of job opportunities, and the initiation of formal and functional education programs for all and most especially the women.

14. The development of a built-in system of evaluation into the program for effective monitoring of the program.

REFERENCES

1. Puffer, R.R., and C.V. Serrano. Birthweight, maternal age, and birth order: Three important determinants in infant mortality. Washington, DC: PAHO Scientific Publication, 1975, no. 294, pp. 38.

2. Mahner, J. Birthweight as a new development indicator, in Birthweight Distribution - an Indicator of Social Development. G. Sterky and L. Mellander (eds). Swedish Agency for Research Cooperative. SAREC/WHO Report 2, 1978, pp.33-39.

3. World Health Organization. The incidence of low birth weight. A critical review of available information. World Health Statistics Quarterly, 33; 197-224, 1980.

4. Bantje, H. A multiple regression analysis of variables influencing birthweight. Trop Geogr Med 38: 123-130, 1986.

5. Davison, D.C. Low birth weight and light-for-dates. Pediatrics in the Tropics: Current Review. R. G. Hendrickse (ed). New York: Oxford University Press, 1981, pp. 27-37.

6. World Health Organization. International Classification of Diseases, 1975, Rev I. Geneva: WHO, 1977.

7. Lechtig, A., S. Margen, and T. Farrell, et al. Low birthweight babies, worldwide incidence, economic cost and program needs. In Perinatal Care in Developing Countries. G. Rooth and L. Engstrom (eds). Uppsala: Perinatal Research Laboratory and WHO, 1977.

8. Petro-Barvazian, A., and M. Behar. Low birthweight – a major global problem. In Distribution – An Indicator of Social Development, SAREC/WHO, 2, 1978, pp. 9-15.

9. Grant, J.P. The State of The World's Children. UNICEF. Oxford University Press, 1989, pp. 96-97.

10. World Health Organization. New Trends and Approaches in the Delivery of Maternal & Child Care in Health Services. WHO Tech Rep no. 6700. Geneva: WHO, 1976. pp. 93-95.

11. Oduntan, S. Olu, and I. Ayeni. Correlates of low birth weights in two Nigerian communities. Trop Geogr Med 220-223, 1976.

12. Harrison, K.A. Childbearing, health and social priorities a survey of 22774 consecutive hospital births in Zaria Northern Nigeria. Brit J Ob Gyn 5: 1-119, 1985.

13. Tafari, N., R. L. Naeye, and A. Gokezie. Effects of maternal undernutrition and heavy physical work during pregnancy on birth weight. Brit J Ob Gyn 87: 22-226, 1980.

14. Fortney, J.A., and J.E. Higgins. The effect of birth interval on perinatal survival and birth weight. Pub Hlth. Lond. 98: 73-83, 1984.

15. Ayeni, O., and S.O. Oduntan. The effects of sex, birthweight, birth order and maternal age on infant mortality in a Nigerian community. Ann Human Biol 5: 353-358, 1978.

16. Harfouche, J.K. Health care problems of the young child in a developing ecological context: Bull WHO 57: 187-403, 1979.

17. Lechting, A., S. Morgen, and T. Farrell, et al. The societal cost of low birth weight. In SAREC/WHO Report, 2, 1978, pp. 55-58.

18. Mangay-Maglacas, A., and H. Pizurki. Problems and Prospects: in the Traditional Birth Attendant in Seven Countries: Case Studies in Utilization and Training. Publ. Health. Paper no. 75, Geneva: WHO,1981, pp. 205–221.

26

INFANT, CHILDHOOD AND ADOLESCENT MORTALITY IN DEVELOPING COUNTRIES

Carlos V. Serrano, M.D., Ph.D.

INTRODUCTION

In developing countries, large segments of the population have little or no access to health services. This situation is worsened by a considerable restriction of resources in the public sector. This challenge imposes increasing administrative demand on the part of health services and greater effective participation of other sectors and the community. According to the evaluation of the degree of accomplishment of the goal of Health for All in the Year 2000 and of the extent of the application of the Primary Health Care strategy, profound changes are indicated in the health systems of most developing countries.[1] One of the basic changes needed is the decentralization and improvement of all aspects of programming and administration in local health systems.[1]

The situation of economic crisis has brought together restrictions in basic services such as health, housing, education, sanitation and transportation. Other forms of adjustments such as the concentration of resources in action programs for control of priority problems such as diarrheal diseases have contributed to limit the transcendental meaning and potential for change of the Primary Health Care Strategy. As a result of the response to crisis, large numbers of persons with increasing risks are seeking assistance in the informal systems.[1]

Assuming that health-fostering in the developing world countries can constitute a powerful motivation element in any social project in which equity is expected, efforts to implement and consolidate the Primary Health Care strategy are a priority.

Health conditions in individuals, families, and societies are the result of the interactions between the biologic, social and ecologic macrosystems as well as the interactions between their own components. The effects of these interactions constitute factors which associate individuals, or groups to one or more health problems (risk factors) or to progress in health through promotion and protection (protective factors). Due to the fact that the macrosystems and their components are not static but very dynamic, the importance of risk and protective factors and, therefore, of health conditions, changes with time and differs according to the places and types of populations.[2]

How vulnerable are the individuals and groups to the effects of risk factors and disease conditions depends to a great extent on their biologic and psychosocial conditions in the moment they are exposed to those factors. This means that their past history is a powerful conditioning factor of risk of protection.

Although death and survival are usually seen through biologic parameters, the psychosocial conditions may be strong determinants of death and survival.

HEALTH CONDITIONS OF CHILDREN

In order to better understand the real meaning of mortality in the early phases of life, brief comments around certain premises, considered universally valid, are thought to be pertinent.

A. Dependence is a constant characteristic that needs to be taken into consideration for health and survival purposes. From conception through the intrauterine life, the health and the survival of the fetus depend greatly on the health of the mother. After birth, the health of the mother and her dedicated care, as well as the adequate environmental conditions and proper feeding of the infant are decisive factors for infant survival.[3] During childhood and adolescence psychosocial factors gain special importance in health and disease.

B. The processes of growth and development prior to and after birth are conditions closely interrelated and very dynamic. Their normality is related to the protective factors and their deviation to risk conditions added to the degree of vulnerability during the intrauterine life, at birth and after.

C. The epidemiologic profiles related to priority problems, considered of priority on the basis of their frequency, seriousness and resolution possibilities, vary in time and place and according to age and group involved. The indicators of health damage such as mortality represent only averages, often times not very realistic, and hide very unfavorable situations of certain populations.

D. Infant, childhood and adolescent mortality has a transcendental meaning which goes beyond the dimension of the biologic wastage. It constitutes a strong indirect indicator of quality of life and psychosocial and physical potential of survivors.

E. The specific mortality rates, in any age, measure only partially the seriousness and complexity of the phenomenon. Death is in fact the result of multicausal and multifactorial complex, which knowledge is necessary for a comprehensive approach in health care with emphasis in prevention.

IMPLICATIONS OF THE PREVIOUS PREMISES

The following statements could describe the meaning of the previous premises:

A. First Premise: Related to dependency character of children:

1. The health care and good nutrition of the mother prior to and during pregnancy are crucial for the health of the child at birth.

2. Fertility regulation with emphasis on child spacing and prevention of pregnancy during early and advanced ages of women, as well as the education for responsible parenthood are necessary measures. The relationships between infant and neonatal mortality, birth order and maternal age are illustrated in Figure 1 (next page). In all groups of maternal age, infant mortality increases with birth order. At the same time, mortality of infants of the youngest group of mothers is higher in the first born and it increases even more in subsequent infants when compared to those born to older mothers.[4]

3. Support for the care of children of mothers working out-of-home and for enforcement of legislation is an increasing necessity.

4. The education of the mother has been shown to exert a great influence in child survival. Table 1 (next page) illustrates the inverse relationship between the degree of instruction of the

Figure 1
Neonatal and Infant Mortality by Birth Order According to Maternal Age, El Salvador Project, Inter-American Investigation of Mortality in Childhood

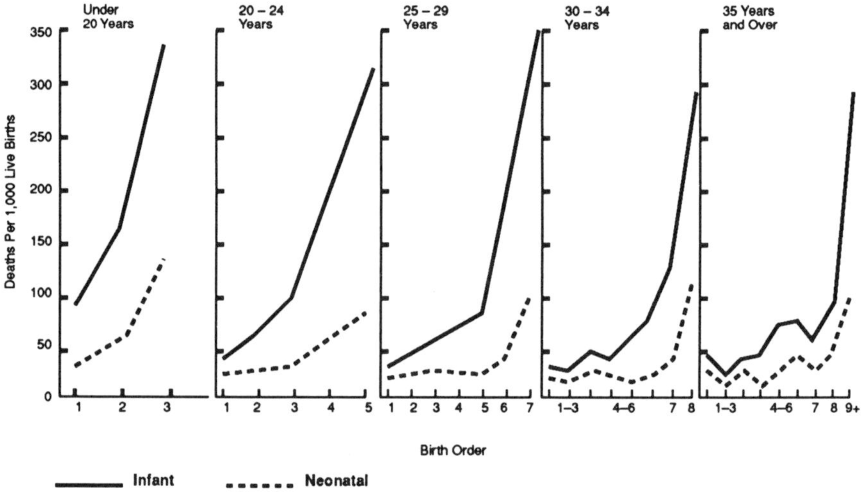

Table 1
Level of Instruction of Mothers Related to Postneonatal Mortality

Areas	Level of Instruction of Mothers of Deceased Children	Per Cent	Postneonatal Mortality
RECIFE	- Less than three years - Secondary /university	68.1 5.3	72.5 3.6
RIBEIRÃO PRETO	- Less than three years - Secondary /university	49.0 9.1	55.5 6.5
SÃO PAULO	- Less than three years - Secondary /university	50.8 8.1	54.8 5.7

Source: Puffer, R.R. C.V. Serrano, *Patterns of Mortality in Childhood*. PAHO, Scient. Pub. 262, 1973

mother and postneonatal mortality in the three Brazilian projects of the Inter-American Investigation of Mortality in Childhood.[3] Therefore, efforts for social promotion of women in terms of increasing rates of literacy and health education are decisive for survival and healthy childhood of developing countries.

5. High coverage and quality of health services with use of risk approach are basic requirements to comply with the principles of efficiency, efficacy and equity of health services delivery.

6. Social participation, and intersectoral action are necessary for early detection of susceptibles and for identification and control of risk factors for promotion of protective factors.

B. Second Premise: Related to characteristics of the processes of growth and development:

1. The evolution of the processes of growth and development are the expression of the health level reached by mothers and children, families and communities. The overall objective of MCH programs is to contribute to satisfy the biologic and psychosocial needs of those processes and, therefore, to the attainment of the following three basic goals:[5]

   a. That every pregnancy be planned and result in the birth of a healthy baby with favorable birthweight and vitality.
   b. That every child progresses through childhood and adolescence with good physical and psychosocial health.
   c. That each woman progresses through the reproductive period in good health and free of sequels.

2. Good nutrition, disease prevention and early diagnosis and treatment, adequate physical and social environments, fertility control, hygienic habits, early stimulation and establishing effective bonds are conditions necessary for normal growth and development.

3. The association of infection and malnutrition is frequently responsible for the initiation of the chain of events leading to severe morbidity and death. The importance of the association is illustrated in Table 2 (next page) – with results of study by Pio[6] which shows that in the case of acute respiratory infections, the incidence may not be affected by the nutritional state but the seriousness and frequency of complications and death may be affected

by the degrees of vulnerability of the child at the onset of the problem.

4. Significant progress is being made in developed and developing countries in reducing infant and early childhood mortality during the period 1960-1987 in selected countries of the world. (Table 3, next page) This reduction has been accompanied by important changes in the profiles of specific mortality. In an increasing number of countries of the world, the perinatal causes of death are the first cause of infant mortality replacing the infectious diseases group (diarrheal diseases the most important). As an example, in the Region of the Americas, 23 out of the 38 countries have the perinatal conditions as the first group of causes of infant mortality.[8] According to data from the same region acute respiratory infections are the second or third cause of infant deaths and the first cause of consultation to services in children under five years of age.[9] Accidents and congenital anomalies are displacing other groups from the first causes of death under five years of age.

5. As reported in a meeting conducted by PAHO,[10] the reduction of mortality indicators is attributed to the following factors:

   a. acceptance and application of the doctrine involved in the Primary Health Care strategy and to qualitative changes in overall and health development models;

Table 2
Annual Incidence of Acute Respiratory Infections (ARI) in Children 0-4 According to Nutritional State. Costa Rica, 1966-1967*

	Normal Weight for Age	Malnourished
Number of children	54	83
Number of ARI episodes	6.15	5.03
Average duration in days	10.92	14.50
Incidence of pneumonia and bronchopneumonia	2	38
Rate per 1000	37.0	457.8

* PIO, A. Et Al. "Follow up of an International Task Force, Sydney, Australia. August 1984 – University Adelaide, Australia, 1985."

Table 3
Infant and Under-5 Mortality Rates of Selected Countries of the World in 1960 and 1987

COUNTRY	INFANT MORTALITY		UNDER 5 YEARS MORTALITY	
	1960	1987	1960	1987
AFGANISTAN	215	173	380	304
ANGOLA	208	169	346	288
HAITI	197	118	294	174
BOLIVIA	167	111	282	176
INDIA	165	100	282	152
GHANA	132	91	224	149
PERU	142	89	233	126
ALGERIA	168	75	270	111
HONDURAS	144	70	232	111
GUATEMALA	125	60	230	103
NICARAGUA	140	64	210	99
ECUADOR	124	64	183	89
BRAZIL	116	64	160	87
EL SALVADOR	142	60	206	87
MEXICO	92	48	140	70
COLOMBIA	93	46	148	69
PARAGUAY	86	42	134	63
CHINA	150	33	202	45
SRI LANKA	70	34	112	45
VENEZUELA	81	36	114	45
ARGENTINA	61	32	75	38
PANAMA	69	23	105	35
URUGUAY	50	27	56	32
USSR	38	25	53	30
CHILE	114	20	142	26
TRINIDAD/TOBAGO	54	20	67	24
COSTA RICA	84	18	121	23
POLAND	62	18	70	19
CUBA	62	15	87	19
USA	26	10	30	13
UNITED KINGDOM	23	9	27	11
CANADA	28	8	33	9
JAPAN	31	5	40	8
SWEDEN	16	6	20	7

b. the development and appropriate application of technologies of great impact in the control of services and the involvement of communities and other sectors;

c. the advances made in scientific knowledge and the experience of the level of health education acquired by populations; and

d. the progress observed in health services, particularly in relation to access. Analysis carried out by Rosero-Bixby[11] of the factors leading to the very significant decline in the rate of infant mortality in Costa Rica, revealed that the extension of Primary Health Care contributed with 41 percent of the reduction; the social and economic progress of the population with 32 percent; the increased access and coverage at the secondary level of complexity of health services with 22 percent, and the control of fertility with 5 percent (Figure 2). The component of control of common infectious diseases (diarrheal diseases, acute respiratory infections and immune preventable diseases) is considered the most effective.

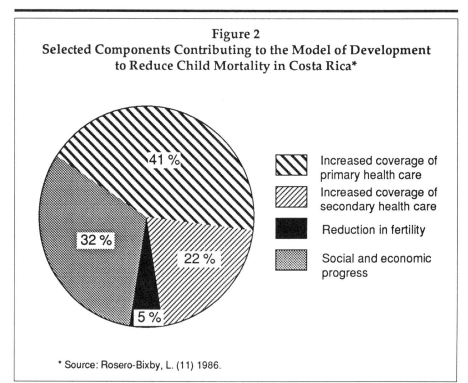

Figure 2
Selected Components Contributing to the Model of Development to Reduce Child Mortality in Costa Rica*

Increased coverage of primary health care

Increased coverage of secondary health care

Reduction in fertility

Social and economic progress

* Source: Rosero-Bixby, L. (11) 1986.

6. Significant advances in the reduction of the so-called "hard" morbidity and mortality, such as the one related to perinatal causes, are also becoming evident. In a recent study by Puffer and Serrano,[12] on patterns of birthweights, favorable changes have been observed in the distribution of live births by birthweight as illustrated in Table 4. As in the case of infant mortality, the reduction in the proportions of live births of low birth weight is attributable to the effect of multiple simultaneous interventions (comprehensive programming), including quantitative and qualitative increments in health actions, education, fertility regulation, better nutrition and social and geographic access to health services.

C. Third Premise: Implications of variations in epidemiologic profiles:

1. The national and international mortality indicators are only overall average values of complex situations, some of them favorable and some unfavorable. They hide important realities and do not permit discrimination of critical risk and problem levels.

2. Another implication is the need for revision and adaptation of strategies and solutions according to the changes in the degree of strength of risk factors to problems and according to changes of frequency of causes of morbidity and mortality.

3. Mortality, as extreme damage to health, is the result of very complex situations in which individual, family and social aspects

Table 4
Progress in Reduction of Low Birthweights
in Four Latin American Countries*

Country	Low Birthweight	
	Per Cent (Year)	Per Cent (Year)
Chile	10.4 (1977)	6.4 (1985)
Costa Rica	9.1 (1970)	6.6 (1984)
Cuba	10.1 (1973)	7.9 (1984)
Uruguay	8.3 (1977)	7.8 (1984)

* Adapted from Puffer, R.R. and C.V. Serrano, *Patterns of Birthweights*, Scient. Pub. - PAHO, 1987.

play roles of variable importance. The levels of mortality obey to positive and negative circumstances occurring in the following dimensions:

a. At the level of the community, a society which has a health culture characterized by solidarity around health, good practices, attitudes and knowledge; good levels of education and economies free of chronic crisis, is in good condition to promote and preserve good health conditions. The role of health and other sectors is to facilitate the capacity for self-care and to promote life styles characterized by healthy behaviors. Users should be in condition to contribute to, create and consolidate effective access and good quality services.

b. In the other extreme, the social and economic policies, if oriented to satisfy biological, psychological and social needs, will contribute to the attainment of the efficiency, efficacy and equity attributes of social sectors, including health.

c. Health services institutions constitute the middle dimension with two main inter-phases: One at the level of the contact of users and providers in which access and quality are desirable goals, and the other within the contact of policy-making process down to the health services at the operational level in which the goals of efficiency, efficacy and equity are the main goals.

4. A conclusion of this premise is that health is a national and not merely a sectoral objective. Therefore, prevention of problems and reduction of mortality are successful when concerted participatory efforts and actions are possible in the various dimensions presented.

D. **Fourth Premise:** Related to the significance of mortality. The following are implications of the premise:

1. The specific rates of mortality, in any age, measure very partial degrees of seriousness and complexity of the phenomenon. Death is usually the effect of multicausal and multifactorial complex whose significance transcends the concept of biological wastage to become a valuable indirect indicator of quality of life and psychosocial potential of survivors.

2. An optimal state of health on the one hand or extreme damage (death or serious sequel) on the other, have a long and rich past history that may go back several generations. In the presence of a child that gets seriously ill or dies, one could ask why this child and why in this moment got sick or died? The answer would be found in the important degree of vulnerability secondary to conditioning factors such as low birthweight or poor nutrition or any other condition which makes him or her more susceptible than other children. Other factors such as ignorance of parents, lack of access to services or exposure to unfavorable environment increase the probability of serious disease and death and are usually associated. So, the combination of both types of factors, conditioning and determining is the rule. The etiologic condition that initiates the chain of events leading to death is the underlying cause and usually is associated to pre-existing (contributory) or added complications or diseases.

3. The degree of development of primordial and primary prevention constitutes the key factor for the reduction of mortality. When the priority axis of work is the primordial and primary prevention through emphasis on fostering factors which protect and promote health (health education, good nutrition, and immunity, sanitation, availability of health services), the result will be not only the prevention of problems, complications, sequelae and death, but the improvement of chances of good quality of life and better accomplishment of psychosocial potential. It will be increasing survival with high quality standards and of human development such as implied in the Primary Health Care philosophy.

E. Fifth Premise:

1. Analyses of mortality in childhood and adolescence which include multiple factors and causes and identification of failures in the various levels of prevention will be very useful for definition of protective and risk factors and diseases, thus avoiding their appearance and the seriousness of diseases and sequelae. Eventually auditing of infant, childhood and adolescent mortality through in-depth study of samples of deaths could be a valuable instrument to monitor the quality of health and other social programs.

2. Psychosocial factors play an increasingly important role in risk-taking behaviors of children, adolescents, and adults. These be-

haviors often contribute to the multi-causality of evolving serious problems such as congenital AIDS, child neglect and abuse, and risk-taking behaviors of adolescents.

3. In most developing countries the high infant and early childhood mortality rates and pressing concerns of development have led health needs of adolescents and young people to be ranked low in priority. Yet, there are grounds for concern in all countries. Most of the majority of deaths occur in otherwise healthy and potentially productive young people.

According to WHO database[13] accidents account for 20 to over 60 percent of deaths of young people (Table 5) and male youths are more affected. A study by PAHO[14] on accidental and violent deaths in 23 Latin American countries showed that homicides were the first cause of death in one country, the second cause in six countries, the third cause in two countries. Suicide was the second cause of death of young people in four countries, although in 10 of the 23 countries it did not appear within the first

Table 5
Accidents as a Percentage of All Causes of Death Among Young Persons 10-24 Years, in Certain Countries

Country	Year	Males	Females
Argentina	1985	37.7	19.0
Chile	1986	17.5	10.1
Cuba	1986	66.9	61.5
USA	1986	51.9	43.7
Isreal	1986	40.3	26.7
Japan	1987	49.2	20.2
Austria	1987	60.5	43.1
Finland	1986	41.6	30.5
Italy	1985	56.8	36.0
United Kingdom	1987	46.5	27.8
Australia	1986	56.8	44.5

Source: WHO Databank

10 causes. Consumption of alcohol and other substances was associated in a significant number of deaths.[15] Pregnancy-related deaths are more important than is apparent. Adolescent girls in the age group 15-17 have a risk of death related to pregnancy 20 to 200 percent higher than older women. In the absence of health care a pregnant girl below 17 years of age has a 5-7 percent chance of pregnancy-related death.[13]

A special observation in relation to the previous premises is the little or no importance given to activities of rehabilitation in the area of rehabilitation and prevention of residual damage in maternal and child programs in the developing countries. The lack of sensitization in relation to residual damage to physical health is evident. When it comes to social and psychological health the situation may be even more serious. This aspect is needing urgent attention in order to minimize the great functional and psychosocial obstacles for a normal growth and development of children and adolescents and for their performance as future adults.

THE RESPONSE

From the issues briefly presented previously, one could envisage that all countries in the world are being subject to a very dynamic state of change. The health and well being of massive groups of populations exposed to this process of change are necessarily affected in positive and/or negative directions. One may recognize that relevant advances for health development of societies have occurred, are taking place, and will continue to evolve. At the same time, it must be recognized that within the same period of time, negative factors have occurred, are taking place and will evolve, thus affecting negatively the development of health and well-being of individuals, families and societies. Examples of the first group of circumstances were given in no. 5 of the implications of the second premise above. Likewise, examples of the second group are:

    a. the serious economic, political and social crisis and the social and social and sanitary debt that it implies;

    b. the insufficient response of sectoral institutions to the increasing needs and demands;

    c. the profound changes observed in the structure and dynamics of the family; and

    d. the voluntary and involuntary massive immigrations intra- and inter-country accompanied by an abrupt enlargement of urban centers with unprotected population groups.

In order to obtain the best benefit from the positive or protective factors and to reduce the consequences of negative factors on the health of vulnerable groups of mothers and children, an adequate response should start with formulation of national and local policies of maternal and child health care programs based on:

a. Emphasis in the contribution of health care to a better quality of life and greater potential for good psychosocial performance of present and future generations.

b. Recognition of the importance of health and development of women in order to optimize their role of best health agents within families and communities.

c. Recognition of the importance of a good organization and function of health services in coordination with services of other sectors in order to be able to respond to the real health needs of the populations. The administrative decentralization and deconcentration of services and the promotion of effective participation of communities are a requirement.

Program formulation and execution should give special attention to the attainment of the following attributes:

a. emphasis in primordial and primary prevention;

b. universal access, at feasible costs;

c. continuity of actions of the various program components in order to facilitate adequacy with the continuum character of the vital cycle; and

d. good quality of service through optimum use of resources and opportunities in all contacts of users with the system.

REFERENCES

1. Pan American Health Organization. The Development and Strengthening of the Local Health Systems. Item 5.6 of the XXXIII Directive Council Meeting. Washington D.C.

2. Serrano, C.V. The Risk Approach and Child Survival. Report of Kellogg MCH Leaders Meeting. Rio de Janeiro, May, 1985. (Spanish)

3. Puffer, R.R., and C.V. Serrano. Patterns of mortality in childhood. Pan American Health Organization. Scientific Publication 262z. Washington DC: PAHO,1973.

4. Puffer, R.R., and C.V.Serrano. Birthweight, maternal age and birth order. Three important determinants of infant mortality. Pan American Health Organization, Scientific Publication 294. Washington DC: PAHO, 1975.

5. Serrano, C.V. Health Care Models and Primary Health Care. Presentation in Meetings on Situation and Perspectives of Infant and Under-5 Mortality in Latin America. Cocoyoc, Morelos, Mexico. October, 1988 (Spanish).

6. Pio, A., J. Leowski, and H.G. Ten Dam. The Magnitude of the Problem of Acute Respiratory Infections. Proceedings of an International Workshop. Sydney, August, 1984. Australia: University of Adelaide Press, 1985.

7. UNICEF. State of the World's Children 1989, pp. 94-95.

8. Guerra de Macedo, C. Infant Mortality in the Americas. Pan American Health Organization. Offset Document.Washington DC: PAHO, 1988.

9. Pan American Health Organization. The Maternal and Child Health Regional Program Offset Document. Washington DC:PAHO, 1985.

10. Pan American Health Organization. Report on the Regional Workshop on Primary Health Care Strategy and Child Mortality. Mexico DF Offset Document. Washington DC: PAHO, 1986.

11. Rosero-Bixby, L. Infant mortality in Costa Rica: Explaining the recent decline. Studies in Family Planning 17:57-65, 1986.

12. Puffer, R.R., and C.V. Serrano. Patterns of Birthweights. Pan American Health Organization. Scientific Publication 504. Washington, DC: PAHO, 1987.

13. World Health Organization. The Health of Youth. Background Document Technical Discussions. May 1989. Geneva: WHO,1989.

14. Pan American Health Organization. Epidemiologic Bulletin 5: no. 2, 1984.

15. Pan American Health Organization. Data Bank of Health of Adults. Regional Program-Accident and Violence (1986-1988). Washington, DC: PAHO.

27

NUTRITION OF CHILDREN UNDER FIVE

SHANTI GHOSH, M.D., F.A.M.S.

Nutrition of young children in most developing countries is far from satisfactory. The reasons are many – poor socio-economic conditions, inadequate care of the mother during pregnancy, maternal malnutrition, short spacing, high fertility, a large number of children under five years, ignorance about feeding, repeated infections and lack of access to health services. (Figure 1, next page) It is obvious therefore that one cannot consider childhood nutrition in isolation.

Across the developing world, 18-20% of babies born have low birth weight (less than 2.5 kg). Some of the Asian countries, especially India and Bangladesh, have a disproportionately larger share of it, up to 30-40%. In Africa, the figure is 10-20%, and in China and Latin America 5-to-10%.[1] These low birth-weight babies account for 30-40% of infant deaths. Those who survive have less than normal physical and possibly mental development. The critical period for the growth and development of brain and other components of the central nervous system appears to begin during the last months of intrauterine life and extends into the early postnatal years. Therefore, nutrition during this period is crucial.

Major causes of low birth-weight babies are maternal malnutrition and anemia during pregnancy, malaria, hypertensive disorders, hard physical work throughout pregnancy and inadequate food intake to compensate for it. Mothers at two extremes of the reproductive period, short spacing and high fertility also contribute to low birth weight. Poor women in developing countries gain 5-6 kg weight during pregnancy, as compared with 10-12 kg weight gain among the better-off women. With repeated pregnancies and short spacing, mothers have no time to recuperate between pregnancies. This phenomenon has been termed maternal depletion syndrome. There is a lack of understanding of the critical relationship between prenatal care and infant mortality. Low birth weight may be a more sensitive indicator than maternal and infant mortality rates for evaluating MCH intervention strategies. Table 1 highlights some of these correlations.

Indeed the problem goes back even further; i.e., the health and nutrition of the young girl, who is discriminated against in many countries. More malnutrition is common among girls and there is discrimination regarding food and access to health services. The girl grows up undernourished and is often married in adolescence, before her pubertal spurt, resulting in a teenage pregnancy, which not only endangers her life, but she does not attain her full

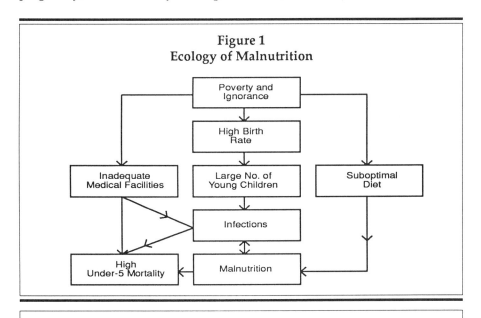

Figure 1
Ecology of Malnutrition

Table 1
Maternal Risk Factors Associated with Low Birth Weight
Risk Factors. Percent Prevalence of Risk Factors

	Birth Weight > 2500 g.		Birth Weight < 2500 g.	
	Urban	Rural	Urban	Rural
Teenage Pregnancy	11.0	28.4	16.9	38.4
Ht. <140 cm.	1.0	0.6	2.9	2.6
Wt. <40 kg.	9.9	18.9	28.8	38.6
Hb. <8 kg.	9.9	17.2	22.5	16.2

(National Institute of Nutrition, Hyderabad, India, 1980)

pubertal growth potential, remains stunted, and in turn gives birth to a low birth-weight baby. In India in 1981, seven percent of girls of 10-14 years and 43% in 15-19 year age group were already married. An estimated 10-15% of births worldwide are to adolescent girls. According to WHO, a non-pregnant weight of less than 38kg and a height of less than 145 cm signify high risk both for the mother and the baby. Many studies in India have shown that about a quarter of women weigh less than 38 kg, and about 12-15% of women between 20-30 years have heights less than 145 cms. Anemia, which is widely prevalent among the adolescent girls, becomes more severe because of early and repeated pregnancies.

A stunted child becomes a small mother, a small mother gives birth to a small baby. Small babies grow less well. Girls who grow less well become small mothers and so the cycle of malnutrition and stunting goes on. The best chance of breaking the cycle of malnutrition and deprivation is through improving children's nutrition in their early years. Figure 2 shows the growth pattern of children in different income groups and with different birth weight.

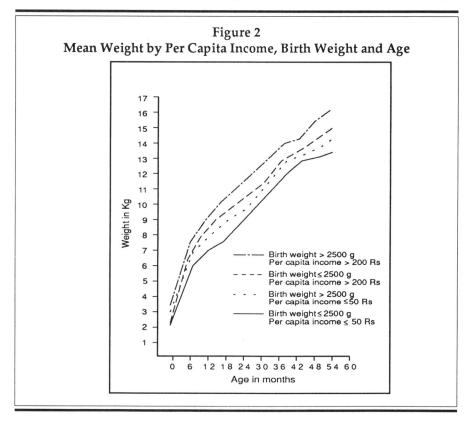

Figure 2
Mean Weight by Per Capita Income, Birth Weight and Age

Malnutrition is the major health problem in the world today. More than half of the next generation is growing up undernourished. Of 850 million children under the age of five, 350 million are estimated to be undernourished.[2]

The outstanding manifestations of under-nutrition in children are: (I) retardation of growth and development; and (II) specific nutritional deficiency signs. Of the latter, protein-energy malnutrition, vitamin A deficiency, iron deficiency and iodine deficiency diseases are the most important.

WHO has compiled results from more than 50 national surveys conducted from 1975. The indications are that prevalence of under-weight children (less than 2 SD weight-for-age) declined between 1975 and 1980 and has been unchanged since then. For Africa as a whole, the average prevalence of under-weight children has been calculated as 24% in 1980 and 25% in 1984. For South Asia, the figure is 65-70% and for South East Asia, 33-34%. In other regions, under-weight is mostly due to stunted growth in height. In South Asia, under-weight also results from a much higher degree of wasting.[1]

Prospective studies in Bangladesh and India have shown the dramatic increased risk of death among malnourished children. The severely malnourished children have a 20 times greater risk of dying than their normal peers.[3] The large PAHO study in Latin America showed malnutrition as an underlying cause in more than 50% of child deaths.

In 1986, over 14 million children died before their fifth birthday, two-thirds of them aged less than one year. Under-five mortality rates in 1987 were more than 150 in some African countries, 152 in India and 45 in China and Sri Lanka.[5] While the immediate cause of death of most of them is infection, malnutrition is a major underlying cause of death, mortality doubling with each lower category of nutritional status. Malnutrition contributes to infectious diseases and infections in turn increase energy demands, decrease food absorption, worsen the level of malnutrition, and a vicious circle begins.

Infections and malnutrition are the common causes of death. There may be 5-10 episodes of illness in a year, each worsening the nutritional status. In a rich country, chances of dying before age one are 1 in 100 while in a developing country the chances are 1 in 5.

Between 1970 and 2000 the number of children in more developed regions will remain almost constant at less than 300 million, while the number is increasing rapidly in spite of high mortality in less developed regions and will be approximately 1700 million by the year 2000.

The health of women and children is threatened by imbalances in distribution and access to resources, by discrimination against women and illiteracy. In every economic setting the children of literate women have a better
chance of survival than those of illiterate women. Educated women tend to
marry later, delay the onset of child bearing and are more likely to practice
family planning. They generally have fewer children with a wider spacing
between births. Women with no schooling on average have almost twice as
many children as those with seven or more years of schooling. Education of
the mother is associated with better child survival. She is the most important
primary health care worker; education gives her better access to information
and improves her status and decision making. Literacy rates among women
are 30-35% in India and 25-40% in the Arab states, Middle South Asia and
Africa.

GROWTH MONITORING

Anthropometric assessment of nutritional status is a scientific diagnostic
tool, in which weight-for-age seems to be the most useful measurement of
nutrition. It is important to start weighing children as soon after birth as
possible (keeping in mind the taboos in some countries about not weighing
the child for the first few months because of a fear of the evil eye) and monitor
growth in a way that mother understands it. Every occasion of growth monitoring becomes a session for communication with the mother, aimed at promoting optimal health in her child. Thus effective growth promotion in contrast to nutrition assessment focuses on the younger age when growth faltering occurs. To be meaningful, mother must be actively involved in it and
understand its significance. The ideal to hope for would be a community-level
growth monitoring and not just a clinic activity.

Data from several countries have shown that growth faltering starts
around 4-6 months and major deviance from normal occurs between six and
eighteen months of life. After 2 years most children grow at the same rate as a
well-nourished population. They remain smaller due to the major deficits that
occurred before age two. So for growth monitoring to have any impact. it
must be started as soon after birth as possible.

The emphasis during the past four decades has been on identifying and
classifying malnutrition into various grades and etiological groups and then
prescribe various regimens to treat it. Growth monitoring on the other hand
aims to monitor the healthy child to try to keep him healthy and prevent
growth faltering by timely advice about feeding and early management of
any infection should it occur. Mothers need to understand and appreciate the

importance of gaining weight, but all healthy children must grow. By charting weight on a suitable growth chart, growth can become visible to the health worker and the mother. Children participating regularly in growth monitoring have higher rates of immunization, more effective breast feeding, more appropriate introductions of weaning foods, and better management of infections, because of health and nutrition education at every contact. Inadequate growth, as shown by the faltering of a growth curve, is one of the first signs of insufficient nutrition and should alert the health worker and mother to consider why food intake has been inadequate and to take the necessary steps.

A view has often been put forward that mother always knows when her child is not growing well. In the beginning, the child usually frets and cries when hungry or ill, but a busy mother does not have enough time or leisure to pay adequate attention to that. Since she sees the child all the time, the early weight loss or lack of weight gain is not noticeable. What is important is the comparison with the child's own earlier weight, rather than what the weight is at one given point of time compared to a standard derived from an entirely normal population.

The often quoted slogan "prevention is better than cure" applies as much to malnutrition as it does to diseases. Therefore it is important that growth monitoring begin as early as possible.

BREAST FEEDING

Breast feeding is the best form of nutrition for the young infant and an important means of spacing births. Almost all women breastfeed their children initially in the developing world, but the length of breast feeding is declining especially in urban areas. "Breast is best" is absolutely true. It provides immunological protection against common childhood illnesses, such as diarrhea and respiratory diseases. It contains the complete range of nutrients necessary to the young infant and is easier to digest than any other kind of milk. Breast milk makes the difference between life and death in a poor household, where there are no facilities for sterilization and refrigeration, clean water is not available, and the cost of buying milk is prohibitive, which may lead parents to dilute the milk formula. As a result, bottle-fed babies are more likely to be malnourished, have more illnesses and are more likely to die compared to breast-fed babies. Both colostrum and mature breast milk contain biologically active substances that guard the infant against infection. The concentration of these substances is highest in the colostrum. Unfortunately, in many countries, there are traditional beliefs against giving colostrum to the baby, often the baby is not put to the breast for up to 2-3 days, and various substitutes such as sugar or honey dissolved in water or diluted animal milk are given. This practice needs to be changed with proper education. The immunological protective agents in human milk include:

- Immunoglobulins, which produce antibodies against specific bacteria and viruses.
- Leucocytes which destroy bacteria and other foreign substances.
- The bifidus factor, which prevents the growth of potentially harmful organisms.

An adequate supply of breast milk satisfies virtually all nutritional needs of an infant for the first four to six months of life. After that, too, breast milk can remain an important source of protein and other nutrients well into the second year.

While the percentage of children initially breast fed is high, the median duration of breastfeeding varies considerably, according to the World Fertility Survey in 28 developing countries, and ranges from 30 months in Bangladesh to less than two months in Costa Rica. In Taiwan and Thailand, over the last decade, the average length of breastfeeding has dropped by about five months. The reason often given for stopping breast feeding or adding animal milk is insufficient breast milk. This may be due to a lack of knowledge regarding breast feeding and there may be a lack of support from the family or health workers. It is ironic that some studies have revealed that breast feeding is more successful when there is no or very little access to health services. Most health workers do not have enough knowledge regarding breast feeding and, at the slightest pretext, advise a change to bottle feeding or at least some addition of milk, when all that was necessary was more frequent suckling. Insufficient suckling is an important factor in the problem of insufficient milk. The reasons for shifting from breast to bottle are trivial and unsound, primarily due to a lack of knowledge and commitment by health personnel. They should be taught that frequent suckling, the pattern of breast feeding in many traditional societies, is necessary to maintain a high level of milk production. It is particularly important in the first few weeks after child birth when lactation is being established. Frequent feeding may also alleviate some common problems like sore and cracked nipples and breast engorgement. Hospital practices of separating mothers and babies and advertising by the milk food companies also contribute to a decline in breast feeding.

Breast-fed babies have lower death rates. A review by the World Health Organization and UNICEF concluded that in the future a decline in breast feeding in developing countries might have a serious, adverse impact on child health in areas where health and other social services are inadequate.

As more women join the work force, there is danger that breast feeding may decline because there are hardly any facilities for keeping the baby at the work place.

BREAST FEEDING AND FERTILITY

Breast feeding delays menstruation, inhibits ovulation and, therefore, reduces the likelihood of conception. In general, the longer a women breast feeds, the longer she will not conceive. Full breast feeding with frequent suckling, night feeding and no other food for the infant for the first few months, delays the return of fertility. Suckling delays the birth of more infants in our world than all contraceptive measures. Frequent suckling results in high levels of plasma prolactin, and ovulation and menstruation do not occur. This increases the supply of milk and also prevents pregnancy. As suckling diminishes, breast milk also diminishes and the protection against pregnancy becomes less. The longer a women breast feeds, the longer the amenorrhoea lasts. A few women may conceive during amenorrhoea. WHO collaborative study on breast feeding conducted in eleven countries gave a range of 1-11% of women who said that their last pregnancy had occurred during a period of postpartum amenorrhoea. By six months, about 20 to 50 percent of women are menstruating and need contraceptives just as much as if they were not breast feeding. An unwanted pregnancy during breast feeding is a proven and serious risk to the health of the mother and eventually to the health of both children. Kwashiorkor, the severest form of malnutrition in children, refers to a disease when a child is weaned too early from the breast because the mother is pregnant again. In a report from Senegal, one-third of the children were weaned because of a new pregnancy. Mortality was higher among those weaned early and probability of death within one year following weaning increased by 50-150%. Avoiding such pregnancies should have high priority for MCH personnel. Breast feeding makes a substantial contribution to birth spacing and fertility control in many areas but for an individual woman it is an unreliable method of family planning. Any shortening of breast feeding will lead to higher fertility unless contraceptive use increases fast enough to counteract this effect.

The choice of a contraceptive has to be considered carefully. Combined estrogen-progestin oral pills decrease milk volume in some cases, but pills with 0.05 mg or less of estrogen do not appear to reduce milk. Progestin-only contraceptives, too, do not seem to have an adverse effect on breast milk. Minute amounts of hormones are transmitted to the infant in breast milk, but no immediate effects have been observed.

INTRODUCTION OF SEMI-SOLIDS

Breast feeding should be continued as long as possible. However, after 4-6 months, breast milk alone may not be sufficient, and so some other food will have to be started in addition. Unfortunately, this is delayed considerably, sometimes due to traditional cultural beliefs (the ceremony of annaprashana in India, when a cereal is given at a particular age) but often due to ignorance. A young child is entirely dependent on his mother or someone else for food, and so this person should have sound knowledge, availability of time and motivation.

The important thing is to remember that the food should not be watery, but energy-dense, and given several times a day because of the small size of the baby's stomach. Most weaning diets in the developing countries are bulky compared to those in the developed countries. Addition of some oil helps to increase energy density as well as makes the food more palatable and less viscous. Another method practiced in some countries is to malt the grain (sprouting, drying, roasting, grinding) which is amylase-rich and reduces the viscosity considerably. It is important not to burden the already over-worked mother with fancy and complicated recipes, but rather advise to modify the family food for the baby. Freshness of food and utmost hygiene should be ensured to prevent infections. A 1-2 year old child needs to eat half as much as his mother. This seems unbelievable to the mother, but is none-the-less true. A great deal of malnutrition is not because the family does not have the food but due to ignorance regarding the child's needs, preference for expensive rather than common family food, and due to infection because of poor hygiene standards.

Of the various nutrients, vitamin A, iron and iodine will be considered here.

Vitamin A

The major problem in terms of numbers affected is in South and East Asia, notably Bangladesh, India and Indonesia. On the basis of WHO data, 34 countries have been identified as having serious vitamin A deficiency problems. Worldwide estimates indicate that there are 700,000 new cases per year among preschool children. Of these, some 60% die and, of the survivors, 25% remain totally blind. This amounts to some 250,000 children going blind or partially blind each year. As a result, some 3 million children under 10 years of age are blind from this cause, over a million of whom are in India.[6]

Approximately 25,000-30,000 children go blind each year in India. And this happens in spite of the fact that the government has a program of administering 200,000 units of vitamin A orally every six months to children between one and five years of age. Prevalence of xerophthalmia varies from 13-16% in different parts of India.

An association between vitamin A deficiency and infections has been reported. Even milder vitamin A deficiency predisposes children to an increased risk of diarrhea and respiratory infections. Studies in Java, Indonesia have shown that vitamin A deficiency may predispose to diarrhea among children. Diarrhea lasts longer and is more severe in malnourished children. Diet containing B-carotene or vitamin A is the most critical factor determining the risk of xerophthalmia. The adequacy of maternal intake and storage is important during the prenatal period of development.

During the first few months of life, breast milk is the primary source of vitamin A. Weaning period is a time of great risk. Faulty feeding practices, taboos, illiteracy, ignorance about normal requirements of infants, coupled with increased demand of vitamin A due to rapid growth, can precipitate xerophthalmia.

IRON DEFICIENCY

Iron deficiency is the most common cause of nutritional anemia in women of reproductive age and in young children. Anemia is due to dietary deficiency of iron, poor absorption, intestinal parasites and in many countries, malaria. Worldwide, anemia is prevalent in 43% of children between 0-4 years. Prevalence in Africa and South Asia is 56% each.[8] In a study in India, 62.8% of children between 1-3 years and 44.0% between 3-5 years had hemoglobin levels less than 10.8 g percent.[9] A later study gave even a higher prevalence rate for Calcutta (96.3%) while it was 66.3% for Hyderabad and 60.9% for Delhi.[10]

IODINE DEFICIENCY

Iodine, which is a component of thyroid hormone, is essential for normal growth and development of the fetus, infant and child, and for the normal physical and mental activity of adults. Iodine deficiency results in goitre, reduced mental function and increased rates of stillbirths and infant mortality. The association of goitre and cretinism with iodine deficiency has been known for a long time; much more prevalent forms of milder mental retardation are now being recognized. Effects of the deficiency are most serious during fetal life and the first two years after birth.

The best known iodine-deficient areas are mountainous, especially the Andes and the Himalayas. However, areas prone to repeated flooding are also iodine deficient. New pockets of deficiency areas are being established. Nearly 200 million people worldwide are thought to have goitre and over 3 million suffer from overt cretinism. Over 50% of these live in South-East Asia. At least 40 million people in South-East Asia are estimated to suffer physical and mental impairment due to iodine deficiency disorders.[11] In India, the population exposed to iodine deficiency is now estimated to be 170 million. Many countries now have a salt-iodating program.

REFERENCES

1. United Nations first report on the world nutrition situation, 1987.

2. Keller, W., and C.M. Fillmore. Prevalence of protein-energy malnutrition. World Health Statistics Quarterly, 36, no. 2, 1983.

3. Chen, U., A.K.M.A. Chowdhary, and S.L. Huffman. Anthropometric assessment of energy-protein malnutrition and subsequent risk of mortality among pre-school children. Am J Clin Nutr 23: 1836-1845, 1980.

4. Puffer, R., and C.V. Serrano. Pattern of mortality in childhood. Sci Publ no. 262. Washington DC: PAHO.

5. The State of the World's Children, UNICEF, 1989.

6. Kuffer, C. World blindness and its prevention. Oxford: Oxford University Press, 1980.

7. Sommer, A. et al. Increased risk of respiratory disease and diarrhea in children with pre-existing mild vitamin A deficiency. Am J Clin Nutr 40:1090-1095, 1984.

8. De Maeyer, E.M. et al. The prevalence of anemia in the world. World Health Statistics Quarterly, 38:302-316. Geneva: WHO, 1985.

9. Indian Council of Medical Research Technical Report No. 26, 1977.

10. Report of ICMR Working Group. Am J Clin Nutr 35:1442, 1982.

11. Clugston, G.A., and K. Bagchi. Tackling iodine deficiency in South-East Asia. World Health Forum, 7: 33-38, 1982.

28

DIARRHEA, INCLUDING ORAL REHYDRATION THERAPY

Nimrod O. Bwibo, M.D., M.P.H.

Diarrhea is defined variously by different people. To the mother, diarrhea is considered subjectively whenever a child passes loose or watery stools. Various investigators tend to use different definitions for diarrhea such as: more than two watery or loose motions in 24 hours; three or more liquid or loose stools in a day; three or more liquid stools in a day.[1] World Health Organization suggests four or more watery stools in 24 hours as the criterion to be used.[2]

Diarrhea is a major public health problem worldwide. The prevalence and incidence of diarrhea vary from area to area, depending upon climatic and environmental factors. The incidence also varies from time to time according to seasonal variations. These factors lead to fluctuations of diarrheal incidence from one year to another. On the whole the prevalence and incidence are much higher in tropical developing countries than in the developed countries; the major factors are the prevailing poor personal hygiene, poor water supply and poor disposal of feces in the developing countries. The point-prevalence found in one study in Indonesia was 8.6 per 1000 population per year when the recall period-prevalence at two weeks was 12.1 per 1000 of population. But the incidence in the study period was 189.4 per 1000 population per year.[2] Feces contaminate water supplies in the developing countries, increasing both the prevalence and incidence of diarrhea. A similar situation prevailed in the developed countries 70 years ago but the situation improved when there was improved sanitation, nutrition and the level of socio-economic status.

Diarrhea occurs either as acute diarrhea or chronic diarrhea. The former has more significance in the causation of mortality than the latter, but both cause severe morbidity.

Acute diarrhea is very common in the first five years of life and the incidence decreases with age. The peak age incidence is 6-12 months. In countries where summer occurs, diarrhea tends to be more common in summer, hence summer diarrhea. In some tropical countries the incidence follows rain season or fly season, but in other countries there is no definite seasonal pattern.[3]

Acute diarrhea lasts from 3-6 days per each episode, and many children in the tropics have 3-7 episodes a year.[1,4] This represents several diarrheal days a year. It is estimated that in one year up to 750 million episodes of diarrhea occur in children below the age of 5 years in Asia, Latin America and Africa. About 4-5 million children die from acute diarrhea. This is estimated as 20 deaths per 1000 population per year in children of less than 2 years of age.[1] Even in developed countries, acute diarrhea is responsible for several admissions to the hospital, ranking second to respiratory disease as the cause of non-surgical admissions. Acute diarrhea is the leading cause of death under 4 years of age and a major cause of under-nutrition.

The direct cause of death in acute diarrheal disease is dehydration and loss of electrolytes. But diarrhea also kills indirectly by causing malnutrition and reducing the body resistance to infections.

Several mechanisms contribute to malnutrition in the course of acute diarrheal disease. During the episode of diarrhea, the child loses not only water but nutrients and electrolytes. Undigested and unabsorbed nutrients are lost through feces. The cumulative effects of all the various episodes of diarrhea lead to malnutrition. Appetite is normally poor during diarrhea. This leads to reduced food intake and hence malnutrition. The custom of withholding food during diarrhea as practiced in India and Bangladesh aggravates nutritional status, leading to undernutrition and eventually to obvious malnutrition.[5] The synergism which exists between malnutrition and infection is well illustrated in the vicious circle between diarrhea and malnutrition. Diarrhea lowers the nutrition status of the child making him susceptible to infection which leads to further diarrhea. The end result is the development of protein-calorie malnutrition such as marasmus and kwashiorkor. Children with poor nutritional status are easily precipitated into malnutrition. Besides, the children with poor nutritional status get severe and prolonged diarrhea with high mortality.

Acute diarrhea is particularly common in the under-two-year-olds and is uncommon in the first few months of infancy, especially in the breast-fed infants. Breast milk protects against diarrhea through several mechanisms. First, breast milk is sterile and hence has no germs that cause diarrhea. Second, breast milk has cellular components and secretory IgA which protect against infective diarrhea. As weaning starts, diarrheal disease begins and increases in scope as the child is exposed to increasing pathogens through the alternative foods and contaminated water. Weaning coincides with the period of declining maternally acquired antibodies leaving the child unprotected. The incidence of diarrhea is less in exclusively breast-fed but is high in bottle-fed infants.

Chronic diarrhea is characterized by a prolonged course. It is common in malnourished children. Pathogens like *Entamoeba histolytica* and *Giardia lamblia* are known to cause chronic diarrhea. This form of diarrhea is more likely to contribute to failure-to-thrive than to death.

PREVENTION

The prevention of diarrhea requires knowledge of the causative agents and their transmission. Improved diagnostic investigations have revealed that many cases of acute diarrhea are caused by viruses; the most important viral cause is rotavirus which causes most of the cases of diarrhea in children aged 6 months to 2 year.[6,7] The other viruses causing diarrhea are Norwalk-like agents. Rotavirus is regularly found in diarrheal cases in the developing countries. But its incidence varies considerably. The discrepancies in the reported incidence are thought to be influenced by factors such as age, nutritional status, socio-economic level of the patient, geographical locality of the socio-economic status and environmental factors.[6]

The bacterial causes of acute diarrhea are Enteropathogenic *Escherichia coli*, (EPEC), Enterotoxigenic *Escherichia coli* (ETEC), *Campylobacter jejuni*, *Yersinia enterocolitica*, salmonella and shigella.[7] In certain countries, *Vibrio cholera* of El Tor strains is a major cause of diarrhea. There are also protozoal causes of diarrhea which include *Entamoeba histolytica*, *Giardia lamblia* and malaria parasites.

These etiological agents for diarrhea, apart from malaria, are transmitted by fecal-oral route, either directly by person to person or indirectly through contaminated food and water. Prevention of the disease is done by interrupting transmission. This is effected by several means, namely: The use of latrines for disposal of feces to reduce the risk of contaminating water, provision of safe water supply which is sterilized to kill any enteropathogens that might be present, improved environmental sanitation to reduce flies which spread the germs, good personal hygiene which reduces person-to-person transmission, improved food hygiene and health education to the community particularly in personal hygiene, food handling and improved home nursing skills.

Breast feeding is an important tool in the prevention of diarrhea. All efforts should be made to promote breast feeding. The dangers of artificial feeding in developing countries are well known. There are no refrigerators to store the milk in a cool environment to avoid multiplication of pathogens. Artificial milk is likely to be contaminated through contaminated water that is used to prepare the milk formula. The best way of avoiding these dangers is breast feeding. Where breast feeding is not possible then sterile techniques for reconstitution of feeding formula and sterilizing feeding bottles must be adhered to. Improved socio-economic status and improved general education are long-term strategies for prevention of diarrhea. Breast milk may not offer complete protection against rotavirus infection as high incidence has been found in breast-fed infants.[8]

Campylobacteriosis and salmonellosis can be spread by direct person to person, by fecal-oral routes and through contaminated water.

Some infections are acquired from animals and animal products; hence animal products, particularly birds' meat, should be handled and prepared scrupulously well to avoid transmission.

Vaccine against rotavirus is being tried. This will be of immense value in the prevention of rotavirus diarrhea if it proves potent. In areas where acute malaria causes diarrhea, control of malaria through control of mosquitoes is an important strategy. Vaccine against malaria parasite will prove a useful tool for prevention of diarrhea due to malaria when it becomes available.

ORAL REHYDRATION THERAPY

Death from diarrheal disease is caused by dehydration; hence dehydration is the factor that is approached in order to save the lives of the children with diarrhea. Dehydration is now effectively managed by administration of Oral Rehydration Solutions (ORS) in the new strategy of Oral Rehydration Therapy (ORT). Oral Rehydration Therapy was first formulated by WHO in 1968 for the treatment of adult patients with cholera. This therapy has now been confirmed for the treatment of diarrhea of all ages and of any cause.[9,12] There are now several commercial preparations of ORS. Many countries also use their locally made cereal-based solutions which are effective. Homemade solutions can also be made using household ingredients.

The WHO recommended composition of ORS is as follows:

Sodium Chloride	3.5Gm.
Sodium bicarbonate	2.5Gm.
Potassium chloride	1.5Gm.
Glucose	20.0Gm.

This comes as a powder and is reconstituted into a solution by dissolving in a litre of clean drinking water. Other sugars are less effective than glucose but should be used according to their availability. Sucrose, the common table sugar, can be used for homemade solutions.

ORT works on the basis that glucose absorption by the bowel remains intact despite the impairment of intestinal absorption during diarrhea and that with absorption of glucose, sodium molecules are simultaneously transported into the vascular compartment while water follows by osmotic pressure.[12]

The mother is the prime person in the administration of ORS. The mother is, therefore, instructed in the correct way of reconstituting ORS into a solution at home and its administration. The mother is also instructed in the correct way of making homemade solutions. ORT is now a primary intervention for the rehydration of diarrhea disease among young children. It can be delivered within the Primary Health Care program with emphasis and responsibility placed onto the mother for its administration as soon as diarrhea starts at home. ORT should also be emphasized at the health center and hospital outpatient clinics and supervised by health auxiliaries as the technique is very simple. It is indicated for mild and moderate dehydration and is recommended that it be started quite early in the course of diarrhea. When started early, ORT prevents the progression of dehydration into severe form; ORT is simple, inexpensive and effective. Unlike intravenous fluids, which it has now virtually replaced, ORT avoids the use of expensive instruments that are required for intravenous fluid administration; it avoids the use of expert health workers as it emphasizes the role of the mother and health auxiliary staff. ORT has saved millions of children's lives since its inception. It is estimated that ORT can save 90-95% of deaths from dehydration.[9] It prevents mild dehydration. When administered effectively, it prevents weight loss which is a feature of diarrhea. When given in conjunction with continued breast feeding, the infant's weight and nutritional status are maintained. It is a very cost-effective strategy.

For ORT to be effective, the patient should be able to drink, must be fully conscious and not in shock. Patients with severe dehydration and in shock are given intravenous (I.V.) fluid therapy instead. Also the few patients that are not improving on ORT should be given the option of I.V. fluid therapy.

Though it is an inexpensive strategy, ORS has its limitations. It has to face serious operational constraints in practical terms at village level. These militate against its full potential and applicability. ORT is also limited in that it cannot reduce morbidity due to diarrhea. The worst limitation is that it has little impact on chronic diarrhea. Bearing these in mind, other interventions are required and these were established in 1978 by World Health Organization in the form of Diarrheal Disease Control Programmes (CDD), with the objective of reducing mortality of children due to diarrhea and preventing deterioration of nutritional status of children in the course of episodes of diarrhea. In this regard, various strategies were established under the CDD programs, namely: effective management of acute diarrhea using ORT; promotion of maternal and child health care by encouraging breast feeding; through promotion of breast feeding; improvement of nutrition during pregnancy and lactation; improvement of personal hygiene; provision of immunization; promotion of environmental health through the use of good water supply; and proper disposal of feces and control of epidemic diarrhea. To date several developing countries have established their own CDD programs whose effectiveness should be evaluated.

REFERENCES

1. Snyder, J.D., and M.H. Merson. The magnitude of the global problem of acute surveillance data. Bull WHO 60:605, 1982.

2. Nazir, M., N. Pardede, and R. Ismail. The incidence of diarrheal diseases and diarrheal diseases-related mortality in rural swampy lowland area of South Sumatra, Indonesia. J Trop Pediatr 31:268, 1985.

3. Khuffash, F.A., and H.A. Majeed. Basic epidemiological aspects of acute gastroenteritis in a regional hospital in Kuwait. Annals of Trop Peds 4:113, 1984.

4. Mohandas, V., J. Unni, and M. Mathew, et al. Aetiology and clinical features of acute childhood diarrhea in an outpatient clinic in Vellore, India. Annals of Trop Peds 7:167, 1987.

5. Khan, M.U., and K. Ahmad. Withdrawal food during diarrheal: Major mechanism of malnutrition following diarrhea in Bangladesh children. J Trop Ped 32:57, 1986.

6. Seth, S.K., W. Al-Nakib, F.A. Khuffash, and H.A. Majeed. Acute diarrheal and rotavirus infection in young children in Kuwait. Annals of Trop Peds 4:117, 1984.

7. Al-Bwardy, M.A.A., S. Ramia, and A.R. Al-Frayh, et al. Bacterial, parasitic and viral enteropathogens associated with diarrhea in Saudi Children. Annals of Trop Peds 8:26, 1988.

8. Malik, A., A. Rattan, M. Ashraf Malik and I. Shukla. Rotavirus diarrheal of infancy and childhood in north Indian town – Epidemiological aspects. J Trop Peds 33:243, 1987.

9. World Health Organization. A manual for the treatment of acute diarrhea. WHO/CDD Series/80.2 Geneva: WHO, 1984.

10. Feachem, R.G., R.C. Hogan, and M.H. Merson. Diarrheal disease control: Reviews of potential interventions. Bull WHO 61:637, 1982.

11. Population Report Series L, no. 2. Oral rehydration therapy (ORT) for childhood diarrhea. Vol. viii no. 6, 1980.

12. Finberg, L., P.A. Harper, and H.E. Harrison, et al. Oral rehydration for diarrhea. J Ped 101:497, 1982.

29

IMMUNIZING THE WORLD'S CHILDREN: PROGRAM AND PROSPECTS

Gregory F. Hayden, M.D.; Carole Chan;
and Ralph H. Henderson, M.D.

PROGRAM ORIGINS: BUILDING THE COALITION

The Expanded Programme on Immunization (EPI) was initiated by the World Health Assembly in 1974. At first sponsored by the World Health Organization (WHO) alone, this program of Member States now operates with a broad-based coalition of United Nations agencies, multi- and bilateral development agencies, private and voluntary groups, and concerned individuals. National statements at meetings of the WHO Executive Board and World Health Assembly over the past decade have reflected strong member support of the EPI. More importantly, many developing countries using the program have achieved spectacular increases in immunization coverage in recent years.

International support has been essential for national progress. The United Nations Children's Fund (UNICEF) has been the major provider of vaccines and other supplies, including the equipment needed to keep vaccines potent as they are transported and stored between the place of manufacture and the place of use (the "cold chain"). The majority of bilateral development agencies and a number of United Nations agencies support the program through contributions to WHO and UNICEF, bilateral contributions made specifically for the EPI, or through cooperation in broader development initiatives.

The World Bank, the United Nations Development Program (UNDP) and the Rockefeller Foundation joined WHO and UNICEF to form the Task Force for Child Survival in 1984. The Task Force has served as an effective catalyst in mobilizing support for immunization and other primary health care initiatives. In particular, it has convened a series of successful meetings, bringing together the heads of the sponsoring agencies along with heads of bilateral development agencies and health ministers from developing countries.

Many other private and voluntary groups also support the program actively. They include the Association for the Promotion of Preventive Medicine, Paris; the International Children's Centre, Paris; Rotary International; and the Save the Children Fund in the Netherlands, the United Kingdom and the USA.

WHO has served as the coordinator and technical authority for the EPI. With collaboration from the Centers for Disease Control (USA), WHO produced prototype training materials which have been used extensively in national programs. These materials have been revised and extended to cover other primary health care interventions (child-spacing and vitamin A supplementation are current examples). WHO established the basic EPI information system which is used mainly to estimate global immunization coverage and disease incidence. WHO also issues technical papers and a quarterly newsletter, *EPI Update*, which serves to disseminate current technical information.

WHO has worked in close collaboration with UNICEF in these efforts and in introducing improved cold-chain methods and materials. During the past decade, the WHO/UNICEF partnership has made available a whole new generation of cold-chain equipment designed to meet the needs of immunization programs in developing countries. UNICEF has been particularly effective in promoting social mobilization and in eliciting financial support. Publication of the annual report on the state of the world's children has brought to the attention of world leaders the problems afflicting children in developing countries and the impact that low-cost interventions – including immunization – can have in promoting child survival and development. UNICEF has helped to publicize the dramatic success of national immunization days in Colombia in 1984, and has encouraged this philosophy and technique worldwide. National immunization days have been an important element in program acceleration activities in many areas.

Because of their basic simplicity, the delivery of immunization services provides an excellent building block for the health infrastructure. Delivering immunization along with other services allows immunization to act in synergy with these other services, maximizing the combined benefits for women and children. When children thrive, parents gain the confidence to limit the number of births to the number of children they desire, and this, in turn, provides further health benefits for mother and child.

The EPI has worked in close collaboration with the WHO Diarrheal Diseases Control Program (CDD) in developing modular training materials which can be integrated and used in a single course. These two programs have worked with the WHO Division of Family Health to develop a teaching module on child-spacing for inclusion in their training courses. In collaboration with the WHO Nutrition unit, the EPI has worked on introducing vitamin A and iodine supplementation within immunization programs serving populations at risk for these deficiencies. These activities have made the EPI an effective promoter of other essential interventions while at the same time reinforcing the priority of immunization through links with other programs.

EPI's achievements have been a major public health success. Immunization services, which reached less than 5% of children in the developing world when the program was established, now reach some 60% with a third dose of either polio or DPT vaccines (Figure 1; Table 1, next page). Each year, immunization in developing countries is preventing almost 250,000 children from becoming paralyzed with poliomyelitis and almost two million deaths from measles, neonatal tetanus and pertussis (Table 2, page 338).

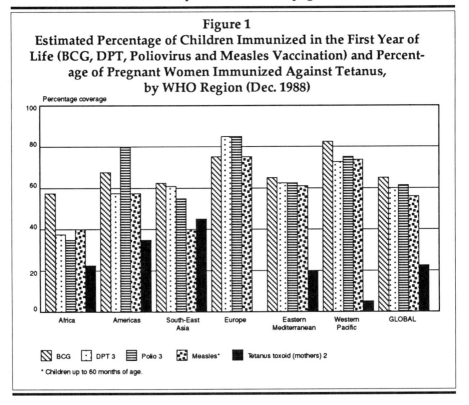

Figure 1
Estimated Percentage of Children Immunized in the First Year of Life (BCG, DPT, Poliovirus and Measles Vaccination) and Percentage of Pregnant Women Immunized Against Tetanus, by WHO Region (Dec. 1988)

Percentage coverage

BCG · DPT 3 ▤ Polio 3 ▨ Measles* ■ Tetanus toxoid (mothers) 2

* Children up to 60 months of age.

Table 1
Estimated Immunization Coverage with BCG, DPT, Poliovirus, Measles, and Tetanus Vaccines (Dec. 1988)

Country[1]	Newborns surviving to 1 year of age (millions)	Cumulative % of infants %	Immunization coverage (%)				Pregnant women
			BCG %	DPT III %	Polio III %	Measles[*] %	Tetanus II %
1. India(a)	22.56	25	72	73	64	44	58
2. Indonesia(a)	5.15	31	74	61	62	55	29
3. Nigeria(b,c)	4.59	36	37	21	21	24	17
4. Bangladesh(b)	4.15	40	14	9	8	6	7
5. Brazil(b)	4.07	45	68	57	90	55	62
6. Pakistan(b)	4 03	49	72	62	62	53	27
7. Mexico (b)	2.68	52	71	62	97	54	42
8. Ethiopia(b,c)	1 99	55	27	16	6	13	7
9. Islamic Republic of Iran(b)	1.98	57	56	74	74	76	12
10. Philippines(b,c)	1.83	59	92	73	73	68	49
11. Viet Nam(b)	1.78	61	68	61	75	60	...
12. Egypt(b)	1.78	63	72	81	81	86	12
13. Thailand(b)	1.44	64	61	48	47	34	38
14. Turkey(b)	1.41	66	34	71	70	50	...
15. Zaire(b)	1.29	67	54	36	36	39	25
16. South Africa	1.28	69	...	...	...	...	...
17. Burma(b)	1.17	70	45	23	13	14	24
18. Kenya(b,s)	1.13	71	86	75	75	60	37
19. United Republic of Tanzania(b,d)	1.07	73	94	81	65	88	54
20. Republic of Korea(b)	0.95	74	95	85	93	95	...
21. Sudan(b)	0.94	75	46	29	29	22	12
22. Algeria(b,s)	0.90	76	95	66	66	59	...
23. Colombia(b)	0.88	77	80	58	82	59	6
24. Morocco(b)	0.85	78	87	78	78	76	33
25. Argentina(b,c)	0.75	78	91	75	85	81	...
Total 25 countries	70.63	78	63	58	58	46	35
Other developing countries	19.46	22	61	48	48	46	25
Subtotal, developing countries (excluding China)	90.09	100	63	55	56	46	33
China(b,s)	19.94		85	75	77	77	...
Total, developing countries (including China)	110.03		67	60	60	52	27
Total, industrialized countries	18.11		59	66	68	76	...
Global total	128.14		66	60	61	55	23

[1] Developing countries ranked by numbers of surviving infants
(a) = 1988 coverage data
(b) = 1987 coverage data
(c) = 1986 coverage data
(d) = 1985 coverage data
(s) = Survey data
(*) Children up to 60 months of age.
... No information available.

Table 2
Estimated Annual Number of Prevented Neonatal Tetanus Deaths,
Prevented Pertussis and Measles Cases and Deaths, and Prevented
Poliomyelitis Cases, in 25 Developing Countries, Excluding China
(Dec. 1988)

	(a) Newborns	(b) Surviving infants	(c) Prevented neonatal tetanus deaths	(d) Prevented pertussis cases	(e) Prevented pertussis deaths	(f) Prevented measles cases	(g) Prevented measles deaths	(h) Prevented poliomyelitis cases
				(in thousands)				
25 largest developing countries	77,176	70,633	274	28,357	325	30,803	918	195
Other developing countries	21,464	19,558	51	6,594	75	8,546	256	45
Total, developing countries	98,640	90,191	325	34,950	400	39,349	1,174	239

(a) Based on 1987 estimated population and crude birth rates.

(b) Based on estimated number of newborns and infant mortality rate.

(c) Based on mortality estimates from surveys or reports, a vaccine efficacy of 0.95 and immunization coverage reported as of December 1988. Countries without data were arbitrarily placed in one of three neonatal tetanus mortality classes: 5, 10 or 15 per thousand live births.

(d) Based on an estimated incidence of 80% of newborns in the absence of an immunization programme, a vaccine efficacy of 0.8 for three doses, and immunization coverage reported as of December 1988.

(e) Based on mortality estimates of one-third of measles deaths, a vaccine efficacy of 0.8 for three doses, and immunization coverage reported as of December 1988.

(f) Based on an incidence estimation of 100% surviving newborns in absence of an immunization programme, a vaccine efficacy of 0.95 and immunization coverage reported as of December 1988.

(g) Based on arbitrary case fatality rates ranging from 2% to 4%, a vaccine efficacy of 0.95 and immunization coverage reported as of December 1988.

(h) Based on an estimated incidence of 5 per 1000 newborns in the absence of an immunization programme, a vaccine efficacy of 0.95 and immunization coverage reported as of December 1988.

When the program was created, few people believed that the goal of providing immunization for all children of the world by 1990 was anything but wishful thinking. Like the global smallpox eradication program before it, however, this initiative has provided a compelling demonstration of what can be accomplished when there is unanimity of purpose. Public health, political and community leaders have made this worldwide program succeed. This progress has been possible because the program is easily understood, inexpensive and relatively easy to implement, and because it brings immediate, highly visible benefits. It is good public health and good politics.

REACHING 1990: THE REMAINING BARRIERS

Can immunization coverage, which took almost 15 years to reach the 50% mark, be boosted to levels of 80% or more by 1990? Can this goal be achieved using methods that will strengthen the other elements of primary health care and that can be sustained in the foreseeable future? The long-term prospects are encouraging because the present coverage level was attained using a health infrastructure which has been built up only since the beginning of the EPI. It was never envisioned that coverage would be expanded by equal increments each year. Rather, it was expected that an initial period of slow growth would be followed by a period of rapid growth. This is, in fact, what has happened.

The program started by emphasizing training, with two major objectives: (1) To enable the development of sound national plans to which external donors could give their support, and (2) to provide a critical mass of competent immunization managers in each country. National programs were encouraged to begin operations in relatively limited areas and then to expand in a phased manner. In this way, problems of logistics as well as those involving training and supervision of peripheral staff could be recognized and solved in the initial areas, and systems permitting effective program expansion could be established or reinforced.

It is only since the mid-1980s that the majority of developing countries have had a core immunization infrastructure that allowed immunization coverage to be increased rapidly in a sustained manner. The emphasis of the global program is now on the acceleration of national programs. Coverage with a third dose of polio and DPT vaccines is lowest in Africa, the region with the least developed health infrastructure (Figure 1), but is increasing rapidly, partly as a result of initiatives begun in conjunction with the African Year of Immunization in 1986.

Unimmunized or partially immunized infants can be found in every country in the developing world. Almost half of all such infants, however, are found in five large countries – India, China, Indonesia, Bangladesh and Nigeria (Figure 2, section A). These five countries have a high commitment to universal childhood immunization, and three (India, China, and Indonesia) already have strong health infrastructures which permit high coverage levels to be reached and sustained. The infrastructures are less well developed in Nigeria and Bangladesh so that coverage levels of 80% or more may not be attained until the next decade, despite acceleration efforts. Experience has shown, however, that considerable progress is possible where the political will is strong.

A smaller but substantial proportion of all incompletely immunized infants reside in the 21 next largest developing countries (Figure 2, section B). In a limited number of these countries, the immunization programs are still in their initial stages. Ethiopia and Burma, for example, have less than 25%

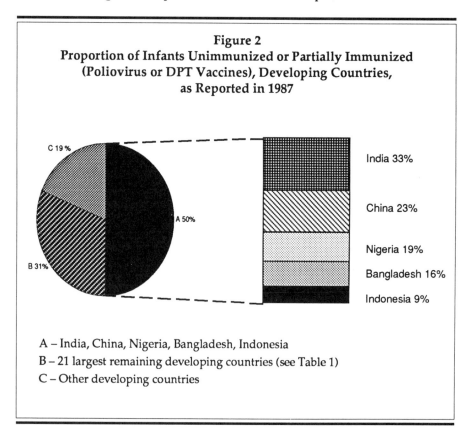

Figure 2
Proportion of Infants Unimmunized or Partially Immunized
(Poliovirus or DPT Vaccines), Developing Countries,
as Reported in 1987

C 19%

A 50%

B 31%

India 33%

China 23%

Nigeria 19%

Bangladesh 16%

Indonesia 9%

A – India, China, Nigeria, Bangladesh, Indonesia
B – 21 largest remaining developing countries (see Table 1)
C – Other developing countries

coverage for a third dose of polio and DPT vaccines. Although these are both considered large countries, together they account for only about 2.5% of developing country newborns as a whole. For this reason, the absolute number of inadequately immunized infants in these countries is much smaller than in the very large countries, such as India and China.

The final group of incompletely immunized infants is scattered among the smaller developing countries (Figure 2, section C). A number of these countries have low coverage rates, but they account for only a very small proportion of all developing country newborns. Efforts to accelerate programs in these countries are urgently needed, but will not be major determinants of coverage rates in the developing world as a whole.

Projections for 1990 forecast: An average increase of some 20% coverage in the five largest developing countries; an increase of some 15% in the 21 remaining large countries (listed in Table 1); and an increase of 15% in the other developing countries. Even with vigorous efforts, however, it will be difficult to surpass a global coverage level of 75% by 1990. As a point of reference, between July 1985 and December 1987, the reported coverage for a third dose of polio or DPT vaccines in developing countries increased by less than 10%.

Nevertheless, the goal of universal childhood immunization remains tantalizingly close to attainment. In almost all countries, more can be done to increase coverage immediately, using the health staff and facilities already in place. Many children who receive a first dose of vaccine fail to return for subsequent doses. A coverage level of 60% for a third dose of polio or DPT vaccine often means that 80% or more of children are in contact with the health system and have received a first dose. With better health education and follow-up, the majority of these children could be fully immunized using the existing staff and facilities.

Many opportunities for immunization are missed. For example, eligible children are often brought for acute illnesses to curative health facilities where immunization is not available. In Gambia, however, most maternal and child health clinics provide integrated curative and preventive care, and immunization coverage has consistently been high. Currently, measles immunization coverage is 75%, which is among the highest rates in Africa. A program review in 1981 revealed that 76% of children immunized against measles had received the vaccine during a visit for acute care, not well-child care. Among those who were eligible but had not yet been immunized, the most common reason was that the clinic attended did not provide immunizations during acute care visits.[2]

The level of measles immunization in developing countries (52%) is lower than that of DPT and polio vaccines. This is in large part due to the very recent introduction of measles vaccine in several large countries of South-East Asia. India, for example, reported measles vaccine coverage of only 1% in 1986. Reported measles coverage in India increased to 44% in 1988, compared to 73% coverage for a third dose of DPT vaccine. It should be possible to raise measles coverage quickly to levels more comparable with those for the third dose of DPT vaccine. The restriction that measles vaccine should not generally be given before the age of nine months (to avoid interference from maternal antibodies) does, however, place an important extra demand on the health services to ensure that eligible children are not lost to follow-up.

Coverage of pregnant women in the developing world with tetanus toxoid is even lower, only 27%. This is particularly disquieting because neonatal tetanus still causes some 750,000 deaths per year, second only to measles among the EPI target diseases (Table 3). The use of every contact with the

Table 3
Estimated Annual Number of Deaths from Neonatal Tetanus, Measles and Pertussis, and Annual Number of Cases of Poliomyelitis in Developing Countries, Excluding China (Dec. 1988)

	Deaths from neonatal tetanus (1)	Deaths from measles (2)	Deaths from pertussis (3)	Total deaths	Cumulative % of total deaths	Poliomyelitis cases (4)	Cumulative % of cases
	(in thousands)				%	(in thousands)	%
25 largest developing countries	590	1,263	402	2,256	79	159	75
Other developing countries	164	330	121	615	21	53	25
Total, developing countries	754	1,593	523	2,871	100	212	100

Note: Using the immunization coverage data in Table 1, the following assumptions were made:

(1)Neonatal tetanus: based on survey data or, in the absence of survey, extrapolated from countries with similar socioeconomic conditions.
(2) Measles: it is assumed that the vaccine efficacy is 95% and that all unimmunized children will contract measles. Coverage is assumed to be "zero" in countries for which data are not available.
(3)Pertussis: it is assumed that the vaccine efficacy is 80% and that 80% of unimmunized children will contract pertussis. Coverage is assumed to be "zero" in countries for which data are not available.
(4)Poliomyelitis: in view of the narrow limits of variation of results of poliomyelitis surveys, and in the absence of an immunization programme, a fixed incidence rate of 5 cases per thousand newborns is used. A vaccine efficacy of 95% is assumed. Coverage is assumed to be "zero" in countries for which data are not available.

health services to provide women of childbearing age with tetanus toxoid will help to improve the coverage, but additional strategies, including special immunization campaigns in certain high-risk areas, will be needed before immunization rates become satisfactory.

While the search for better immunization strategies continues, most national programs should give priority to improving the performance of existing staff and health facilities. This calls for intensified training with particular emphasis on assigning responsibility for every essential task and providing supervision to ensure that these tasks are carried out.

Community action is also needed. Members of the community can identify eligible children and direct them to the immunization services. They can also exert the pressure required to make these services available at times and places convenient to the community. An aroused community can exert political pressure so that a comprehensive array of primary health care services, including immunization, will be available. Other forms of community mobilization may also be appropriate. For example, national immunization days have been very successful in a number of countries. Special care must be taken, however, that acceleration efforts are compatible with sustainability. Unless the accelerated activities strengthen the permanent health care delivery mechanisms, they may actually exert a negative influence on health services development.

The increase and maintenance of immunization coverage in many developing countries depend on augmenting and sustaining outside financial support. If immunization is to be a permanent service of the health care delivery infrastructure, many developing countries will require continuing support well into the next century. A number of studies in the early 1980s estimated a global cost of US$5.00-15.00 per fully immunized child.[3] Cost variations in individual programs remain substantial, but an average figure of US$10 per fully immunized child seems reasonable when estimating future program costs. The following assumptions were used in calculating the annual program cost for the latter half of the 1990s.

1. US$10 cost per fully immunized child for a population of 50 million children immunized yearly with a third dose of polio or DPT vaccines: total cost, US$500 million per year.

2. External share of total costs, 30%: external cost, US$50 million/ year.

3. Double the above costs to account for full coverage: total cost, US$100 million/year; external cost, US$300 million/year.

4. Double the costs again to include use of new vaccines and popu-
    lation growth: total cost US$2,000 million/year; external cost,
    US$600 million/year.

The figure of US$600 million per year is a generous estimate of what
outside support might be required during the next decade, but is minuscule
compared with other international development costs. At the 1984 meeting at
which the Task Force for Child Survival was formed, international development agencies gave the assurance that, if the developing countries placed immunization high on their list of national priorities, funds would not be lacking. Up to now, external funding for the EPI has kept pace with the needs, and
prospects remain optimistic for the continuing availability of external support.

TOWARDS THE YEAR 2000

Although the year 1990 was chosen as the first target date for the EPI, it
was never intended that the program be terminated, because high immunization coverage will have to be continued. There are also other tasks for the EPI
in the 1990s, and preparations for these are already under way. The five major
areas of action that will be pursued during the coming decade are: full use of
existing vaccines; disease control; introduction of new or improved vaccines;
promotion of other primary health care interventions; and research and development.

FULL USE OF EXISTING VACCINES

Not all countries will have attained satisfactory immunization rates by
1990. Even within countries with satisfactory coverage rates, there are likely
to be pockets of poorly immunized individuals. Efforts will be continued to
accelerate progress during the coming decade to ensure that no child or
woman of childbearing age is denied the benefits of immunization. A related
challenge is to ensure that high coverage levels are sustained.

DISEASE CONTROL

The primary concern of the EPI is not immunization but disease control,
using immunization as the strategy. Disease control will be given even higher
priority during the 1990s, with special efforts being centered on poliomyelitis,
measles and neonatal tetanus.

Global poliomyelitis eradication by the year 2000 was adopted as a target
in May 1988 by the Forty-first World Health Assembly. Eradication targets for

or before the year 2000 had previously been designated by the American, European and Western Pacific Regions of WHO, and the case for global eradication was recently summarized.[4] A world without poliomyelitis would be a fitting gift from the twentieth to the twenty-first century. Poliomyelitis eradication presents an enormous challenge, however, and calls for sustained political determination as well as increased financial and technical support. This initiative requires not only achieving and sustaining high levels of immunization coverage throughout the world, but also markedly improving disease surveillance, using both clinical and laboratory methods, and improving the control and investigation of outbreaks. These requirements make poliomyelitis eradication an excellent means for strengthening national immunization programs on a wide front.

Despite the successes of the EPI, measles continues to kill more than 1.5 million children each year (Table 3). Even with better coverage, cases may continue to pose problems among infants under 9 months, the currently recommended age of immunization. Research is already under way to evaluate strains of measles vaccine (such as the Yugoslavian Edmonston-Zagreb strain) which can perhaps be administered effectively at earlier ages. At the same time, immunization strategies are being examined to see what opportunities might be available to bring this highly infectious and lethal disease under better control with the vaccine strains now in widespread use. The program has set the target of reducing the incidence of reported measles in all countries to below 40 cases per 100,000 population by 1995, a reduction of over 90% from pre-EPI levels.

The drive to control neonatal tetanus provides a direct link between those concerned with immunization and those concerned with a safe motherhood, for tetanus immunization and clean delivery practices are both effective in preventing this disease. The EPI target is to eliminate neonatal tetanus by 1995.

INTRODUCING NEW OR IMPROVED VACCINES

One of the goals in establishing the EPI was to put in place a delivery system capable of using the new vaccines resulting from current investments in research and development. Already, individual countries are adding, or are considering adding, vaccines such as yellow fever, hepatitis B and Japanese B encephalitis vaccines to their national programs. It is hoped that rotavirus vaccines and improved vaccines against typhoid, shigella and cholera may become available during the coming decade. Leprosy vaccine is currently undergoing field trials, and active research is continuing on vaccine against many other diseases.

Vaccines now used in the EPI are being improved. New manufacturing techniques have permitted the introduction of an improved inactivated polio vaccine, and oral polio vaccines with a diminished potential to cause paralysis and better efficacy in tropical environments are a realistic possibility. A less reactogenic vaccine against pertussis is being actively evaluated, and the Edmonston-Zagreb strain of measles vaccine is being tested among 4 to 6 month-old infants. During the 1990s, the EPI will continue to advocate the widespread application of new or improved vaccines of public health significance.

PROMOTING OTHER PRIMARY HEALTH CARE PRACTICES

The program's coverage of infants and their mothers makes it imperative to promote other primary health care practices which are compatible with the EPI delivery system and which can also contribute to the health of these individuals. These practices include improved maternal and child nutrition, diarrheal disease control, appropriate birth-spacing, and vitamin A and iodine supplementation in selected populations.

RESEARCH AND DEVELOPMENT

Research and development will be a major EPI priority in the 1990s. When the program was first established, it was believed that the available vaccines, equipment, and knowledge about immunization were already sufficient to make it a success. The main emphasis was therefore placed on the application of existing knowledge. Even so, research and development have been a part of the EPI from the beginning because it quickly became apparent that the materials and methods that had served the industrialized countries so well had to be adapted for use in the developing countries. Equipment for the cold chain was improved, time/temperature monitors for vaccines were introduced, more efficient immunization schedules were proposed, and a more appropriate policy regarding contraindications to immunization was adopted.[5]

The subjects and areas for research and development are, however, multiplying. In part, this is due to the advent of new vaccines and new technologies, but it is also due to the steady growth of immunization programs in developing countries, which has revealed many of the limits of our current knowledge of immunization. Important questions have been raised concerning the approaches needed to ensure optimal control of the EPI target diseases.

The EPI will therefore focus on applied research encompassing biotechnology and epidemiology, which will complement the more basic research being carried out through other WHO programs (including the WHO Vaccine Development Program, the WHO Basic Vaccinology Program, the UNDP/World Bank/WHO Special Program for Research Training in Tropical Diseases, the Special Program of Research Development and Research Training in Human Reproduction, and the Diarrheal Diseases Control Program). Research and development activities of the EPI will play an essential role in guiding program actions over the coming decade.

CONCLUSION

The EPI has been a major public health success. Immunization services were virtually non-existent in developing countries in 1974, but in less than 15 years, a public health revolution has quietly taken place. National immunization services are now providing some 60% of infants in developing countries with a third dose of either polio or DPT vaccines, thereby preventing each year about 250,000 children from becoming paralyzed with poliomyelitis and almost two million deaths from measles, neonatal tetanus and pertussis. Social value systems have been changed so that immunization is now recognized as a high priority by both national and international leaders. EPI provides a compelling demonstration of what can be accomplished when there is unanimity of purpose. Such unanimity has been possible because the program is inexpensive, easily understood, and relatively easy to implement, and because it brings immediate, highly visible benefits.

Present estimates suggest, however, that only 75% of infants in developing countries will be covered by 1990. Efforts to better that figure must be continued beyond that year in order to: accelerate progress in countries which have still not attained full coverage; sustain full immunization coverage in the remaining countries; and eliminate EPI's target diseases as public health problems. EPI can be used as a springboard for the promotion and delivery of other primary health care interventions, and represents an important stepping stone toward the goal of health for all by the year 2000. EPI must pursue research and development in support of these activities, and introduce new vaccines as soon as they become appropriate for public health use.

REFERENCES

1. Grant, J.P. The State of the World's Children 1988. New York: Oxford University Press, 1988 (published for UNICEF).

2. Expanded Programme on Immunization. Programme evaluation. Weekly Epidemiological Record 56:276-278, 1981.

3. Henderson, R.H. Vaccine-preventable diseases of children: The problem. In: Protecting the world's children: Vaccines and immunization. Bellagio Conf, 13-15 Mar 1984. New York: Rockefeller Found, 1984, pp. 1-15.

4. Hirman, A.R., et al. The case for global eradication of poliomyelitis. Bulletin of the World Health Organization 65:835-840,1987.

5. Galazka, A.M., et al. Indications and contraindications for vaccines used in the Expanded Programme on Immunization. Bull WHO 62:357-366, 1984.

30

ACUTE RESPIRATORY INFECTIONS

LATA KUMAR, M.D.;
B.N.S. WALIA, M.D., D.C.H., F.A.M.S.;
SURJIT SINGH, M.D.

Acute respiratory infections (ARI) are responsible for high morbidity in children all over the world. Mortality due to ARI is unacceptably high in developing countries where the figure may reach 1000 or more per 100,000 live-births, compared to 30-40 per 100,000 live-births in industrialized nations.[1-5] Poverty, malnutrition, ignorance, lack of and underutilization of health facilities, and predominance of bacterial etiology of pneumonia are considered responsible for this difference.[6,7]

ARI comprise approximately 50% of all illness in children under 5 years of age and 30% in children in the age group 5-12 yrs.[8] Approximately 30% of all outpatient consultations and 25% of all admissions in pediatric units of developing countries are for ARI.[6,7] Most infections are limited to the upper respiratory tract, but about 5% involve the lower respiratory tract. The latter are potentially fatal. While the incidence of ARI is almost the same the world over (i.e., 5-7 episodes per child per year in urban areas and 3-5 in rural areas), mortality rates per 100,000 population are high in Africa (103.2) and Asia (87.2) as compared to North America (30.5).[9-12] Considerable variation exists in proportion of deaths from ARI to deaths from all causes in various age groups in different parts of the world.[12]

CLASSIFICATION OF ARI

ARI can be classified on anatomical bases as upper respiratory infection (URI: common colds, sinusitis, pharyngitis, tonsillitis, otitis media), laryngotracheobronchitis and epiglottitis, acute bronchitis, bronchiolitis and pneumonia.[8]

However, this traditional classification is not helpful for management-oriented decisions at the field level, especially in developing countries. An expert group of the World Health Organization (WHO) has proposed that ARI be classified on the basis of clinical severity as mild, moderate or severe based on 3 simple clinical manifestations: respiratory rate > 50/minute, presence of chest indrawing, and inability to drink (vide infra).[13]

ETIOLOGY AND CLINICAL MANAGEMENT OF ARI

Most of the ARI are restricted to the upper respiratory tract. Well over 90% of these are caused by viruses.[8] Most pneumonia on the other hand is of bacterial etiology in developing countries.[6,7] The viral and bacterial etiologic agents of common ARI are listed in Table 1 (next page).

A. **Common Cold (Coryza):** The clinical picture resulting from different etiologic agents is not pathognomonic. However, the influenza and the para-influenza viruses cause a severe illness whereas the illness caused by rhinovirus is milder.[8] Treatment is supportive.

B. **Acute Otitis Media:** It is generally agreed that appropriate antimicrobial therapy should be instituted for all cases of otitis media, even though some authors opine that the infection may be self-limiting.[14,15] Viruses are being isolated increasingly from middle ear effusions and they have been shown to cause direct mucosal damage.[16] Antimicrobials (amoxicillin/co-trimoxazole) should be given for 10-14 days. Most children have significant improvement within 48-72 hours of initiation of therapy. Persistence of severe otalgia, fever and signs of toxicity indicate the need for prompt tympanocentesis and a change in antimicrobial therapy if necessary.[17] Antihistamines and decongestants do not assist resolution of acute otitis media, but may produce unpleasant side effects like drowsiness, irritability and restlessness.

C. **Acute Sinusitis:** Diagnosis of sinusitis, though infrequently made due to lack of specific signs and symptoms, is entertained in 0.5-5.0% of cases presenting as acute upper respiratory infections.[18] Antimicrobial therapy in acute sinusitis is necessary because it reduces the chances of orbital and intracranial complications and helps in the rapid resolution of infection.[19] However, if there is persistence of pain or fever, sinus aspiration is indicated.

D. **Sore Throat (Acute Pharyngitis/Tonsillitis):** An overwhelming majority of sore throats are viral in origin. Throat swab isolation rates of beta-hemolytic streptococcus (BHS) group A, in children with sore throats vary from 10-33%, but are commonly reported as approximately 15%.[20] In viral sore throats the lymph nodes are usually firmer and tenderness is less marked. Petechiae and follicular pus spots on fauces favor bacterial etiology. BHS infection has

Table 1
ARI of Viral Origin

COMMON COLD (CORYZA):	rhinovirus, adenovirus, enteroviruses, influenza & para-influenza viruses.
ACUTE SINUSITIS & ACUTE OTITIS MEDIA:	(Same as above)
SORE-THROAT:	adenovirus, influenzavirus, enteroviruses, parainfluenza virus, coxsackie virus
INFECTIOUS CROUP: (mainly laryngotracheitis)	parainfluenza virus, adenovirus
BRONCHIOLITIS:	respiratory syncitial virus
PNEUMONIA:	respiratory syncitial virus, parainfluenza virus, influenza virus, rhinovirus

ARI of Bacterial Origin

ACUTE SINUSITIS & ACUTE OTITIS MEDIA:	*Streptococcus pneumoniae, Hemophilus influenza, Branhamella catarrhalis.*
SORE THROAT:	Beta Hemolytic *Streptococcus* Gr.A
INFECTIOUS CROUP:	*Corynebacterium diphtheria, Hemophilus influenza, Staphylococcus aureus* (diphteria, epiglottitis, bacterial tracheitis)
PERTUSSIS:	*Bordetella pertussis**
PNEUMONIA:	*Streptoccus pneumoniae, Hemophilus influenza, Staphylococcus aureus.*

*Vaccine preventable but continue to occur in developing countries due to inadequate immunization coverage.

a more acute onset, whereas involvement of other mucous membranes (e.g., nose, eye) is more common in viral infections.[21] However, distinction between the two may, at times, be difficult if not impossible. In the tropics BHS infection may develop in children younger than four years.The drug of choice is penicillin and duration of therapy at least 10 days.[22] Shorter courses of therapy fail to eradicate the organism and predispose to recurrences of infection. In a prospective evaluation of the prescribing practices of various categories of doctors, we found that there was widespread ignorance as regards the choice of antimicrobial agent and duration of therapy in BHS sore throat. Less than 12% of the consultant pediatricians were aware of the mandatory 10-day antimicrobial therapy on questionnaire analysis, while the responses on prescription audit were even less.[23] The widespread fear of anaphylactic reaction hampers the greater acceptance of penicillin as agent of choice. We would like to emphasize that these reactions occur in less than 1 out of 10,000 injections and need not be fatal if resuscitation is prompt.

E. **Infectious Croup:** The croup syndrome is a life-threatening emergency characterized by inspiratory stridor, cough and hoarseness. Acute laryngotracheitis, epiglottitis, diphtheria and bacterial tracheitis are the important causes of infectious croup, of which the latter three need specific antimicrobial therapy. Maintenance of adequate airway is of paramount importance.

F. **Pertussis:** Pertussis remains an important respiratory illness in developing countries. Antimicrobials (e.g., erythromycin, chloramphenicol, tetracycline) are indicated during the catarrhal stage to abort/attenuate the attack and during the paroxysmal stage to render the patient noninfectious.It has been the general belief that antimicrobials do not affect the course or severity of disease once the patients have reached paroxysmal stage. A recent study, however, has shown that administration of erythromycin to children with pertussis up to 14 days from onset (most of them having reached paroxysmal stage), reduced the number of whoops as compared to placebo-treated groups.[24] Some recommend the use of salbutamol (0.3-0.5mg/kg/day) in life-threatening croup.[25]

G. **Bronchiolitis:** Bronchiolitis is a common acute lower respiratory tract infection of the small airways seen in children 2 months - 2 years of age. Respiratory syncytial virus (RSV) is the main etiologic agent but other viruses (e.g., adenovirus) can also produce this syndrome. Supportive care is sufficient. In severe cases ventilatory support may be required. An antiviral drug, ribavirin, has shown promising results and may be indicated in cases where bronchiolitis affects a pulmonary cripple or an infant suffering from congenital heart disease.[26]

H. **Pneumonia:** Most pneumonia occurring in developed countries of the world is attributed to non-bacterial agents of which viruses are the most important.[6,7] In the developing countries, on the other hand, bacterial infections are responsible for at least two-thirds of all cases of pneumonia.[6,7] This information is based on data from lung aspirates obtained from hospitalized children in seven countries – Brazil, Chile, Gambia, India, Nigeria, Papua New Guinea and the Philippines. *Streptococcus pneumoniae* (pneumococcus) and *Hemophilus influenza (H.influenza)* were the most common isolates.[27] Our data indicate that in India *Staphylococcus aureus (Staph aureus)* is also a common causative organism in children, especially in pneumonias that follow infections like influenza and measles.[28]

Precise contribution of bacteria in the etiology of pneumonia is difficult to determine for many reasons. Isolation rates of the etiologic organisms in blood culture are low. Culture of a bacterial pathogen from the upper respiratory tract is no evidence that the organism is responsible for pneumonia. Lung puncture is not routinely indicated in most cases. Rapid diagnostic tests (latex agglutination, coagglutination) are expensive and not easily available.[6,7]

Penicillin serum levels achieved after procaine penicillin administration once a day are effective against pneumococcus (even against strains with reduced sensitivity to penicillin, MIC 0.1-1 mcg/ml) and *H.influenza* (MIC usually 0.1-1 mcg/ml).[13] Procaine penicillin, therefore, is the agent of choice for treatment of pneumonia at any level of primary health care services. When intramuscular agents are not feasible, an oral antimicrobial may be selected. Co-trimoxazole is preferred because it is effective against pneumococcus, *H.influenza* and *Staph aureus*, is cheap, can be given twice a day and is well tolerated.[13] However, it has not been used very frequently in neonates and young infants. Use of co-trimoxazole may induce resistance to antimalarials such as sulfadoxine and pyrimethamine in endemic malarial areas. Amoxicillin (or ampicillin) is the drug of second choice because it is less effective and more expensive than co-trimoxazole. Oral phenoxymethyl penicillin (penicillin-V) has little effect on *H.influenza* and, therefore, is not recommended.

At present most staphylococcal infections (90-95%), whether community-acquired or hospital-acquired, are caused by organisms resistant to penicillin. Therefore, initiation of therapy should be with the semisynthetic beta-lactamase resistant penicillin (i.e., methicillin, nafcillin or oxacillin).[21] Simultaneous administration of gentamicin for the first 2-3 days may have some synergistic effect.

I. **Measles:** Measles continues to be the most common exanthem in developing countries. The average annual incidence of measles in children under 5 years of age is about 150 cases per 1000 children. The average case fatality rate is 2-3% (range 1-16%), of which 30-50% is due to pneumonia.[29] There is an urgent need for systematic studies to identify causative bacteria of post-measles pneumonia. In our experience *Staph aureus* is the most common recognizable bacterial invader in such patients.[28-30]

SUPPORTIVE THERAPY IN ARI

Supportive therapy may be required in some cases of ARI.[13] Evidence as regards its effectiveness has not been tested by controlled trials. Therefore, ineffective supportive measures (e.g., steam, cough suppressants, expectorants, nasal decongestants, mucolytics, anti-histamines) need not be encouraged. However, care should be taken to ensure that fluid intake is adequate and breast feeding is continued; avoid forced feeding. The child should be nursed in a neutral environmental temperature. Paracetamol (10-15 mg/kg/dose orally) should be given every 6 hours if axillary temperature exceeds 38.5°C. Sponging with cold water is best avoided. Oxygen is administered (by intranasal catheter or mask) if respiratory rate is more than 70 per minute, or if child has a wheeze or cyanosis.[13]

THE WHO STANDARD CASE MANAGEMENT PROTOCOL AND THE ARI PROGRAM

It is obvious that if the high mortality due to pneumonia in developing countries is to be reduced, the diagnosis and treatment must be available in the primary health care setting.[13] The WHO Program for the control of ARI was established in 1982 when the 35th World Health Assembly adopted resolution 35.25 approving the organizations' Seventh General Program of Work, covering the period 1984-89. Because of the enormous global impact of ARI, first priority has been assigned to the problem of high mortality among young children in the least developed countries. The overall objectives of the program are to reduce the morbidity and mortality from ARI, the major emphasis being on the prevention of death from pneumonia. There has been a growing recognition in recent years that ARI control must be an essential part of primary health care and child survival programs.[31]

The WHO and UNICEF have recommended ARI control programs comprising health education, standard case management (with objective of reducing mortality on short-term basis) and immunization. Standard case management consists of discrimination of severity, use of antimicrobials in moderate cases at village level and referral of severe cases (Table 2, next page; and Table 3, page 357). These recommendations for case management were based on the results of two pioneering studies.[32,33] Leventhal studied clinical signs and chest x-ray findings in American children with respiratory illness.[32] Shann took up pediatric outpatients with cough in Papua New Guinea.[33] The findings of these 2 studies in very different populations were very similar – tachypnea was the best clinical predictor of pneumonia and a history of rapid breathing was almost as good as actually counting the respiratory rate. In the Papua New Guinea study a respiratory rate of more than 50/minute was found to be the best definition of tachypnea. Evidence from the latter study also suggested that chest indrawing indicated more reliably (than tachypnea, fever or crepitations), which children need admission to the hospital.

Expert groups to the WHO have prepared technical guidelines on case management, training modules, educational aids and an operational manual for program managers. Since 1987, a number of countries have established national ARI control programs, formulated technical policies, and begun the requisite training of their health staff.

The program has two main components: Health Services Component (comprising control strategies, development of materials for program implementation, planning and implementation of national ARI control, training, monitoring and evaluation), and Research Component (comprising intervention trials, clinical and etiologic studies, indoor air pollution studies and vaccine development). The former is concerned with application of already available methods and strategies for the treatment and prevention of ARI in children while the latter is directed at discovering new and better methods and approaches for control.

Training modules for senior managers and mid-level managers have been developed and field-tested in several countries. Their incorporation and integration with immunization and diarrheal disease control programs have also been tested. Our institution participated in field testing of this material developed by WHO.

INTERVENTION STUDIES IN ARI

When the WHO initiated the ARI program, it was widely believed that little could be done to reduce childhood mortality from pneumonia in developing countries. In 1982, a group of epidemiologists convened by WHO formulated a design for research into the feasibility and impact on childhood mortality of a prototype ARI intervention that could be carried out by community health workers following a standard case management protocol.(Table 4, page 358) This protocol based the management of a child with cough on three signs: inability to drink, chest indrawing and fast breathing. Further work showed that tachypnea is the best indicator for initiating antimicrobials while chest indrawing is the best indicator for inpatient treatment.[32,33]

Table 2
ARI Classification to be Applied by the Community Health Worker
(less than 6 months training)

MILD ARI
- Cough, hoarseness, wheeze or fever with no fast breathing (less than 50/min)
- Stridor that goes away when the child is at rest (not crying or upset)
- Red throat with or without exudate
- Blocked or runny nose
- Earache or ear discharge (can be referred to first health care facility)

Treatment: Supportive measures only. No antimicrobials

MODERATE ARI
- Fast breathing (over 50/min), with cough, wheeze or fever but no chest indrawing

Treatment: Antimicrobials at home plus supportive measures

SEVERE ARI
- Cough or wheeze, plus chest indrawing
- Cough, plus chest indrawing
- Cough with wheeze, plus very fast breathing (over 70/min)

Treatment: Referral and antimicrobials

Two projects, one in Punjab (India) and the other in Papua New Guinea, had provided a basis for this work. Experience in both projects suggested that antimicrobial treatment of pneumonia in the community by primary health care workers could lower case fatality rates.[34,35]

Ten intervention studies were initiated between 1983 and 1985. These studies have all shown that the case management protocol is simple enough to be understood and applied by community health workers and that it can significantly reduce the mortality rates from pneumonia in children. In all studies, total mortality was also reduced.[31]

TRAINING OF HEALTH WORKERS

Results of the intervention studies show that the signs and symptoms of moderate/severe ARI can be taught with ease to health workers and even the

---

Table 3
ARI Classification to be Applied at the First Referral Health Facility

MILD ARI:
- Cough, hoarseness, wheeze or fever, with no fast breathing (less than 50/min)
- Stridor that goes away when the child is at rest (not crying or upset)
- Red throat
- Blocked or runny nose
- Ear discharge for more than 2 weeks

Treatment: Give supportive treatment. No antimicrobials

MODERATE ARI:
- Cough & fast breathing (over 50/min), with no chest indrawing
- Wheeze and fast breathing between 50-70 per minute
- Red ear drum, or ear discharge for less than 2 weeks (or earache, if no otoscope available)
- Purulent pharyngitis with large, tender lymph nodes in the neck

Treatment: Antimicrobials at home plus supportive therapy

SEVERE ARI:
- Cough & chest indrawing but no wheeze
- Wheeze & very fast breathing (over 70/min)

Treatment: Admit & give benzyl penicillin.

VERY SEVERE ARI:
- Cough or wheeze with cyanosis or not able to drink

Treatment: Admit and give chloramphenicol. Give oxygen if child is cyanosed, or has wheeze with respiratory rate over 70/min.

Table 4
Intervention Studies in ARI*

Location	Study Design	Baseline IMR[1]	Intervention Besides Case Management		Case Detection		Pneumonia Treatment		
			Immunization	CDD[2]	Case Finding	ARI Maternal Education	Primary Treatment	First Line Drug	Referral Care
Haryana, India Low birth weight study – 1982-84	Concurrent control	106	Increased	Started	Active	Yes	CHW[3]	Oral Penicillin	None
Jumla, Nepal 1986-87	Concurrent control	200	Remained Low	Absent	Active	Yes	CHW	Co-Tri-moxazole	None
Abbottabad, Pakistan 1985-87	Concurrent control	90-100	Increased	Started	Active	Yes	CHW or Clinic	Co-Tri-moxazole	Poor Access
Bohol, Philippines 1984-87	Concurrent control	49-63	Increased	Present	Passive	No	Clinic only	Co-Tri-moxazole	Yes
Bagamoyo, Tanzania 1983-87	Concurrent control	137	Increased	Started	Passive	Yes	CHW or Clinic	Co-Tri-moxazole	Yes
Kathmandu, Nepal 1984-87	Before & After	162	Increased	Started	Active	Yes	CHW	Ampicillin	Limited Utilization
Kediri, Indonesia 1986-87	Before & After	154	Increased	Present	Active	Yes	CHW	Co-Tri-moxale	Poor Access
Haryana, India 1985-87	Concurrent control	100	Increased	Present	Active	Yes	CHW	Co-Tri-moxazole	Yes

* Modified from: Case management of acute respiratory infections in children: Intervention Studies. WHO/ARI/88.2

1. Infant Mortality Rate
2. Control of Diarrheal Disease
3. Community Health Worker

mothers.[31] The adoption of this approach enables the transfer of skills and knowledge to health auxiliaries with no need for a stethoscope, chest x-ray or laboratory investigations. Standard case management has demonstrated that community health workers can identify and treat moderate ARI and refer severe ARI. The Haryana study[36] clearly shows that the health workers' use of antimicrobials in ARI was rational. In mild ARI the usage rate of co-trimoxazole was less than 2%, while in moderate ARI the usage rate was as high as 88.8%. In severe ARI, however, the use of co-trimoxazole was variable because many of these children were either referred or treated with other antimicrobials. It was also demonstrated that the drug was being used in correct dose and for an appropriate duration.[36]

The integration of ARI programs with MCH services would require minimal additional inputs, and is likely to enhance considerably the capability and credibility of the health workers in the community. The evaluation of this program can be combined successfully with immunization and control of diarrheal disease.

PREVENTION OF ARI

Though the standard case management approach is effective in significantly reducing ARI mortality, long-term control of morbidity and further reduction in mortality is possible only through prevention of ARI. However, the existing data base for initiating concrete preventive measures is not as sound as for control of mortality through appropriate case management. Environmental and host factors have been incriminated.[7,29] Some of these are well defined and amendable to simple interventions (e.g., control of atmospheric pollution). Most of the studies on prevention of ARI are not controlled for various confounding variables.

Among the vaccine-preventable serious ARI, the benefits of diphtheria, pertussis and measles immunization are well established.[29] It has been calculated that measles immunization at 9-11 months of age, with 80-90% coverage and 90% seroconversion rate, can avert 59-67% of measles cases and deaths, and 20-25% of ARI deaths in children under 5 years of age.[29] The two newer vaccines (23-valent pneumococcal polysaccharide vaccine and *H. influenza* type "b" vaccine) however, are not very effective in producing a sustained immune response in the population most at risk, i.e., preschool children. Moreover, there is evidence that a significant proportion of pneumonia due to *H. influenza* in the developing countries may be caused by non-typable strains which would, in any case, not be covered by the conventional vaccine.[6,7,35] Exciting possibilities to improve the immunogenicity of these vaccines in younger children are under study.

Breast feeding has been promoted as an effective intervention reducing ARI morbidity and mortality.[29] As far as malnutrition is concerned, those with moderate and severe forms have a 15-19 times increased risk of acquiring moderate/severe ARI and a 4-13 times increased risk of ARI-associated death.[29] Vitamin A deficiency also predisposes preschool children to 1.8 times increased risk of ARI.[37] Similarly, low birth weight (LBW) is a risk factor as regards mortality from ARI.[38] And as the incidence of LBW babies is high in developing countries, efforts directed towards LBW reduction would indirectly help reduce ARI mortality. Infants should not be taken to congregations and fairs as this increases risk of exposure to infected individuals. Harmful practices like instillation of oil in nostrils and feeding of butter oil (ghee) may lead to lipoid pneumonia and should be avoided.

Studies from the West show that air pollution was associated with an increased incidence of acute lower respiratory tract infection.[29] Similarly, indoor air pollution secondary to use of biomass fuels (e.g., wood, cattle dung, crop residue) for cooking has been reported by some workers to be a contributory cause in ARI.[7,8,29] Our studies, however, do not support these latter findings.[39] Data from developed countries also indicate that passive smoking may predispose a child to respiratory illness. Children of parents who smoke in the house have a 1.5-2.0 times increased risk of bronchitis and pneumonia in comparison to children of non-smoking parents.[8] Overcrowding has also been related to a high incidence of ARI. It is obvious that most of these factors are intimately related to the socioeconomic milieu of the population and simple, specific interventions may not always be possible.

REFERENCES

1. Denny, F.W., and F.A. Loda. Acute respiratory infections are the leading cause of death in children in developing countries. Am J Trop Med Hyg 35:1,1986.

2. Cockburn, W.C., and F. Assad. Some observations on the communicable disease as public health problem. Bull WHO:1,1973.

3. Bulla, W., and K.L. Hitze. Acute respiratory infections: A review. Bull WHO 56:481,1978.

4. World Health Organization. Clinical management of acute respiratory infections in children – A WHO memorandum. Bull WHO 59:707,1981.

5. Pio, A. Acute respiratory infections in children in developing countries: An international point of view. Ped Inf Dis J 5:179, 1986.

6. Kumar, L. Acute respiratory infection: Current status. Indian Ped 25:595,1988.

7. Stansfield, S.M. Acute respiratory infections in the developing world: Strategies for prevention, treatment and control. Ped Inf Dis J 6:622, 1987.

8. Phelan, P.D., L.I. Landau, and A. Olinsky. Respiratory illness in children. Oxford: Blackwell Scientific Publications, 1988, pp. 29-50.

9. Datta-Banik, N.D., R. Krishna, and S.I.S. Mane, et al. A longitudinal study of morbidity and mortality pattern of children under the age of five years in an urban community. Indian J Med Res 57:948, 1969.

10. Kamath, K.R., and R.A.Feldman, et al. Infection and disease in a group of South Indian families. II General morbidity patterns in families and family members. Am J Epi 89:375,1969.

11. Gupta, K.B., and B.N.S. Walia. A longitudinal study of morbidity in children in a rural area of Punjab. Indian J Ped 47:297, 1980.

12. Narain, J.P. Epidemiology of acute respiratory infections. Indian J Ped 54:153, 1987.

13. World Health Organization. Case management of acute respiratory infections in children in developing countries. Report of a Working Group Meeting. Geneva: WHO, Apr 3-6, 1984.

14. Van Buchen, F.L., J.H.M. Dunk, and M.S. Vant Hof. Therapy of acute otitis media; myringotomy, antibiotics or neither. Lancet 2:983, 1981.

15. McCracken, G.H. Antimicrobial therapy for acute otitis media. Ped Inf Dis 3:383, 1984.

16. Nelson, J.D. Changing trends in the microbiology and management of acute otitis media and sinusitis. Ped Inf Dis 5:749, 1986.

17. Bluestone, C.D. Update on antimicrobial therapy for otitis media and sinusitis in children. Cutis 36:7, 1985.

18. Siegel, J.D. Diagnosis and management of acute sinusitis in children. Ped Inf Dis 6:95, 1987.

19. Wald, E.R. Acute sinusitis in children. Ped Inf Dis 2:61, 1983.

20. Holmberg, S.D., and G.A. Faich. Streptococcal pharyngitis and acute rheumatic fever in Rhode Island. JAMA 250:2307, 1983.

21. Kumar, L., and V. Kumar. Clinical management of acute respiratory infections in children. Indian Ped 21:64, 1984.

22. Congeni, B.L. An approach to the child with pharyngitis. Primary Care 8: 571, 1981.

23. Singh, S., L. Kumar, and V. Kumar. Prescribing practices in childhood sore throat. Indian Ped 25; 1149, 1988.

24. Berquist, S.O., S. Bernander, and H. Dahnsjo, et al. Erythromycin in the treatment of pertussis: A study of bacteriologic and clinical effects. Ped Inf Dis 6:458, 1987.

25. Krantz, I., S.R. Norrby, B. Trollfors, and V.S. Salbutamol. Placebo for treatment of pertussis. Ped Inf Dis 4: 438, 1985.

26. Pollock, I. Treatment of respiratory syncytial virus infections. Indian J Ped 54:613, 1987.

27. Shann, F. Etiology of severe pneumonia in children in developing countries. Ped Inf Dis 5:247, 1986.

28. Kumar, L., V. Kumar, and S.K. Mitra, et al. Styaphylococcal lung disease in children. Indian Ped 11; 793, 1974.

29. Singhi, S., and P. Singhi. Prevention of acute respiratory infections. Indian J Ped 54: 161, 1987.

30. Kumar, L. Severe acute lower respiratory tract infection: Etiology and management. Indian J Ped 54: 189, 1987.

31. World Health Organization. Programme for the control of acute respiratory infections. 1987 Programme Report. WHO/ARI/88.1.

32. Leventhal, J.M. Clinical predictors of pneumonia as a guide to ordering chest roentgenograms. Clin Ped 21:730, 1982.

33. Shann, F., K. Hart, and D. Thomas. Acute lower respiratory tract infection in children: Possible criteria for selection of patients for antibiotic therapy and hospital admission. Bull WHO 62: 749, 1984.

34. McCord, C., and A.A. Kielmann. A successful programme for medical auxiliaries treating childhood diarrhoea and pneumonia. Trop Doctor 8: 220, 1978.

35. Shann, F., M. Gratten, and S. Germer, et al. Aetiology of pneumonia in children in Goroka Hospital, Papau New Guinea. Lancet 2: 537, 1984.

36. Kumar, V., N. Raina, and A. Kaur. Acute respiratory infections: Control intervention trials in children in Haryana, India. Unpublished data.

37. Sommer, A., J. Katz, and I. Tarwotjo. Increased risk of respiratory disease and diarrhoea in children with pre-existing mild vitamin A deficiency. Am J Clin Nutr 40:1090, 1984.

38. Datta, N. Acute respiratory infections in low birth-weight infants. Indian J Ped 54:171, 1987.

39. Walia, B.N.S., S.K. Gambhir, and S. Singhi, et al. Socio-economic and ecologic correlates of acute respiratory infections in pre-school children. Indian Ped 25;607, 1988.

31

CHILD SURVIVAL

F. JOHN BENNETT, M.B., CH.B., D.P.H., F.F.C.M.

INTRODUCTION

"Child Survival" is a call to action – an attempt to arouse the world to end its apathy toward the needless suffering and death of millions of children. It has become the battle cry of so many programs and projects that now it can be called a movement. The movement has in fact raised the awareness of the world, and of governments, but as yet awareness is less in communities and individuals to the plight of small children dying of conditions which are preventable; preventable if only there were a universal concern by adults and a conscious realization of their power to do something to improve survival rates.

This concept of "Child Survival" started gaining momentum with analysis of figures of infant deaths at the beginning of the 1980s decade. James Grant,[1] the executive director of UNICEF, later described the situation in *The State of the World's Children* 1981-82 as "another year of quiet emergency, of 40,000 children quietly dying each day; of 100 million children quietly going to sleep hungry at night; of ten million children quietly becoming disabled in mind or body; of 200 million 6-11 year-old children quietly watching other children go to school; of one-fifth of the world's people quietly struggling for life itself." The evidence no longer confined to statistical terms was now being couched in journalist's dramatic language to bring home the fact that something drastic was needed. Nothing short of a revolution was needed, a revolution in man's feelings for children – a child survival revolution. Analysis clearly showed that deaths were largely due to diarrheal disease and consequent dehydration; immunizable diseases, especially measles; and malnutrition.

This idea of a revolution then gathered strength from the fact that effective techniques were already available. These were *Growth* monitoring, *Oral* rehydration therapy, *Breast* feeding and *Immunization;* the acronym, GOBI, was coined. Cynics however said "survival for what - for disability, malnutrition?" and so the concept of child survival was extended to "Child Survival and Development (CSD)." Many pediatricians, however, prefer to think of their objective as "Child Health" and not "Child Survival." In 1984 the now well-known annual UNICEF document,[2] *State of the World's Children,* declared that worldwide support had been gathering behind the idea of a revolution which could save the lives of seven million children each year and protect health and growth of millions more and help slow population growth.

The word "revolution" added in 1983 to make the slogan "Child Survival and Development Revolution" was soon dropped. However, the concept has grown and become more revolutionary as it gathers more weapons and allies and even questions the policies and philosophy of international development systems such as the International Monetary Fund. However, as the loan repayments and spending on arms increase, more political will or determination will be required to give Child Survival the necessary priority for funds. Criticism of the acronym GOBI and of the strategy of a limited number of potentially vertical programs was made as it was felt to be cutting across the Primary Health Care integrated approach, even though integration of EPI/ CDD/MCH/FP/EDP are not as integrated as was hoped. To increase the development as well as the survival elements and broaden the approach, 3 F's were added – food supplementation (which soon gave way to the better aim of food security), family spacing, and female education; although these were recognized as more costly and more difficult.

MORTALITY AND SURVIVAL: WHICH CHILDREN DIE?

Child mortality (divided into infants and 1-4 year-old children) and geographic inequalities are usually stressed first in drawing attention to the plight of children. Child Survival targets have been established by international organizations and by individual donor-sponsored programs and projects and by many countries, districts and municipalities, for example, countries in 1980 with an infant mortality rate of 100 or above to reduce their IMR to 50 by the year 2000. Figures for 1985[3] bring out the reality: Of every 100 children born in Africa, 12 die before age 1 and 20 before age 5. Figures for Asia were 10 and 15, respectively, and for developed countries between one and two. Of the 10 million infants who died in 1985, 25% were in Africa, 48% in Asia, and only 3% in developed countries. Of the 5 million dying aged 1-4 years, 31% were in Africa, 49% in Asia, and 0.8% in developed countries. Fifty-three percent of all deaths in Africa in 1985 were children under 5. The corresponding figure for developed countries was 3%. The percentage of the world's births in 1985 by region was 17.7% Africa, 36.1% Asia, 7.5% Near East, 15.3% China, 9.7% Latin America and Caribbean, and 13.7% developed countries. Percentages will decrease by the year 2000 for all countries except Africa, which will rise to 21.7%. The risk of a child dying has been shown to be generally higher in rural areas than in urban areas, and is much increased for children of rural uneducated agricultural parents; for example, in Senegal[3] the percentage of children dying before 5 years of urban educated professional parents is 4.2 and is 26.7 for children of rural uneducated agricultural parents. In parts of Africa a proportion of the infant and child deaths can be attributed to war, destabilization, insecurity, refugee situations and droughts.

CAUSES OF DEATHS

For any Child Survival program to have a rational basis, the causes of under-5's deaths must be determined. The 1988 State of the World's Children[4] gives a breakdown for the 14 million child deaths as follows: diarrheal disease, 5 million (mostly due to dehydration); malaria, 1 million; measles, 1.9 million; acute respiratory infections, 2.9 million (0.6 million due to whooping cough); neonatal tetanus, 0.8 million; other causes, 2.4 million, of which many could be prevented by prenatal care, breast feeding and nutrition education. Malnutrition is a contributing cause in approximately one-third of all child deaths.

COMPONENTS

A large proportion of the "Child Survival" programs in the world is assisted by donor funds. Some of the well known programs are assisted by UNICEF or though UNICEF with funds sought for this purpose from bilateral or other sources. USAID has been assisting many through its African Child Survival Initiative "Combating Childhood Communicable Diseases (CCCD)" and through assistance to private voluntary organizations for Child Survival projects. A Task Force for Child Survival has also been created (by UNICEF and Interaction) and with sponsoring agencies (WHO, UNICEF, World Bank, UNDP and Rockefeller Foundation). It has held a series of conferences,[5,6] the first at Bellagio, Italy. The recent consensus view on components in child survival includes:

- Immunization	and in many programs:
- Growth monitoring	- Drinking water
- Oral Rehydration	- Acute Respiratory Infections (ARI)
- Breast feeding	- AIDS control

- Female education   - Malaria
- Family planning   - Vitamin A Supplementation
- Food security   - Iodine Deficiency Disorders

The processes or strategies whereby these can be initiated, achieved, or sustained have become prominent components recently as it has become clear that they are essential. These have now included: education and communication (IEC), mobilization and "grand alliances," accelerated immunization coverage and campaign tactics, community involvement, and cost recovery for sustainability.

COUNTRY PROGRAMS

Programs are determined by the country's disease and mortality pattern and the existing health infrastructure and emphasis of programs. In many developing countries dependent on donor support, the thrust may have been biased or skewed toward donor interests such as family planning or diarrheal disease control or newsworthy campaigns.

PROCESSES INVOLVED

The initial phase of any Child Survival program should be a detailed situation analysis of the mortality and morbidity of mothers and children. This should analyze differentials due to socio-economic status, education, rural/urban areas, ecological and cultural areas of the country, access to and utilization of health services, and differences in disease pattern. Most countries by now have many ongoing projects – often initiated by private voluntary organization (PVO),[8] donor or local government. These should also be assessed in the situation analysis and an effort made to move on from projects to district or city programs and hence to a national program. Child Survival activities require intensive detailed planning based on the situation analysis. This plan must, for each intervention, have objectives, strategies, targets, indicators and details of activities all making optimal use of resources available. One of the problems has been the relative isolation and vertical nature of some of the component interventions in Child Survival. Immunization is delivered through the EPI program, diarrheal disease control through a CDD program, family planning through a Family Planning program. All are essential elements of a Primary Health Care program and many actions take place within Maternal and Child Health Clinics. The technology is often initiated through a vertical program and some aspects, e.g., the cold-chain for immunization, are most easily standardized and monitored through a vertical hierarchy of personnel. Real integration of the components of Child Survival might be achieved through the new district emphasis for primary health care (PHC). Districts with a PHC subcommittee of the district development committee can have a task-force to help plan, implement, monitor and evaluate Child Survival, and to expand it to a wider program for Child Health.

MOBILIZATION AND INFORMATION, EDUCATION AND COMMUNICATION (IEC)

One of the dilemmas of accelerating Child Survival activities is that this can conflict with the slower process of community involvement for PHC, building up community awareness, involvement and ownership or strengthening of leadership and committees, and training of community health workers. This is a slow process. It can be disrupted by hasty social mobilization if this has an emphasis on compliance and mere participation in a program planned and managed outside the community in a way which is often not replicable or sustainable. Accelerated programs which aim at lifting a stagnating program up to a higher plateau of coverage by mobilizing leadership and resources within the community through a process of carefully prepared communication of researched messages is one of the means by which some countries have made great progress in child survival. Social mobilization harnesses the energy of groups in the community for joint action – these may be religious or women's groups, cooperatives, clans, a political party together with their leadership. Recently UNICEF has enlisted the skill in communication of artists, singers, musicians, authors and journalists and has also linked the intellectuals in universities with the movement. The top pediatricians, obstetricians, and medical teachers in a country should all be actively involved in disseminating the most cost-effective technical solutions to the local problems of child survival. The teacher-training colleges, primary and secondary schools and adult literacy classes all require changes in curriculum if they are to be involved in education for health and child survival. Involvement of the mass media should lead to a coordinated barrage of information through television, radio and press in all the local languages with messages prepared in the manner of social marketing if behavior is to be altered.

COMMUNITY INVOLVEMENT, COST RECOVERY AND SUSTAINABILITY

Community involvement should be the basis of child survival and development programs. If communities do not internalize the problem and its solutions as their own, then no amount of foreign aid will permanently improve survival. Child Survival is related to local political will influenced by community pressures and demands, and to what people do for themselves. Queing up for shots is mere compliance, with no guarantee that the proper full schedule of immunization has been understood. When the community plans the outreach clinic from the health center, pays for the fuel, provides lunch for the health workers, mobilizes all children for the immunizations they need, and ensures minimal dropouts, then that community can be said to be involved, as they have taken over aspects of planning, management and monitoring. To do so, communities need financial resources as well as the human resources which they have but which also need further training. UNICEF and WHO have recently formulated a "Bamako Initiative"[9] in which essential drugs with cost recovery will be managed by communities who will establish revolving funds and then use the profits generated for sustaining community health and development activity. The initiative will also make more accessible essential drugs for child survival.

METHOD-SPECIFIC INTERVENTION – IMMUNIZATION

The WHO EPI program has set the standards for the world and countries now have established and maintained cold chain, and use quality-controlled vaccines usually on the same accepted schedule. This has been slightly modified over the years based on accumulated scientific evidence and field experience. The most universally used schedule includes tetanus toxoid for pregnant mothers and all women in child-bearing age; the number of spaced doses might be five to ensure 99% protection of neonates.[10] The schedule also includes four (or even more) doses of oral polio vaccine and 3 doses of diphtheria/tetanus vaccine, both of these starting now at 6 weeks of age. In some parts of the world child survival and development programs would include immunization against hepatitis B, rubella and encephalitis but these all add to the costs. Immunization programs have not been without difficulty or anxieties – lack of fuel has led to trials and use of solar-powered refrigerators, fear of HIV transmission has led to steam pressure sterilization and reusable plastic syringes. Mobile clinics with their high cost per immunized child have given way, except in some nomadic populations, to outreach clinics often carried out using bicycles for transport. Monitoring and periodic evaluation (both national and district level) have enabled targets to be defined and have given justification to the pleas for acceleration and community mobilization.

NUTRITIONAL IMPROVEMENT

Three of the original child survival and development interventions are directly related to improvement of nutritional status – growth monitoring, breast feeding and family food supplementation. Oral rehydration, immunization, family planning and education of women also have very great impact on nutrition and this is one of the features of Child Survival activities, that they should all be synergistic. Growth monitoring usually by regular measurement of weight-for-age is the most frequently employed measure and in many programs this, when analyzed collectively, can become the basis for nutritional surveillance of an area liable to food shortage. Weight-for-height as a measure of wasting is used in many programs dealing with refugees or with communities in semi-arid areas prone to drought or seasonal shortages. Height or length for age is used to show stunting or chronic undernutrition which is an aspect of child development which can be overlooked. In many developing countries breast feeding is only a problem of the educated working urban women, but Child Survival should ensure that existing high levels of breast feeding are not undermined by powdered milk companies and their advertising – hence the need for continued monitoring of the international code for marketing of breast milk substitutes. Breast feeding, besides its obvious nutritional value, is an important measure to diminish both diarrheal disease and respiratory infections, and improve child spacing. Two additional CSD activities now to be found in areas of deficiency are vitamin A and iodine administration. The former in the form of food and nutrition education with capsules, and the latter either as repository injections, capsules or as iodated salt. These two interventions are introduced if epidemiological surveys show that there are deficiencies (often only in localized districts or areas of a country). Biochemical tests can also be carried out. These signs elicited in surveys, however, draw attention to specific organs (eye and thyroid) but the effects of mild deficiency are now known to be more serious. Vitamin A deficiency is associated with high mortality and morbidity from respiratory infections and diarrheal disease,[11] and iodine deficiency disorders include retarded growth and development.[12]

ORAL REHYDRATION AND DIARRHEAL DISEASE CONTROL

Oral rehydration is merely one of the four strategies of diarrheal disease control and is aimed at reduction of mortality. As it became clear that diarrheal morbidity of 2-6 episodes per year contributed to poor growth and development, it became necessary also to increase emphasis on clean water and sanitation. Breast feeding, improved weaning practices, and food hygiene, as well as measles immunization, are other preventive measures which decrease diarrheal disease morbidity and have been included in educational approaches to CSD. Oral rehydration has been incorporated into curricula for training all health workers. Doctors and pediatricians have had to have special orientation, and international workshops have helped to emphasize the saving of life now possible. Many health units and hospitals have set up rehydration corners where mothers can be shown how to give the oral rehydration solution made up from the standard WHO/UNICEF formula. There is no problem with this in health units – the problem comes when deciding what to advocate in the home. UNICEF/WHO in a joint statement advocated the use of home fluids and incomplete salt and sugar formula for prevention of dehydration in the home and the use of the full-formula sachets where clinical dehydration has commenced. Salt and sugar home-made solution has in some countries become controversial since many surveys have found it is often made up with high concentration of sodium chloride and could be dangerous. Moreover, in many developing countries salt and sugar are not available in homes nor are accurate measures for the water, the salt, and sugar. Emphasis is now placed on home treatment with ricewater, maize or other gruel or whatever fluid is available.

FAMILY PLANNING

Many countries, especially in Africa, prefer the term child-spacing as it is closer to traditionally accepted methods and has less association with population control. However, child spacing to obtain a longer birth interval has only some of the benefits of family planning, which also aims at planning when to start the family, how many to have and when to stop, each with particular benefits to mothers and children. In Africa teenage pregnancy is a big problem, with girls becoming pregnant while they are still growing themselves and then having low birth-weight babies with lower chances of survival. Total number of births per woman in the region of 8-9 also carry nutritional and other implications; as with increasing economic problems it is now difficult to feed and educate a family of this size. Family planning is being propagated by two main thrusts – first, information, education, and communication to increase knowledge and change attitudes and increase the number of clients; and second, making services more accessible and acceptable. The former activity often had a poor start in countries until there was political support. The service thrust often was confined to family planning associations or NGOs before political support allowed it to become a routine part of the maternal and child health services. Family planning should then be available as one of the daily activities of every MCH clinic/health center or dispensary. Community-based distribution of contraception through trained community health workers or trained traditional birth attendants is also one of the ways which brings certain contraceptives to the homes of rural mothers who otherwise have difficulty in obtaining supplies. In countries in Asia incentive family planning has been used (e.g., in India) and disincentives for a larger family (e.g., China) have been prominent measures to obtain high rates of acceptors. Husbands, wives and adolescent children all need family planning knowledge and the messages should not be only on methods, services, and physiology but must include the newer information about Child Survival and Development benefits as well as economic benefits. Child Survival is in itself a motivating factor for acceptance of family planning.

ACUTE RESPIRATORY INFECTIONS

Bacterial pneumonia responsive to antibiotics is a major cause of child mortality in the developing world. Although measles and whooping cough immunization, and breast feeding are also activities that could reduce ARI deaths, it is early recognition and prompt antibiotic treatment of severe respiratory infection that will make an impact on this cause of death – often the top cause. Low birth-weight babies deserve specific attention for in them ARIs are particularly lethal. ARIs are a good example of a condition requiring high quality curative care. The problem is first, late diagnosis and second, lack of the correct management with appropriate drugs, although both aspects have relatively simple technology available. Parents, community health workers, and workers in dispensaries and health centers can be trained in the algorithms worked out by WHO which help to differentiate mild, moderate, and severe respiratory infections each with definite lines of management. An IEC program can alert parents to the signs and symptoms of ARI and enlist their cooperation in early diagnosis and seeking help. Help can be provided closer at hand by equipping community health workers or dispensary workers with the necessary drugs and training.

MALARIA

Malaria in many developing countries causes many infant and young child deaths through a variety of mechanisms. A pregnant mother (especially primigravida) who has malaria may develop severe anemia, have fever, lose weight, and have a placenta with parasites so that she delivers a low birth-weight baby and possibly has poor lactation. Such babies have higher mortality even if they do not then start having malaria, and later develop severe anemia or cerebral malaria. In areas with seasonal peaks of malaria, these may coincide with the rains when mother is working in the fields and frequently ill and the baby is having malaria and diarrhea and being cared for poorly by siblings. Adequate malaria interventions are difficult and mostly stop at early treatment of cases and prophylaxis in pregnancy. Vector control and environmental improvement are usually too expensive but one recent rediscovery is the value of mosquito nets as a preventive measure for infants and toddlers.

Early treatment is facilitated by community education and by providing trained community health workers with chloroquine. Unfortunately chloroquine-resistant malaria is now widespread and second-line drugs are more expensive and often less available. The CCCD programmes in Africa have included monitoring of chloroquine resistance, also.

AIDS

The latest threat to survival of children in developing countries is the human immunodeficiency virus (HIV) which could seriously increase the infant and child mortality in spite of gains made by interventions such as immunization. In some antenatal clinics in a few countries, 4% of women are now HIV-positive and a proportion of these women, perhaps 30-50%, will have infants developing AIDS. The preventive measures that need to be taken are basically the same for all sexually transmitted diseases (STD) although other STD can at least be treated. An IEC campaign has to be launched with even more determination than for immunization, to enable children and adolescents to develop correct behavior, and adults to modify their behavior toward having one faithful sexual partner or using condoms when this is not done. This has to be coupled with a sympathetic and carefully planned system of counseling for all identified virus carriers including advice on family planning as necessary. Untested blood transfusions and use of unsterile equipment still pose a problem in some poorer countries and these two methods of transmission also need to be blocked.

RESULTS AND EVALUATION

It is because monitoring and evaluation have been such an integral part of Child Survival programs that the results to date are already known. The clear definition of objectives, targets and indicators has also been of great assistance. Those countries with satisfactory monitoring managed to set up functioning health information systems and often have sentinel reporting health units. Evaluation was in many countries done by teams with participation from government, NGOs, WHO, UNICEF and health staff from other neighboring countries. Projects with a good information system have good management and are likely to publish good results. Poor results are published infrequently. Participatory evaluation in PHC and for components of Child Survival has become a standard procedure and there are now several manuals on the process.[13,14] Model sets of indicators for GOBI have been prepared.[15]

IMMUNIZATION

The percentage of children fully immunized within countries or globally over time has been an important feature of evaluation but more important are calculations of illness prevented and deaths averted. Graphs of decreasing cases notified and of decreasing case fatality are now commonplace. EPI country reviews and coverage surveys have followed standardized methodologies developed by WHO and the reviews have often been broadened to cover a wide range of inputs, outputs, and processes as well as quality assessment. Cost-effectiveness studies not only of immunization but of growth monitoring and oral rehydration as well as other aspects of MCH or PHC are also being done. In 1980 total child deaths from immunizable diseases were 5,255,000. By 1988 it was stated that more than 3 million children were killed in the previous 12 months by measles, tetanus, and whooping cough, and another 200,000 disabled by polio.[16] In 1982 UNICEF supplied 129.7 million doses of all EPI vaccines and by 1986 this had risen to 494.0 million doses. Immunization coverage of 12 month-old children in Africa (which has the lowest coverage rates) was 17% for polio and 27% for measles in 1982 and rose to 36% and 38%, respectively, by 1986.

These gains toward an objective of Universal Coverage of Immunization 1990 were achieved by social mobilization and PHC activities of many countries. The evaluation of immunization coverage is done by comparing the doses administered in relation to the calculated number of children under 1 year, or by a standard survey method to look at the immunization records of a random sample of children of the right age in the population. Evaluation of impact is done by estimating cases or deaths averted or by analysis of reported cases and deaths. Efficacy of vaccines and drop-out rates provide some measures of quality of services. An example of an intensive Child Survival acceleration program is that of Botswana[17] which has a small population of 1.2 million people in a very large country. In 1986 the national coverage rate for full immunization was 76% and subsequently in two years of very intensive activity this was raised to 82% with individual antigen coverage as follows: BCG, 98%; DPT/OPV 1, 96%; DPT/OPV 2, 94%; DPT/OPV 3, 89%; Measles, 83%; and TT 78% for mothers. A door-to-door channeling/survey strategy was used which combined social mobilization with project evaluation done with community involvement (school children, leaders, parents). In 1987 in Botswana, 34,027 cases and 1021 deaths from measles were prevented. Measles vaccine efficacy was found to be 70%, which was, however, less than expected. This example was chosen as it shows that the last difficult push above 75% to over 80% can be achieved although it means achieving individual antigen levels in the 90% range.

GROWTH MONITORING

Growth monitoring and promotion have had a lot of evaluation and been assessed from the point of view of the instruments (availability and suitability of scales and growth cards), of the process (the involvement, education, understanding, behavioral change of mothers, and the incorporation of routine child care), and of the impact on nutritional status. It is also used for growth surveillance of a community or district. The key activities of growth monitoring must take place early before there is faltering or malnutrition so that the mother becomes concerned with monitoring good growth and the activity is a preventive and educational one rather than a curative or rehabilitative one. Although some programs are coupled with food supplementation if growth is faltering (e.g., in Botswana which is a drought-prone country), many now aim at encouraging mothers to make optimal use of family resources and to think in terms of establishing family food security. It has been observed that when supplementation is a part of a program, it soon becomes the focus and the monitoring becomes of less importance.

Growth monitoring is usually done using a chart which is coupled with immunization and treatment records. Children with growth charts are more likely to have immunizations and mothers who have been taught about prevention and management of conditions such as diarrhea. These other activities also have a great impact on nutrition. Women and communities organizing growth monitoring are also usually involved in other development activities. Thus there has been impressive improvement in nutrition of children in the Jamkhed program over 10 years which was attributed to community participation and the fact that growth monitoring was part of an overall strategy for PHC and rural development.[18] In the Iringa Nutrition Program in Tanzania[19] (with support from WHO/UNICEF) severe malnutrition in 1987 had dropped to a level one-third of that found at the start of activities in 1984. Communities were involved in weighing children and in recording and analyzing results. The results were attributed to better mobilization of local resources from families, communities and local authorities. The monitoring with growth charts made the problem of poor growth visible at all levels and hence it was easier to discuss, analyze, and act upon. There was improved understanding of the causes of child deaths and malnutrition.

VITAMIN A DEFICIENCY

The results of incorporating Vitamin A supplementation in deficient areas should be a drop in mortality and morbidity from respiratory illness and diarrhea as well as a change in occurrences of blindness due to keratomalacia.[11] Evaluation is usually directed at determining inputs (capsules administered, high risk groups, e.g., measles cases, protected) and processes (the smooth incorporation of the supplementation into PHC/MCH programs and of the nutrition educational process for families) and impact as measured in terms of reduction of eye signs, blindness and morbidity and mortality.

IODINE DEFICIENCY

The most dramatic results of increasing the intake of iodine by adding it to salt have already occurred in developed countries such as U.S.A., Switzerland, and England. It is now countries such as Bangladesh, China, and India with enormous goitrous populations that will demonstrate the biggest changes from a preventive program of iodating salt. China, for example, reduced the prevalence of goitre in Jixian county from 65% in 1978 to 4% in 1986 and no children have been born with cretinism, although there was previously a high rate of mental retardation.[20] New Guinea has already shown the efficacy of injection of iodized oil in pregnancy. Evaluation can now be done by staining a special absorbent paper with cord blood and determining thyroxine levels in newborns. This neonatal hypothyroid screening can show the prevalence of newborn children who are hypothyroid. Other methods of evaluation are by estimating urinary iodine and goitre-prevalence surveys. In any control program monitoring is required of the level of iodine in salt or of the regularity and coverage of iodized oil injections (every 3 years) or capsules (1-2 years).

ORAL REHYDRATION

The results of oral rehydration in diarrheal disease control programs are usually expressed in certain input indicators as well as outcome and impact indicators. Diarrheal disease-specific death rates, diarrheal disease case fatality rates, % of episodes treated with ORT, % of population with access to ORS and with knowledge and skills in use are some of the measures. The results of this intervention have been described in a voluminous literature – WHO Diarrhoea Disease Control Programme, UNICEF publications, yearly conferences such as ICORT proceedings,[21] and journals so that it is difficult to select the most telling results. Twenty percent of children with diarrhea are now treated with either ORS or homemade solutions, and ORT may be preventing more than 600,000 deaths a year. The efficacy of ORS in preventing death had been well illustrated in a controlled study in Costa Rica as early as 1980 when sachets were distributed to mothers; after 1 year there was a 50% reduction of infant diarrhea deaths in 20 municipalities, but no change in remaining municipalities where the intervention was not used.[22]

FAMILY PLANNING (FP)

The impact of family planning is on fetal wastage, perinatal mortality, infant mortality, child mortality, maternal mortality as well as on maternal and infant morbidity. Impact can also be measured on population effects and socio-economic status both of which have implications for child survival. Lengthening of the birth interval is the most important factor for preventing both infant and child deaths. Other measures of success of family planning relate to the availability of services and to their use, which is also related to changes in knowledge and attitudes. Kenya is an example of a country with a very high rate of natural increase (3.8% per annum) and a total fertility rate of 7.7. It was, however, the first country in Africa to accept an official population policy and has had family planning services for twenty years. These services are now given by a family planning association, and also as a routine part of MCH services in 1800 places; clients are encouraged by a special cadre of field workers. Non-government health organizations have also started programs of community-based distribution. User rates increased from 7% in 1979 to 15% in 1984. In one well-managed Kenyan NGO program in Chogoria, 98% of women knew at least one method, current use was 42% among married women, and total fertility had decreased to 5.2. This FP program took place within the context of a broad PHC program. Differentials in total fertility are very marked in Kenya: 8.5 for women with no education, 5.4 for those with 9 years or more of education. There have been few of the newer Child Survival programs which have documented their family planning programs in relation to child survival and development. Fortunately surveys such as the World Fertility Survey and Family Formation and health surveys have provided good evidence of the benefits of increased birth interval and the adverse additive effect of short prebirth and short postbirth intervals in increasing the under-5 death rate.

ACUTE RESPIRATORY INFECTION (ARI)

Control of ARI as a newcomer to the set of child-survival interventions is still largely at the research stage. Ten intervention studies were started between 1983 and 1985 but four did not proceed. All of the studies showed that the case management of ARI can be carried out by community health workers and can lead to significant reduction of mortality due to ARI in children. In Haryana State, India, standard case management with oral penicillin was given to low birth-weight infants recognized to have moderate or severe ARI by trained health workers.[24] This led to a significant lowering of case fatality rates to 8.7% in the intervention area as compared with 24.5% in the control area. In Kathmandu Valley, Nepal, trained lay reporters first established a baseline of ARI-specific infant mortality rates; then case management inter-vention was introduced by PHC workers using oral ampicillin as a first-line drug for moderate and severe ARI cases and chloramphenicol as the second-line drug. The baseline in 1984 was over 50 deaths per 1000 live births and this was reduced to 5 in 1986.[25] These results were from projects, and sustainabil-ity and lack of problems from increased use of antibiotics still have to be demonstrated.

MALARIA

Although malaria is one of the most important causes of morbidity and mortality in endemic areas, control programs in most countries of Africa and many other areas have had little success. This is due to increasing resistance to chloroquine, and problems of cost and insecticide resistance in vector control. The malaria case fatality rate in Zaire has shown an alarming rise from 2 per 100 cases in 1984 to 5 in 1987.[26] Anemia due to malaria has also apparently increased in many countries of Africa, indicating failure of effective interven-tions. Ten of the 12 CCCD programmes in Africa in malarious areas have carried out drug sensitivity studies. Although decreased sensitivity to chloro-quine is now widespread, the drug is used as first-line treatment as it still usually decreases parasitemia and lowers temperature. Unfortunately as there is increasing resistance of *Plasmodium falciparum*, the cost of antimalarial drugs in Africa will rise almost ten-fold in the next four years.[27] The number of CHW trained in the use of chloroquine for treatment (now usually over a 3-day period) has increased. However, as it is also suggested that use of chloroquine at community level will lead to selection of more resistant stains of parasite, there is controversy about the widespread use of the drug by CHW. The drug is often available in shops and kiosks in many countries but it is better that the CHW at least make a presumptive diagnosis and give adequate and correct dosage related to age. It is especially these aspects of more definitive diagno-sis and of correct drug use which need careful consideration and monitoring.

AIDS

Data on the impact of interventions on AIDS in relation to women and children in developing countries are few. Most information relates to inputs on training, information, education and communication, distribution of con-doms, sterilization of syringes, needles and equipment, and to testing of blood for transfusion. Unfortunately information on prevalence rates of HIV infec-tion usually shows increases; except in one study[28] on prostitutes in Nairobi who were taught the use of condoms for their clients. Notification rates for

AIDS in most developing countries continue to show a depressing increase especially alarming in countries such as those in eastern Africa where funds have already been available for a massive IEC program.

CONCLUSIONS

Child Survival and Development programs or activities have produced a very good effect on country awareness of the priority that must be placed on prevention of infant and child mortality, morbidity and disability. These programs have mobilized public opinion and created an increased demand for better services. The interventions for child survival and development have also been studied and refined. Technologies and methods of delivery have improved following implementation of the findings of operations research. However, an emphasis on donor assistance and programs elaborated without community involvement have been all too frequent. This might stifle community initiative and also lead to attempts to meet a rigid schedule with unrealistic targets which is in conflict with the slow pace of community sensitization and involvement leading to sustainability. Some programs are now being made aware of the inadequacies of concentrating on a few interventions at the expense of a broader PHC approach. On the other hand the Child Survival and Development approach has proved to be a spearhead for PHC development and has given it a focus leading to recognizable measurable achievements. When diarrheal disease management is shown to be adequate or to have improved, then realization of the continued frequency of diarrheal episodes forces programs to put more effort into water and sanitation. Similarly "safe motherhood" activities which lead to improved perinatal and neonatal survival also come into prominence. Child Survival and Development programs are thus becoming less uniform and more responsive to local needs and they are constantly expanding and consolidating activities due to operations research and increasing community awareness and more vocal demands. It is the Child Survival program approach which has made the attainment of "Universal Coverage of Immunization" feasible, and which has made oral rehydration and growth monitoring essential components of all child health activities.

REFERENCES

1. Grant, J.P. The State of the World's Children 1981-82. New York: UNICEF, 1982, p.11.

2. Grant, J.P. The State of the World's Children 1984. Oxford: Oxford University Press, 1983, pp. 1-10.

3. Galways, K., B. Wolff, and R. Sturgis. Child survival: Risks and the road to health. Columbia, MD: Institute for Research Development/Westinghouse, 1987, pp. 3-7, p. 47.

4. Grant, J.P. The State of the World's Children 1988. Oxford: Oxford University Press, 1988, p. 3.

5. Halstead, S.B., J.A. Walsh, and K.S. Warren (eds). Good Health at Low Cost. Conference Report. New York:Rockefeller Foundation, 1985, p. 248.

6. Task Force for Child Survival. Protecting the World's Children. Bellagio II at Cartegena. New York: Rockefeller Foundation, 1986, pp. 230.

7. World Health Organization. Discussion Paper – Selected Primary Health Care Interventions. JD/EPI/80/1 Geneva: WHO, 1980.

8. The Johns Hopkins University School of Hygiene and Public Health, Institute for International Programs. PVO Child Survival, Summary of Lessons Learned and Recommendations, PVO Child Survival Support Program. Baltimore, MD: JHU, 1988, pp. 1-38.

9. Grant, J.P. Towards Maternal and Child Health Care for All: A Bamako Initiative in Report of Thirty-seventh Session of the WHO Regional Committee for Africa held in Bamako Republic of Mali. Brazzaville: WHO, 1987, pp. 77-89.

10. World Health Organization. Expanded Programme on Immunization Update 1988 Neonatal Tetanus. Geneva: WHO, 1988.

11. Sommer, A., J. Katz, and I. Tarwotjo. Increased risk of respiratory disease and diarrhea in children with pre-existing mild vitamin A deficiency. Am J Clin Nutr. vol. 40, Nov 1984.

12. Lancet editorial: From endemic goitre to iodine deficiency disorders. Lancet, 12 Nov 1983.

13. Feuerstein, M-T. Partners in Evaluation. London: Macmillan, 1986.

14. Rugh, J. Self Evaluation. Oklahoma City: World Neighbours.

15. LeSar, J., M.D. Mitchell, and R. Northrup, et al. Monitoring and evaluation of child survival programs. In Cash, et al. The GOBI-FFF Programme. Beckenham: Croom Helm, 1987, pp. 173-204.

16. Grant, J.P. The State of the World's Children 1988. Oxford: Oxford University Press, 1988, p 2.

17. Ndambi, I.O., and S. Madema. The Botswana Universal Child Immunization Project A: A Status Report 1988. Gaborone, Botswana: Ministry of
Health, 1988.

18. Arole, M. A comprehensive approach to community welfare: Growth
monitoring and the role of women in Jamkhed. Indian J Ped (suppl) 55,
100-105, 1988.

19. WHO/UNICEF Joint Support for Improvement of Nutrition in the United
Republic of Tanzania. Report of a mid-term review by external evaluation
team. Dar es Salaam: UNICEF, Mar 1986.

20. Grant, J.P. The State of the World's Children 1987. Oxford: Oxford University Press, 1987, p. 82.

21. Agency for International Development: ICORT II Proceedings – 2d International Conference on Oral Rehydration Therapy. Washington DC:
USAID, 1985.

22. Mata, L. The evolution of diarrhoeal diseases and malnutrition in Costa
Rica. Assignment Children 61/62. Geneva: UNICEF, 1983, pp. 125-224.

23. Kenya Ministry of Health. Kenya Contraceptive Prevalence Survey. Nairobi: Ministry of Health, 1984.

24. Datta, N., and L. Rumar, et al. Application of case management to the
control of acute respiratory infections in low birth-weight infants: A feasibility study. Bull WHO 65(1):77-82, 1987.

25. Pandey, M.R., P.R. Sharma, and G.M. Shakya. Nepal: Impact of a pilot
ARI control program. ARI News no. 6, 1986, p. 4.

26. Agency for International Development. African Child Survival Initiative.
Combating Childhood Communicable Diseases. Annual Report. Atlanta:.
Centers for Disease Control, 1987, p. 24.

27. Agency for International Development. African Child Survival Initiative.
Annual Report. Atlanta: USAID, 1986, p. 11.

28. Ngugi, E.N., et al. Prevention of transmission of human immunodeficiency virus in Africa: Effectiveness of condom promotion and health
education among prostitutes. Lancet, pp. 887 - 890, 15 Oct 1988.

32

THE IMPLEMENTATION OF THE RISK APPROACH IN MATERNAL AND CHILD HEALTH SERVICES

ANNA ALISJABANA, M.D.

I. INTRODUCTION

Considerable efforts have already been made to develop health care services and yet still in many populations access to health care is limited, especially for pregnant mothers and their newborn infants. This is also true for Indonesia, a country with +180 million population scattered over 3000 islands. One of the major problems is then how to use most effectively the health resources available in order to reach a maximum effect.

The concept of risk is important in MCH programs. The ability to predict a birth of a jeopardized infant before its delivery means that decisions about optimal management of the pregnancy can be made and that the chances of a favorable outcome can be increased. Neonatal morbidity is significantly reduced (and the cost of hospitalization approximately halved) if patients are referred before delivery rather than after.[1] Many attempts have been made to develop an index for scoring high-risk pregnancies. Risk scoring is based mostly on a compilation of several risk variables with a given weight, and may be useful for health care providers with a certain level of education. However, in most developing countries, traditional health providers (such as traditional birth attendants:TBA) are illiterate and of old age. Hence a screening method using risk scoring will be difficult to conduct. Some modification appropriate to the sociocultural conditions in Indonesia has to be made.

The risk approach strategy aims to improve health care for all, but give special attention to those individuals or groups with greater needs. The main objective is to find the best match for the patient's needs using the appropriate and available health services and skills required for that problem.[2,3]

Therefore, the purpose of this chapter is to present the analysis of risk variables. The validity of an indicator is assessed in terms of its capacity to "predict" risk of perinatal outcome and low birth weight. The result of the Perinatal Mortality and Morbidity and LBW Survey in Ujung-Berung (a district in a rural area in West-Java, one of the most populated provinces of Indonesia with a total population of +32 million) will be used. This chapter will also present the major steps in the implementation of the Risk Approach Health Intervention strategy, an ongoing research project in Tanjungsari, a rural district adjacent to Ujung-Berung.

II. MEASURE OF RISK

Risk is a measure of the probability or chance of a future unwanted health outcome. The risk approach to health intervention uses this measurement of risk as an indicator of the need for health care. Those risk factors that are causally related to the outcome can, if removed, reduce the risk for the unwanted health outcome. Other factors may only be indicators of risk or are not amenable to change by interventions (such as age and parity).[2,3] One of the most common indicators of risk in epidemiology is the absolute risk or the incidence of the unwanted outcome in a given period of time in the population at risk. This measures the occurrence of the outcome in both those with and without the risk factors. Another measurement used is the relative risk which is the ratio of the incidence of the unwanted health outcome in the population with and without the risk factor. The relative risk can also be considered as the strength of the association between the risk factor and the outcome. It gives an indication of the excess risk for the outcome in the population with the risk factor.

The relative risk is an important measure in deciding which risk factors should be used in an intervention to identify individuals or groups for treatment or for referral or other services. These are the vital components of the risk approach strategy.

III. THE PREPARATION PHASE: AN EPIDEMIOLOGICAL STUDY TO MEASURE RELATIVE RISK

Data from an epidemiological study in a rural district (Ujung-Berung) adjacent to the intervention area Tanjungsari provided the baseline data. The data were collected from a Perinatal Mortality and Morbidity Study conducted in 1978-1980. A cohort of pregnant women was followed within a period of 18 months to study the natural history of pregnancy. During the study period a total of 2335 infants were born. The total population was 40,787 people and the birth rate 3.8%. Perinatal mortality was 45 per thousand births and the incidence of low birth weight was 14.7%.[4]

Table 1, and Table 2 (next page), list some maternal risk factors for poor perinatal outcome and low birth weight which are individual characteristics or aspects of reproductive history. Some factors are based on physical examination and include abnormal fetal presentation, evidence of twins, maternal weight and height.

Table 1
Summary Table of Relative Risk Associated with Perinatal Deaths
(Longitudinal Survey Ujung-Berung 1978-1980).

Risk factors	Perinatal Deaths	Number of Births	Relative Risk	X^2-value
Age mother (<u><20</u> vs 20+)	56	1,306	1.28	6.67*
Parity (<u>>6</u> vs 1-6)	56	1,306	1.17	0.27 NS
Birth interval (<u><18 month</u> vs 18 months+)	42	1,024	2.76	8.29*
Plurality (<u>Twins</u> vs singletons)	104	2,335	4.14	18.34*
Sex (<u>male</u> vs female)	95	2,289	0.91	0.20 NS
Mothers occupation (<u>yes</u> vs no)	58	1,306	0.97	0.002 NS
Mothers education (<u>no</u> vs yes)	56	1,306	0.72	0.39 NS
Betel chewing of mother (<u>yes</u> vs no)	103	2,310	1.64	1.98 NS
Smoking of mother (<u>yes</u> vs no)	103	2,312	0.31	3.02 NS
Antenatal care visits (<u>none</u> vs 1 or more)	56	1,303	0.84	0.39 NS
Family Planning (no vs yes)	57	1,282	2.53	2.75 NS
Birth attendant (<u>untrained</u> vs trained)	92	2,035	1.15	0.38 NS
Previous Medical History (<u>unsatisfactory physical</u>/satisfactory).	57	1.291	1.78	2.20 NS
Weight of the mother (<u>less than</u> 50 kg. vs ≥ 50 kg.)	56	1.06	1.08	0.09 NS
Presentation of fetus (<u>breech</u> vs cephalic)	104	2,333	5.70	48.35*

*Significant at P < 0.05.

Table 2
Risk Factors and Relative Risk of Pregnant Women in
Ujung-Berung (1978-1980) for Low Birthweight

Risk factor	Prevalence all births	LBW %	Total Births	Relative Risk	X^2-value
Biological factors					
Sex (female vs male)	49.2	17.2	2,335	1.42	9.4*
Plurality(Twins vs Singleton)	1.9	76.1	2,342	5.65	141.1*
Age (<20 vs >20+)	18.8	22.2	2,345	1.69	23.7*
Parity (first vs 2+)	22.4	24.5	2,339	2.06	52.1*
Socio-economic factors					
Education (yes vs no)	9.4	13.1	2,335	1.67	6.0*
Employment (yes v no)	7.4	22.4	2,335	1.58	8.8*
No. persons/HH (2 vs 3+)	5.8	21.5	2,335	1.49	5.1*
Sleeping area (1.5m² /person vs more)	67.0	14.3	2,260	0.90	0.9 NS
Medical history:					
Previous Malaria (yes vs no)	—	24.1	1,829	1.64	5.7*
Previous Urine Tr.Inf. (UTI) (yes vs no)	—	28.3	1,829	1.77	3.1 NS
Complication during labor and delivery					
Presentation (breech vs vertex)	2.5	33.9	2,335	2.3	16.2*
Complications (all causes prior to delivery) (yes vs no)	3.3	50.6	2,335	3.7	80.0*
Complications (all causes during labor)(yes vs no)	5.9	15.1	2,335	1.04	0.04 NS
Utilization of Health services					
Antenatal care (none vs yes)	52.5	15.4	2,316	1.09	0.84 NS
Family planning (no vs yes)	86.8	15.1	2,300	1.18	1.03 NS
TBA (untr. vs trained)	58.9	16.2	2,035	1.35	6.01*
Birth attendant (trained TBA vs Midwife)	28.4	12.0	881	1.05	0.05 NS

*Significant at P<0.05.

IV. THE RISK APPROACH AS AN INTERVENTION STUDY TO IMPROVE MCH SERVICES

Four issues have to be considered if the risk approach will be used in an intervention survey for Perinatal Health.

A. WHO IS AT RISK OF A POOR PREGNANCY OUTCOME?

In the baseline survey poor outcome means perinatal death or the delivery of a LBW infant. The result of the epidemiological study will provide the answer to this question. The relative risk and the attributable risks of the target population will permit predictions of who is at risk. These measures of risk will provide an indication of how much of a reduction in the unwanted outcome is possible by successfully implementing an intervention.

Risk factors identified during pregnancy and their relative risk for perinatal outcome can be seen in Table 1. It shows the number of perinatal deaths, the perinatal mortality rate and the number of births it has been calculated on, the relative risk and the value of X^2.

The perinatal mortality is highest in mothers under 20 years of age, then decreases to rise again from 35 years on. The relative risk of being aged less than 20 years is 1.28, meaning that the risk of a perinatal death is 28% higher in mothers aged less than 20 compared to others of 20 years and over. The perinatal mortality increases also with increasing birth order with the highest PMR in parities 1 and ≥ 7. Short birth interval (<18 months) and very long birth intervals increase the risk of mortality. Twins were found to have significantly higher PMR than singletons. The PMR for singleton males was lower than for singleton females. The opposite was found for early neonatal deaths, which showed a lower mortality rate for females.

In rural communities in Indonesia most deliveries are assisted by traditional birth attendants, either trained or untrained. The result shows that trained TBAs have a slightly lower, though statistically not significant, PMR compared to untrained TBAs.

Surprisingly, risk factors such as occupation, education, socio-economic condition and certain health-related habits (such as betel chewing) revealed any statistically significant association with the risk condition being present or absent. This relative lack of variability may point to the fact that within villages in the survey area, living conditions and sociocultural factors do not differ widely.

Daily habits such as smoking, betel chewing and previous breast feeding were not significantly associated with the risk of having a low birth-weight infant.

B. HOW WILL THE RISK STATUS OF THE PREGNANT MOTHERS BE DETERMINED?

There are several ways to determine the overall risk of the pregnant mother for a poor perinatal outcome. One of them is by giving a different score or weight depending on the different degrees of risk associated with the factors. Cut-off points for the total score can be used to determine whether the women should deliver at home or by a midwife or by a doctor in the hospital. The next possibility is by using the cut-off point for some risk variables easily detectable by illiterate TBAs. In the latter, single variables will be used rather than combined scores for several variables. For each single variable the cut-off point for referral was calculated for its sensitivity and specificity as can be seen in Table 3 for maternal nutritional variables.

The scoring system may misclassify women. If too many women are falsely classified as high risk, this may result in an unnecessary use of the already limited resources. On the other hand if not enough high-risk women are identified, the intervention will have little impact on the unwanted health outcome. As can be seen in Table 3, a relatively low sensitivity is found for all nutritional variables of mothers delivering a low birth-weight infant, meaning that those who are screened are those who are really in need of referral. A relatively high specificity means that those cases not referred most probably will not deliver a low birth-weight infant. In the survey area as in most

Table 3
Anthropometric variables to identify women at risk for LBW
(singletons)

Variable	Risk Criteria%	PPV %	Sens %	Spec. %	F.P.	F.N.	RR
Weight (30 wks)	<45 kg. 13.2	21.8	24.3	87.5	78.1	11.0	1.9*
Height	<145 cm 9.5	18.8	13.8	90.8	81.1	11.4	1.5*
MUAC	<22 cm 30.6	17.6	47.6	62.6	82.9	11.8	1.4*

MUAC= Mid-upper-arm-circumference. * Significant P <0.05.

developing countries, the ratio of health center to population ranges from 1:30,000 to 1:100,000 or more. A large number of referrals would create an overload, therefore a low sensitivity will create fewer problems.

C. WHO WILL IDENTIFY THE HIGH-RISK PREGNANT WOMEN?

In the survey area more than 80% of deliveries are attended by TBAs, who are old, illiterate and resistant to change. Therefore, identification of single-risk variables as can be seen in Tables 1, 2 and 3 instead of a risk scoring system is more applicable and acceptable in this situation.[5] Defining risk factors based on epidemiological studies alone is not enough. To have a working referral system, the risk factor has to be in agreement with the perception of the TBA as well as of the pregnant woman herself. A pilot survey to study this behavior found that risk factors such as age and parity were not considered a risk by the community. On the other hand the result also shows women in the survey area had at least one risk factor. There was an average of 1.73 risk factors for every women at risk.[4] To refer all these cases will certainly result in an overload to the health center. Therefore, the more specific and selective factors have to be defined. Risk factors directly related to a fatal outcome will have the first priority. Risk factors easy to identify are the nutritional risk variables and therefore, are in the second place, while biological and social risk factors have a lower priority.

When working with traditional birth attendants these procedures may need to be presented in pictorial form. Even though these action cards may seem very simple to those who work at more sophisticated levels of the health care system, they may make a big difference to the level of care for village women. In the risk approach some questions about the existing health care system and perinatal referral system have to be answered.[3]

1. What proportion of the high-risk population use antenatal care services at different levels of the health care system?
2. What health manpower is available at the community health center?
3. What are the resources available at the district hospital?

In rural areas of Indonesia it is likely that the traditional birth attendants who attend 80-90% of deliveries will need to be trained to do preliminary screening with further risk assessments being done by the community health center midwives. Preliminary results show that the majority of pregnant women visit the health center for pregnancy confirmation at about 3-5 weeks of pregnancy.

D. WHAT ACTION IS TO BE TAKEN WHEN HIGH-RISK PREGNANCIES ARE IDENTIFIED?

The actions to be taken will be influenced by the health care resources available, the costs of the intervention and its acceptability to the women concerned. A definition of the tasks that are to be performed at each level of the health care system will also be needed. An example for the actions at each level from community to hospital can be seen in Table 4.

Table 4
Detection(D), Managenent(M) and/or Action(A) of some risk factors at each level of Health Services. Calculated on 2000 pregnant women in Tanjungsari, West Java.

Risk factor	Outcome of risk	Women/ community	TBA	HC/doctor (midwife)	Hospital Obstetrician	Expected workload
Height <145 cm	Prev. 11:.5 LBW:±19% PMR:40%	D:+ A:Utilization of health-services	D:+ A:ANC refer if complication	D:+ A:pelvic ex. -if normal back to TBA -if abnormal refer to hospital.	D:+ A:Diagnosis/ management	±230 cases
Weight <45 kg	Prev:15.6 LBW:23.7 PMR:49%	D:+ A:Health ed. + suppl. feeding	D:+ A:Health ed. Refer for cause Follow-up ANC	D:+ A. Diagnosis Terapi refer for causes Follow-up ANC Delivery at HC.	D:+ A Diagnosis primer/ secundair -terapi	±310 cases
Breech	Prev: 2.4 LBW:33.9% PMR:228%	D:- A:-	D:+ A:referral for delivery.	D:+ A.-ANC Delivery -First parity referral Hosp.	D:+ A:delivery First parity. (SC).	±48 cases
Antenatal Bleeding	Prev: 0.4% LBW:12.5% PMR:875%	D:+ A:direct to HC/Hosp. Drink lot of fluids.	D:+ A:refer mild to HC. severe to hosp.	D:+ A:diagnosis managernent severe hosp.	D:+ A:diagnosis: -proper management. (SC).	±8 cases.

V. THE MEASUREMENT OF THE EFFECTIVENESS
OF THE RISK INTERVENTION

Components of the risk strategy have been monitored on an ongoing basis in terms of its feasibility, relative importance and whether it would produce the desired outcome. Frequent meetings were held at district level in order to solve local problems. Meetings were held with the pregnant women to discuss the importance of a specially designed reporting and action card, the Mother and Child Card, the meanings of special codes in the care for immediate referral to health centers or hospital with the TBA as well as the pregnant women and the community. Meetings were also organized with the village heads and women's groups to motivate them to support the pregnant woman and her family in case a referral is needed. Several discussions were held on how the neighborhood could cooperate in collecting funds for hospitalization.

Continuous monitoring and evaluation of the risk intervention are needed to examine whether the intervention is applicable and acceptable. To be able to do so, some questions have to be answered:

1. Is the risk screening valid?
2. Are the new tasks feasible?
3. Does the strategy need modification?
4. Does new intervention decrease the level of unwanted health outcomes?

At each level of the health care system, changes in the proportion of high-risk women seen should be measured, whether the match between risk factor and risk management at each level is appropriate. To measure the level of reduction in the unwanted perinatal outcomes, an effective registration system for vital events is important. Vital registration systems in Indonesia are not complete; each department has its own registration system and may vary in their quality by province. A system of simple and effective demographic surveillance will need to be developed to assess the impact of the intervention.

VII. PROBLEMS IN THE IMPLEMENTATION
OF THE RISK CONCEPT

If one aims at an overall coverage of the high-risk groups, in an area where more than 80% of deliveries are attended by TBAs, then it is important to incorporate TBAs into the formal health care system. TBA training has been directed more or less toward improving their clinical skills in order to have safe maternal and child health care. Problems arise mostly in identifying and reporting and recording the condition of mother and child. The older TBAs had problems in identifying pictures showing risk factors. To increase the knowledge of TBAs, regular refresher meetings and supervision are necessary.

More attention has to be given to change women and community perceptions of risk/perception and action may not go necessarily hand-in-hand as expected. Changing behavior certainly may need more time and may be an area for further research. This can be seen in their response to referral: Although their perceptions of risk are more or less in agreement, response to referral is influenced by their sociocultural background.

During the preliminary stage of the survey, there are some people who felt that by training TBAs and enabling them to utilize primary health care methods is devaluating the work done by midwives. This claim seems to be unfounded, because in the Risk Approach Strategy the health center midwife and doctor are both central in the design, implementation and supervision of the project. In many rural areas, TBAs are not invading the midwives' territory, because most of the people are poor and cannot afford to pay the high cost of a midwife or doctor. Concern was expressed by the health personnel to include curative care in the training module of the TBA training.

Acknowledgement: The author gratefully acknowledges financial support for this study provided by the Sophia Stichting Rotterdam, EEC Contract no. TSD-M-361.B(B), WHO-SEARO and the Ford Foundation project no. 870-0714. Statistical assistance was given by Dr. R. Peeters from the Antwerp University, Belgium.

REFERENCES

1. Fortney, J.A., and E.W. Whitehorne. The development of an index of high-risk pregnancy. Am J Obstet Gyn 501-507, 1982.

2. Backett, E.M., et al. The risk approach in health care. Geneva: World Health Organization, 1984 (Public Health Papers, no. 76).

3. Dibley, M. The use of epidemiology and risk approach in the development of perinatal health care system. Proceedings of the National Workshop on Safe Birth and Perinatal Health Care Promotion. H. Pratomo, G.H. Wiknjosastro, and E. Sirman (eds). Cipanas 19-21 Juni. 1987 7.R.F.

4. Alisjabana, A., E. Surotio-Hamzah, and S. Tanuwidjaja, et al. Perinatal mortality & morbidity and LBW: Final report V. The pregnancy outcome. Unpublished report, 1983.

5. Lechtig, A., H. Delgado, and C. Yarbrough, et al. A simple assessment of the risk of low birth weight to select women for nutritional intervention. Am J Obstet Gyn. 25:34, 1987.

6. Alisjabana, A., R. Peeters, and M. Meheus. Traditional birth attendants can identify mothers and infants at risk. World Health Forum 6: 240-242, 1986.

7. Peeters, R.F., S. Tanuwidjaja, and A.Z. Meheus. Knowledge, attitudes and practices of traditional birth attendants in rural West-Java. An ethnographic survey. ESOC Publicatie NR. 2 University of Antwerp, 1987.

33

THE UNDER-FIVES CLINIC

DAVID MORLEY, M.D.

Each year, in the North, there is an average annual expenditure of over $500 and, in many countries, over $1,000 for every child on health care. In the South, the expenditure is in the region of 2% of these sums and those countries who spend more than $10 are fortunate. The yearly shifts of capital and the changes in the health expenditure in poor countries in the last decade are shown in Figure 1 (next page).

The concept of an Under-Fives Clinic was developed in the late 1950s in the Wesley Guide Hospital, Ilesha, then the Western State of Nigeria, to provide appropriate health care for children within this resource restriction. At that time and, to some extent, now, most doctors give much greater time and thought to the management of illness among in-patients than for out-patient or ambulatory care. The Under-Fives Clinic was also one of the first attempts to provide a balanced, preventive and curative care to all those children who attended. It is this last issue that most doctors and nurses find difficult. The concept of separating curative and preventive care still persists and is difficult to replace with a more appropriate care such as the Under-Fives Clinic. The original description of the Under-Fives Clinic[1] describes a specific clinic as it was developed in Nigeria. The present chapter will attempt to update this experience in the light of a wider knowledge of child health and how this can be best improved with limited resources.

THE NAME "UNDER-FIVES CLINIC"

This has frequently been criticized. Some have said that it is the under-threes in whom the greatest mortality occurs and others have suggested that it should be under six or under seven as, for example, in the Philippines where children do not go to school until after six, they have been called Under-Six

393

Clinics. The original reason for giving this name is to try and imply that all health care to this age group child is given through these clinics. Unfortunately, in so many countries, "child welfare" does not include the immediate treatment of acute conditions which are so common and of immediate concern to the mother. Wherever individuals come for health care there is a tendency to separate them into groups; in countries of the South the first division is usually between men and women. However, small children have a special need to be separated off. Small children bear the greatest brunt of illness. The time between the start of an illness and its fatal outcome may be short, and relatively simple measures such as immunization are more cost-effective than in any other age group. For this reason, the separating of small children under five and developing a rational program for their comprehensive care must be a priority in health care systems.

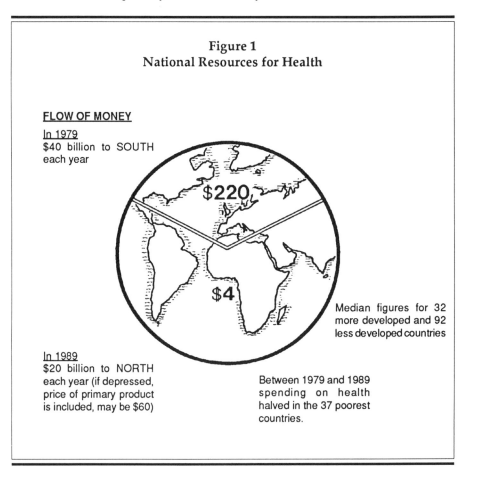

Figure 1
National Resources for Health

FLOW OF MONEY

In 1979
$40 billion to SOUTH each year

$220

$4

Median figures for 32 more developed and 92 less developed countries

In 1989
$20 billion to NORTH each year (if depressed, price of primary product is included, may be $60)

Between 1979 and 1989 spending on health halved in the 37 poorest countries.

THE OBJECTIVE: BALANCING NEEDS WITH RESOURCES

The need is vast. If all children, including the poorest, are to have services available, then the mother is unlikely to be able to travel more than 5 km. Equity demands that, as far as possible, the child living in a remote area of the country will get an equivalent service to children living in the capital city. Unfortunately, in the latter, there are likely to be many unemployed or under-employed doctors and also strong political pressures leading to more costly services which are similar to those found in countries of the North. If children are to receive appropriate care, then it will need to be provided by other than doctors. In the original Under-Fives Clinic, the care was provided by nurses who had undertaken a simple but very practical training in local small hospitals.

OBJECTIVES OF THE UNDER-FIVES CLINIC

The clinic will aim to reach all the children of the area, including specifically the poorest, who carry the greatest burden of illness in a society and are likely to be sick one day in every three (Figure 2). These children are the least likely to be brought, first because the mother is less organized and less likely

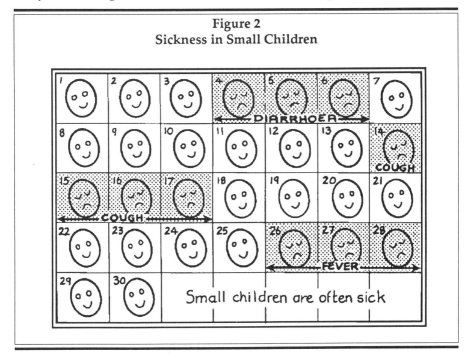

Figure 2
Sickness in Small Children

to have even primary education. Her pride will often mean that she will not bring the child because her clothing and the child's clothing are likely to be poor and her lack of washing facilities may mean the child is not clean. Unfortunately, the workers in the clinic who come from the better-off groups in a society are likely to criticize such mothers and, as a result, they will not return again. Areas where such mothers live need to be a priority for home visits when their growth charts can be checked and the family encouraged to bring the child if they have not attended over the last few months.

All the mothers, but particularly the mothers of the poorest, have very many calls on their time and every effort should be made to reduce the time spent in a clinic by regular study of the lines of flow through a clinic and what steps can be taken to reduce any waiting or delays.

SIMPLE, COMPREHENSIVE, LOW COST, CURATIVE CARE

The vast majority of those attending an Under-Fives Clinic come with common upper respiratory, gastrointestinal or skin infections. The majority of these are self-limiting and the mother needs encouragement and help in how to care for and, most important, to shorten the illness. Management of minor episodes of acute diarrhea is important, using whatever system of oral rehydration has been established in the area. The staff need to be reminded that only one child in a hundred with diarrhea is likely to have a fatal disease and this child cannot be recognized from the other 99. However, treatment of the other 99 is equally important to minimize the effect on the child and particularly to ensure that the episode of diarrhea has as little effect on the nutrition and growth of the child as possible.

The staff must be expert at counting children's respirations to identify those breathing faster than 50 per minute and they must all observe and discuss any children who arrive with rib recession and other signs of respiratory difficulty until they are all very familiar with such early signs which are necessary in the recognition of pneumonia.

PREVENTIVE STEPS

For a variety of reasons, the mother will look on the Under-Fives Clinic first of all as a place where she can get sympathetic and effective treatment for the common illnesses of her children. However, as mentioned already, many of these episodes will be mild and these can be used as occasions on which immunization and other preventive steps can be taken. The World Health Organization and International Pediatric Association agree that illness is not a reason for delaying immunization unless the child is so sick that it needs to be admitted to the hospital. If an immunization is due, it should be given. The decision to delay an immunization is a serious one and should be made only by the doctor in charge.

Training in oral rehydration takes time, and convincing mothers to use this whenever their child suffers from diarrhea takes even longer. However, in some countries the majority of children attending with diarrhea have now had some oral rehydration and the mothers need support and encouragement in using this simple technique.

Support for breastfeeding should be routine during the first two years of life. This is particularly important in societies where there may be pressures on the mother to use a feeding bottle and breast milk substitutes. Research in East Africa suggested that around 50% of mothers do have some difficulty in establishing and maintaining breastfeeding. Discussions on how to overcome difficulties that arise and how to help mothers should be a priority in the ongoing training of staff.

Weighing is now established around the world in most clinics seeing children. Unfortunately, entering the weight on the weight chart is less satisfactorily performed and achieving a proper understanding of the meaning of the growth curve by the mother is even less frequent. It is possible that, with the introduction of the TALC direct recording scale and weighing near or around the home, the understanding and value of the weight chart may be greatly improved (Figure 3, next page). These scales may also reduce the frequency of attendance at a clinic, as it is hoped some woman with further training within the community, such as a community health worker, would be involved in the weighing. She would also be responsible for encouraging a discussion which would involve the grandmother and father and others in the family and among the neighbors who are more likely to be influential in decision-making than a young mother. This is necessary, as so many of the decisions to be made to improve a child's nutrition are not those that can be easily made by a young mother. For example, she may need to have more time for breastfeeding or alternatively, if she is going out to the fields and leaving an older child behind, there may be a need for the grandmother or someone else to give the child an extra meal or meals through the day.

THE ROLE OF WOMEN IN THE UNDER-FIVE CLINIC

Mothers who themselves have successfully brought up children in a clinic are much more likely to be listened to by other mothers and are also more likely to provide practical advice and support to young mothers in the difficult problems they have in child rearing within a community. For this reason, the best workers in Under-Five Clinics will be mothers who are respected and can give practical advice. There may be a place for young men to be involved in the weighing and in clerking and crowd control in larger clinics, but the most valuable workers will be those who have had intimate experience of child rearing within the local community.

WHERE SHOULD UNDER-FIVES CLINICS BE SITED?

There is much research to show that mothers will not travel much more than 5 km, particularly if they have a toddler and a young baby and, for many mothers, 5 km may be too far. For this reason, Under-Five Clinics should be held as close as possible to the homes of the mothers.

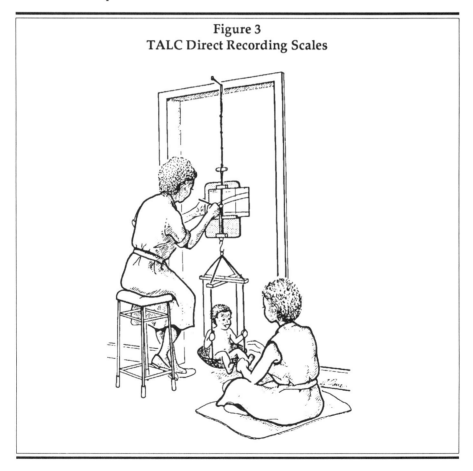

Figure 3
TALC Direct Recording Scales

Under-Five Clinics should also be present in all hospitals and all children under five should be directed at first to such clinics. A hospital where children are seen in other out-patient areas than the Under-Fives Clinics cannot claim to have a true Under-Fives Clinic, and children attending other units will clearly miss out on opportunities for preventive services such as immunization and growth monitoring. As already mentioned, the Under-Fives Clinics to be found at the teaching hospital should work very similarly in their operation to those in the remote areas of the country. The Under-Fives Clinic should be a good opportunity for medical students and others to learn how to work with colleagues with less training, and learn from their long practical experience.

THE DESIGN OF UNDER-FIVES CLINICS

More often than not, Under-Five Clinics will have to be run in buildings which exist already and have been modified. If a new building can be developed, then this should be along the lines suggested in Figure 4. The following is a possible checklist to consider in either a new building or alteration of an existing building:

- Will the waiting area be large enough and capable of extension if numbers increase, as is likely?

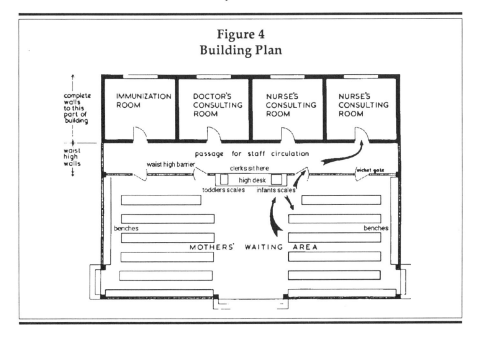

Figure 4
Building Plan

- If weather permits, can the waiting area be open-sided to encourage air flow and decrease the chances of droplet-borne cross infections?
- Is a water tap readily available? Are there washing facilities and toilets which can be maintained and are not frightening to children?
- Is the seating 30-35 cm high so that mothers can comfortably have a child on their lap? (Figure 5)
- Is the seating of clerks for registration sufficiently high so that their eye level is that of a standing mother?
- Can children be weighed in the waiting area?
- Can a waiting area be modified for health education? Space for records has not been included as it is assumed that home-based records will be used. However, arrangements may be necessary for storing records such as X-rays.
- Can the waiting area be separated from the staff circulation area, particularly the plan should make sure that mothers with their children will not be crowding around doorways? In Figure 4, the waiting area is separated from the service area by a waist-high barrier, which, as it were, does not shut the mothers and their children out but prevents crowding.

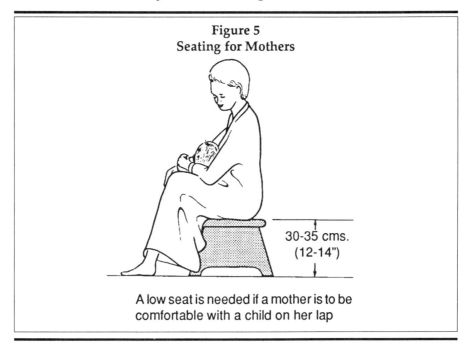

Figure 5
Seating for Mothers

30-35 cms.
(12-14")

A low seat is needed if a mother is to be comfortable with a child on her lap

WEEKLY STAFF CONSULTATION

Once a week, all the staff, including those responsible for cleaning, should if possible be assembled for a discussion session. This should be used for problem-solving and further training of all staff. The staff should consider particularly how the care they provide to mothers can be improved with existing resources.

In this meeting, the junior members of the Under-Fives Clinic team should be encouraged to make suggestions for improvement and, if at all possible, these should at least be tried out.

All staff should be encouraged to try to recognize the very ill child and be encouraged to bring such children without delay to the senior member of staff present.

TRAINING THE STAFF IN THE UNDER-FIVES CLINIC

The senior worker in the clinic has a greater responsibility for training. This should be at least as important a responsibility as the diagnosis and treatment of the more complex conditions that are referred. The traditional pattern of a consultation between a doctor and a mother and child is not suited to the majority of consultations in the Under-Fives Clinic. The doctor's time should be too precious and the conditions brought are, for the most part, simple and repetitive and can be better cared for by well-trained auxiliaries or nurses. Experience has shown that 9 out of 10 children can be well cared for by locally trained individuals and only about 10% require referral to a senior worker. However, the locally trained nurse should also be involved in such consultations. In this way, they can receive further training and supervision in their work. In this variety of consultation (Figure 6), the doctor takes care to

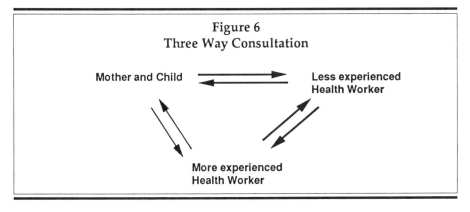

Figure 6
Three Way Consultation

Mother and Child   **Less experienced Health Worker**

More experienced Health Worker

treat the nurse or auxiliary as an equal colleague in front of the mother and child and, in this way, the mother and the child will have respect for the locally trained worker and will be happy for the majority of consultations to be undertaken by them. The locally trained workers will use a standard treatment regime and, wherever possible, the doctor will follow the same regime so that the mother does not feel that she is getting different and "better" treatment by seeing the doctor or senior worker.

REFERENCES

1. Morley, D.C. The under-five clinic. Chapter in Medical Care in Developing Countries. Maurice King (ed). London: O.U.P.,1966.

34

DAY CARE OF CHILDREN IN DEVELOPING COUNTRIES

O.P. Ghai, M.D. and M.M.A. Faridi,M.D., D.C.H.

Increasing numbers of women all over the world are joining the work force. Economic compulsions, escalating cost of living and rising expectations of people from the modern technological advances force mothers to take up jobs outside their homes, for supplementing family income and achieving better living standard. Family structure is fast changing from the extended to nuclear families. A large proportion of children are nowadays reared by a single parent, who could be either the mother or the father. Stay-at-home mother is becoming more and more rare in the rapidly changing social milieu. In the year 1980 about 47 percent of mothers with children less than 6 years old and 42 percent of those with children 3 years old were working in the U.S.A. It is estimated that both the parents of almost 70 percent of children will be working outside their homes by the year 2000. About 16 percent of all children 3 years of age had a single parent in the U.S.A. More than half of the latter were working for their living. Reliable data on the proportion of working mothers are not available in many developing countries. The problem in these societies is probably as acute, if not worse, with women ploughing and harvesting the fields, along with the men. These women are not recorded in the statistics as working mothers, because they do not get financial compensation from outside the family. Many poor women work as unskilled migrant laborers at construction sites and as domestic help often at lower wages than their male counterparts. More and more women from middle class families are taking up office and professional jobs in many developing countries. Besides being producers, processors and distributors of food to their families, women have a dual productive and economic role as unpaid helpers at home and in fields and as paid workers outside the home.

403

In the early 1980s, about 50% of working women in India were unpaid helpers in the family's vocation. This social change has brought into focus the need for good quality substitute care for children, while their parents were at work and could not look after them. Euphemistically the word "day care" appears less unjust, less compulsive and more in line with the modern way of life, compared with the term "substitute care" in the presence of a mother. The latter term fosters a feeling of guilt, since the mother leaves a crying unwilling child in the center. The objective of "day-care" is to provide a healthful environment for the child, so that there is little interruption in the parental activities. Day-care services are being increasingly sought by working mothers. Their need always outstrips the available resources in all developing countries.

TYPES OF DAY CARE

A. Most day-care programs for infants, toddlers, and 3 year-olds are essentially "custodial" in nature. Children are taken care of for a few hours every day. They are protected from injury and encouraged to play. Either the mother comes to breastfeed the baby or the child is fed by the caretaker at the appointed time. Medical care is provided in most organized establishments for day-care. Generally, the quality of care in the custodial type of day-care is not of the optimal standard.

B. "Developmental day care or preschool programs" focus on children between 3-6 years of age. These programs take care of the child during the day and are not located in the child's home. These are comprehensive enough to stimulate the personality and optimal physical, nutritional, cognitive and emotional development of the child. Some programs also involve parents in day-to-day activities .

ORGANIZATIONAL ASPECTS

A. Informal day care: In almost all countries of the world, including the industrialized societies, day care is often provided informally, when children are entrusted to the care of untrained personnel, while parents go outside the house for work. This is either provided at the home of the child, or in the house of a baby-sitter or a relative. In many developing countries an elder sibling often a girl, looks after the younger sibling. This elder sibling may not be sent to school because of social and financial constraints. In some families, grandparents provide substitute care for the child.

B. Formal day care. This may be provided in a residential or non-residential setting.

   1. Day-Care Homes. These provide day care to a group of children from at least two families. These could be "family day-care homes" for 2-6 children in the same locality or in a relative's home. In "group day care" a larger group of 7 to 14 children from the same neighborhood is taken care of by a housewife in her own home. These day-care homes have sprung up without any regulation or licensing in large metropolitan areas. Children participate in group play. The worker in charge of the facility provides custodial care.

   2. Day-Care Centers. Day-care centers are meant for a group of 15 or more children of variable ages, kept in one or two rooms and looked after by one or more adults. These could be full time establishments providing day care for 30 hours a week or be part time for 10/20 hours per week.

Informal family day care is the most prevalent type of substitute care provided all over the world. These provide a reasonably good milieu for optimal physical and emotional growth of younger children. Ratio of child-care staff per child is higher in family day-care homes compared with that in the day-care centers. These are generally not regulated or linked to any sponsoring agency and are therefore less expensive. Medical care of the child is often left to the individual family.

Day-care centers are established in the organized or unorganized (unregulated) sectors. Government and voluntary (non-profit) organizations are increasingly getting involved in initiating and developing these services. Some day-care centers are also run by profit-making firms.

The first nursery in the U.S.A. was established by a voluntary women's organization in 1854. Many day-care centers were subsequently supported by the government of U.S.A. during the years following the First World War and during the Thirties (the years of great depression). Countries such as Israel, Denmark, European Common Market and socialist countries have made significant investment in building up day-care facilities for children. In India a movement for establishing mobile creches for the care of children of migrant women labor at construction sites was started in the voluntary sector. The Government of India encourages and supports industrial establishments for setting up creches for working mothers. All organizations employing more than 50 women are required by law to set up a creche or day-care center.

The "Integrated Child Development Services Program" was started by the Government of India in 1975. Day-care Centers (anganwadis) for children between 3-6 years were established in the rural areas, tribal districts and urban slums. The program is now being rapidly expanded to cover most parts of the country. Children are looked after by an anganwadi teacher and a helper. They are given environmental stimulation, pre-school education and a nutritious diet. They receive regular medical check-ups and preventive and promotional health care. Indian Council of Child Welfare and other voluntary agencies supported by the Department of Social Welfare train workers for day-care centers.[3]

PROBLEMS OF DAY-CARE

Few systematic studies of day-care regarding its impact on the physical and health aspects, socio-behavioral implications and cost have been carried out. National Day-care Center Study[1,2] showed that when the size of the group of children in day-care was small and the staff of the day-care center was trained, developmental outcome of such children was better. Quality of day care suffers when there is poor monitoring of the services offered and trained staff is not available. There is a risk of sexual and other types of child abuse. Acute shortage of day-care facilities compared to the demand, low salaries of child-care providers, lack of standard policy of admission/exclusion of sick child, and paucity of scientific data on the long-term effects of day-care are some of the other areas which deserve careful consideration in the management of day-care.

ACUTE DAY-CARE ILLNESSES[4,5]

Infants and children in day care are at high risk of morbidity due to acute infective illnesses. Outbreaks of gastroenteritis do occur in all types of child-care settings. The incidence is generally low in the family day-care homes compared with that in day-care centers. Epidemics may occur as a result of child-to-child transmission through fecal-oral route. About 50 percent reduction in the cases of diarrhea may be achieved, if the day-care staff and older children practice hand-washing before taking food and after going to the toilet. Risk of respiratory infections is significantly more in the day-care centers than in the day-care homes. Stangert[6] reported the frequency of hospitalization due to respiratory tract infection at 2 percent and 5 percent in the home reared and day-care children, respectively. Day-care centers may facilitate spread of Hepatitis A and meningitis due to *Hemophilus influenzae* or meningococci, among day-care children, staff and their household members. Acquisition of cytomegalovirus infection and duration of excretion of the virus are significantly higher in full-time day-care children. They can transmit infection to pregnant women of the day-care staff and other contacts.

Care of the sick child in day care is another important aspect requiring consideration. Exclusion of the sick child from the day-care center does not always prevent further spread of the disease but definitely taxes the parents, since they miss their work and lose their wages. Medication is often not carried out correctly in proper doses and intervals in the day-care setting. It is better to prescribe a drug in once- or twice-a-day regimen in the form of chewable tablets or sachets. It is best to avoid giving medication during day-care hours.

SOCIO-BEHAVIORAL IMPLICATIONS

Infants should grow and develop in a loving, caring and stimulating milieu. The younger the child the more critical is the environment for his/her emotional and cognitive development. For millions of children the substitute care may not always be optimal. Available evidence does not suggest significant adverse psychosocial effects on children attending day-care facilities. Children who have been in group care early in life are more assertive, aggressive and peer-oriented rather than adult-oriented. They socialize adequately in the long run. Parent-child attachment is not affected by substitute care.

Gender of the child also modifies the psychosocial effect of day care. According to Moore, home-cared boys are self-controlled, more mature and show socially conforming behavior while day-care boys are less conforming and more demanding. Effect on girls is less consistent but they exhibit increased imitation.

Risk of health hazards with good medical supervision of day care is minimal. Well organized day care, e.g., as in Government of India-sponsored Integrated Child Development Services Program, provides a good developmental package for the child such as preventive health care, prophylactic immunization and early detection of deviation from normal growth pattern besides health promotion, nutritional support and environmental stimulation for good cognitive, personality and emotional development.

HOW TO CHOOSE A DAY-CARE CENTER

The mother should be encouraged to visit various day-care centers near her home, observe their physical facilities, play equipment, play area, safety provisions, equipment for storage of food, medical facilities, telephone, referral arrangements, etc. Decision about keeping her child should also take into account the monthly cost or fees, which should be affordable by the family.

ROLE OF FAMILY DOCTOR OR A PEDIATRICIAN

Family doctor or a pediatrician may be consulted by the parents regarding advantages and hazards of day care. She may seek doctor's advice on the choice of a day-care center. A doctor may be requested to provide preventive and therapeutic services for children in the creche or day-care facility. He may also act as consultant to one or more day-care centers regarding planning of services. A subcommittee of the American Academy of Pediatrics 1980 gave guidelines for establishment of day-care centers for children.

REGULATION OF DAY-CARE CENTERS

Day-care home and most of the day-care centers in the developing countries are in the unorganized sector without proper licensing, regulation and monitoring. These do not provide any developmental stimulation to the child and unless properly supervised could be potential health hazards. Neglect of safety provisions could result in irreversible damage to the child or may have even a fatal outcome. Pediatricians should seek and motivate decision makers to increase the availability of day care of children of needy mothers but ensure that these services are duly licensed and properly monitored to give good development experiences to the child.

As early as 1895, the Health Department of New York City was responsible by law for regulating sanitation and disease prevention in all centers providing group day care to young children. In 1985 "Model Child Care Standard Act" was developed by the Federal Government to improve the nation's child care program. This act provides the following safeguards.

1. Parent visit and participation. To allow unrestricted access of the parents to child-care program and to give guidelines to parents to check sexual abuse of their children.
2. Employment history checks of the staff and other background screening should be mandatory.
3. Staff qualification requirements and job classification to encourage employment of qualified staff and to ensure availability of trained care providers.

4. Probationary period was provided for the new staff.

5. Staff training, development, supervision and evaluation, training in the prevention, detection and reporting of the suspected case of child abuse was desired.

6. Staff ratio was determined. Staff-child ratio was determined with the increasing need for day care and likely expansion of services in the future.

Parents, pediatricians, day-care providers, public health personnel, nutritionists and teachers should come together to act as pressure groups to promote community and state interest in the welfare of children and passage of relevant legal provisions.

REFERENCES

1. The National Day-care Home Study. Cambridge, Mass: Abt Associates. 1981.

2. U.S. Department of Health and Human Services. Final Report of the National Day-care Study. DHMS Pub No. 80-30287. Washington, DC: U.S. Govt. Printing Office, 1981.

3. An analysis of the situation of children in India. UNICEF Regional office for South Central Asia. New Delhi: UNICEF, 1984.

4. Haskins, R., and J. Kotch. Day care and illness, evidence, cost and public policy. Peds 77 (supp):951-82, 1986.

5. Lemp, G.W., W.E. Woodward, and L.K. Pickering, et al. The relationship of staff to the incidence of diarrhea in day-care centres. Am J Epi 120:750-56, 1984.

6. Stangert, K. Respiratory illness in preschool children with different forms of day care. Peds 57: 191-196, 1976.

7. Moore, T. Exclusive early mothering and its alternative: The outcome to adolescence. Scan J Psychol 16: 255-272, 1975.

35

SCHOOL HEALTH SERVICES: RATIONALE

Y.C. MATHUR, M.D., AND AJIT KUMAR, M.D.

INTRODUCTION

School children constitute a significant portion of the population. By virtue of their numbers, children are entitled to a major share of the community health services. During this period, there are rapid physical, mental and emotional changes; hence there is a great need for health supervision and guidelines. School health services provide an excellent opportunity for early detection of defects and diseases which may in later life stand in the way of attaining full health and ability. The school-going child experiences group living outside the home, learns to adjust in the community and is exposed to hazards of infection in a mixed community.

HISTORY

School health services were introduced first by the French in 1883[1] which made the school authorities responsible for the sanitary conditions of the school building and for the health of children. Later, these types of services were introduced in other Western European countries. In the Eastern Bloc, it was first introduced in U.S.S.R. in 1871. In the developing countries, school health services are in infancy.

U.K.: School health services are provided both in clinics and in schools by local health/education authorities with grants from the Ministry of Education. Free treatment is provided to the children under the National Health Scheme. School health services continue to have a separate identity organized by local education authorities and designed to develop and maintain the physical and mental wellbeing of children who are being educated in public schools:

410

- Well maintained records and free treatment;
- Good dental service, child guidance clinic for each region, good health education (immunization, nutrition, adolescent problems, sex education, smoking, drugs);
- Special services for handicapped children. Physical, mental and cognitive handicaps, if necessary, are sent to special schools;
- School nutrition; 200 ml. milk is given to children up to 7 years of age. Mid-day meal given at subsidized prices and freely for needy children.

U.S.S.R.: They have well developed service from birth until the child completes education. All schools having more than 800 pupils have a full time doctor/nurse/dentist. It is a well developed service which was initiated in 1871.

FRANCE: The French were the first to develop school health service in 1883. The French Ministry for National Education has a department of school and university health which includes a central coordinating body, supervisory body, supervisory doctors, regional doctors and departmental doctors. School health services cover all school-age children including college and university students.

JAPAN: Health services are regarded as an integral part of school education. Each school has a doctor, nurse, dentist and a pharmacist. Health services are conducted by cooperative efforts of the school/Ministry of Education, Health Centers and other medical agencies.

U.S.A.: The responsibility for determining and operating the school health may be shared by the local school board and local health department services. Medical, nursing and other health personnel for school health services are provided with major emphasis on health appraisal, health education, immunization, sex education, child guidance and nutrition supplementation.

PHILIPPINES: School health services operate on a division or city level administered by the Bureau of Public Schools and the Department of Education.

SRI LANKA: There is a government Department of Health and Sanitary Services which provides school medical services under the direction of the school medical officer.

PAKISTAN: There is no separate organization to look after the school children; regular health centers are entrusted with this responsibility.

BANGLADESH/NEPAL/MAURITIUS/MALDIVES: School health services are not well developed.

INDIA: School health services were started in 1909 in Baroda City. Supplementary feeding of school children to improve their health and school enrollment was begun in Trivandrum in 1910. In Andhra Pradesh state, school medical inspection was started in 1935 during the Nizam's regime and was confined mostly to Hyderabad. Bhore committee in 1946 noted that school health services were practically non-existent even in places which were in a primitive state. In 1953, the Secondary Education Committee emphasized the need for medical examination for pupils and school feeding. In 1960, the Government of India constituted a school health committee to assess the standards of health and nutrition status of school children and suggest ways and means to improve them. In 1974, the National Policy for Children was adopted by the Indian government; it laid emphasis in areas such as child health, nutrition, immunization and welfare of handicapped children. Integrated Child Development Services looks after pre-school children while school health services look after school children.

In Andhra Pradesh state where school medical inspection was started in 1935 in Hyderabad, later Central Referral School Health Clinics were started at Hyderabad, Vishakapatnam, Tirupati which are attached to pediatric teaching hospitals. In 1985 Comprehensive School Health Services were established involving all school health children up to 5th grade, and students staying in dormitories with check-up twice a year with referral and follow-up services.

National Task Force on school health services was constituted in 1981. On the recommendation of the Task Force, intensive pilot projects were started in 1982 in 25 selected blocks.

1. To study morbidity pattern and nutritional status,
2. To study volume and type of acute and chronic morbid conditions requiring referral facilities,
3. To study the feasibility of entrusting the school teacher with responsibility relating to health status of school children, and
4. To strengthen health education in order to have better results from the scheme.

Health status of the children of a nation is a highly reliable index of health of the population. The needs of the children and our duties toward this are enshrined in our constitution. The constitution of India provides for the care and protection of children in Article 24 under Fundamental Rights, and in Articles 39 and 45 under directive principles. Besides constitutional provisions there exist a number of legislative provisions to safeguard the interest of children.

A clear, consistent national policy was absent until the adoption of National Policy for the Child in 1974; children constitute 25% of our population. Government of India expressed a keen concern for the adoption of a national policy since children are supremely important and a valuable asset to the nation; their nature and solicitude are of great significance for the development of human resources. India is also a party of the United Nation's Declaration of Rights for Children. This policy suggests and requires the State to provide adequate services to children, both before and after birth, and through the period of growth to ensure their full physical, mental and social development.

MORBIDITY PATTERNS

Anthropometry: Children (4-16) belonging to higher socio-economic groups have growth similar to Western standards (All-India Public School Data); lower socio-economic group — lower than better-off in spite of supplementary nutrition indicating the effect of early malnutrition (Punjab Primary School Children).

Nutritional problems: 40-50% of school-going children are under weight and 25% under-height. Sarat, et al.[11] have reported delay in the appearance of postnatal centers of ossification as compared to Western children. Avathel et al.[6] reported anemia of less than 10g in 12.9%. There was gross deficiency of protein intake, B complex deficiency is 5%, vitamin A deficiency is 2.7%, phrynoderma in 2.4%. Nutritional deficiency (34.19%) of all grades of malnutrition. Different studies indicate a preponderance of cereal-based diet. Insufficient intake of protective foods like milk, meat, and cereal is shown. Incidence of scabies was reported high in rural areas ranging between 8-11.8%.

Eye problems constitute about 8%, Xerosis, 14-20.4%, refractive error in 60%, and 13% infections.

Upper respiratory tract infections – 8-13%

ENT problems:

Tonsillitis – 5-6%
URIs – 8-13%

Hearing impairment – 1-2%

Dental problems:

Dental caries are common – 10.3-50%
Malocclusion – 10%
Need for oral prophylaxis – 90% of children.

SET UP OF SCHOOL HEALTH SERVICES:

Central Referral Clinic:	Peripheral School Health Staff:
A Vehicle	Pediatrician
Driver and Cleaner	Health Visitor
Statistician	Health Inspector
Pediatrician	Pharmacist
Dental Surgeon	
Ophthalmologist	
ENT Surgeon	
Public Health Nurses	

IMPORTANCE OF SCHOOL HEALTH SERVICES:

- School children constitute a large segment of population in any country.
- Well-defined target group at one place, with the help of teachers so that their health status, growth and development can be monitored easily.
- Children learn healthy habits in school based on the health education received at school from teachers and other health professionals and thus spread the message of healthy living in the community where they live and grow.
- A child who is not well cannot derive the full advantage of the education imparted at school.
- Early detection of defects in growth and development, vision, hearing, speech, and behavioural problems; correction will help the child to overcome the handicap and thus contribute better to the community where he lives.

AIMS/OBJECTIVES:

1. Promotion of positive health by periodic medical inspection of school children.
2. Early diagnosis and treatment of disease, institution of remedial measures to correct the defects observed during medical inspection and follow-up.
3. Control of communicable diseases by immunization.
4. Ensuring proper environment, sanitation in school, including attention to housing facilities, protected water supply, drainage,

disposal of waste, hygienic environment where mid-day meals are prepared and served.

5. Health education to impart knowledge and develop health attitude and habits to fight superstition, misconcepts, beliefs and fads which are likely to affect health, and make maximum use of available health services.
6. First aid and emergency care.
7. Improvement of nutritional status of school children by way of health education, supplementary nutrition, mid-day meals, etc.
8. Promotion of appropriate social and emotional behaviour and correction of behavioural problems with the help of child guidance clinics.
9. Detection and proper guidance to physical and mentally handicapped children.
10. Awareness of health problems of national importance, ways and means of prevention and population-control education, nutritional, communicable diseases, immunization, etc.

Objectives can be achieved by a Comprehensive School Health Service program as follows:

1. Curative Services: Out-patient management, hospitalization and rehabilitation
2. Preventive Services: TAB Vaccine; Diphtheria and Tetanus; Poliomyelitis; Nutrition/Supplementation/Iron and Folic Acid; Vitamin A supplementation.
3. Health Education: Periodic refresher courses in health education to teacher/paramedical staff. Health Education incorporated into the school syllabus. Parent interviews.
4. Research: Field surveys.
5. Statistics: Proper maintenance of records.
6. To promote child- to- child health program.

ACTIVITIES OF SCHOOL HEALTH SERVICES:

- Periodic health check-up of school children.
- Remedial measures and follow-up.
- ENT/Skin problems screening and treatment.
- Mental Health: Cognitive handicaps, juvenile delinquency, behavioural problems, smoking/drug addiction; hence, needs a child guidance clinic to correct these children.
- Growth monitoring: Physical development to be monitored.

- Handicapped children to be given special attention so that the child is able to attain his full potential.

HEALTH EDUCATION IS THE MOST IMPORTANT ASPECT:

1. Because of the growing documented linkages between health status of children and their educational achievement.
2. Because of the concurrent development, benefits that occur as a result of educating school-age children in basic health knowledge skills and practices.
3. Because schools themselves are an important channel of communication for health education, messages and distribution point for health services.
4. Because of the relationship that needs to be strengthened between school learning and out-of-school student community health/behaviour.

SUBJECTS TO BE COVERED

1. Personal hygiene – emphasis is on skin, hair, teeth, eyes, nose, ear and clothing. Attention to posture while sitting in the classroom.
2. Environmental hygiene – School/Home/Community.
3. Importance of protected water supply/sanitary lavatories.
4. Immunization services and their importance.
5. Nutritive value of foods and their effective use.
6. Population education, sex education.
7. Bad effects of smoking and drug addiction.

Health education is imparted by teacher as a part of school curriculum and as general knowledge and by periodic visits of health professionals.

ROLE OF SCHOOL TEACHER IN SCHOOL HEALTH SERVICES:

- Recording height/weight/vision/hearing test at regular intervals.
- Daily observation of children with a view to spotting any deviation from normal health.
- To maintain health record of the child and other family members.
- To assist and follow-up of children with defects/handicap and ensure that they follow the advice given by doctors.

- To assist health professionals in the course of medical examination of children.
- To give first aid and care during emergency, like injuries, bleeding, loss of consciousness, convulsions, etc.
- To educate parents regarding importance of school health services.
- Health and nutrition education through parent-teacher association and to the school children as a part of school syllabus.

School Health Services should, therefore, be encouraged all over the world, more so in the developing countries to prevent morbidity and mortality and for early detection and prevention of diseases.

REFERENCES

1. Van der Vynckt, S. UNICEF School Health Education Report. Feb 1985.

2. National Policy for Children. Government of India, Ministry of Education & Social Welfare, Department of Social Welfare. New Delhi: Ministry of Ed and S.W., Jan 1974, p. 1.

3. Annual Report 1980-81, Government of India, Ministry of Health & Family Welfare.

4. Kurup, S. Editorial. Health care of school children. Indian Peds, vol. X, no. 9, Sept 1973.

5. Gangadharam, M., et al. School health service programme in Kerala – A rural study. Indian Peds, vol.XIV, no. 8, p. 603.

6. Avthwale, N.B. School health services and medical examination of school children. Ind J Child Health, 8:387, 1959.

7. Shah, P.M., and P.M. Udani. Medical examination of rural school children in Palgarh Taluk. Indian Peds, 5: 343,1968.

8. Prakash, S.A., et al. Survey of school children in Achampet rural study. Indian Peds, 8:497, 1973.

9. Rao, R.B.H., et al. Nutritional health survey of school children. Indian J Peds, 28:39, 1961.

10. Agarwal, R.N., and P.C. AMunwani. Physical growth of Indian school children. Khadga, D.K. Agarwal, vol. 7, no. 3, p. 146, 1970.

11. Sarat, S., et al. Skeletal growth in school children. vol. 7, no. 2, 1970, p. 98.

12. Nagaraja Rao, D.N., et al. A comprehensive study of school children in twin cities of Hyderabad and Secunderabad. Indian Peds, vol. XI, no. 8, p. 567.

13. Primary school children in rural Punjab. Nutrition & Anthropometric Profile. Indian Ped, vol. 12, no. 11, 1975.

14. Rao, B.R.H., et al. (Vellore) Nutritional health status – Survey of school children. Indian J Peds 281:203, 1961.

15. Vijayaraghavan, K. Growth & Development of Indian Infant & Children. Publication of NIN, Hyderabad.

16. Rao, R.B.H. Nutritional and health status survey of school children. Indian J Ped 28: 39, 1961.

17. Santhana Krishnan, B.R., D. Shanmukham, and Chandrasekharan. School health programme in Madras City. Ind Ped 11:44, 1974.

18. Rao, R.B.H. Nutritional and health status survey of school children. Ind J Ped 28:39, 1961.

19. Rajammal, et al. Diet and eating practices of school children in Coimbatore. Indian J Ped 35: 350, 1968.

20. Dietary Allowances for Indians. Special Report Series no. 60, I, CMR. 1958.

21. Park, J.E., and K. Park. School Health Service Textbook of Preventive Social Medicine. 11th ed. 1986, p. 376.

22. Central Health Education Bureau. Report of Seminar on School Health Services. New Delhi, 1965.

36

SCHOOL HEALTH SERVICES: OVERVIEW

Anne-Marie Masse-Raimbault, M.D.

According to the different legislations, in most developing countries children aged 6-7 to 12-14 are supposed to go to school, but in reality, millions of them do not have access to schooling for many reasons. Scarcity of facilities and school teachers; population growth and the present worldwide economic crisis; poor financial capacities of families for school charges (school fees, text books, school uniforms); or inappropriate curricula have negative bearings on the attitudes of families toward education and particularly regarding access to girls' schooling.

For example, in Niger in 1986 primary school enrollment ratio was 37% of boys and 20% of girls.

In addition, many countries experience a very high drop-out rate in primary education. In Argentina, for example, 66 out of 100 pupils do not enjoy the benefit of a full cycle of primary education.

In a few countries, some structures such as creches, day-care centers, day nurseries, nursery schools, kindergartens, have been created for younger children aged 2-3 to 6-7. Most of them are located in cities. These different names correspond to differences in the provided services and in the educational objectives.

A small percentage of students, often from the better-off families, attending secondary schools and university can be added to school and pre-school children.

Though these school structures are heterogeneous, they gather an important percentage of children in every country. All of them are very eager to know about their health and the health of every member of the community where they live.

Should school be a privileged place where children should be guided "to build" their health through learning about health and getting into good health habits?

Pre-school and school-age are the stages in the course of which the child builds the foundations of his(her) knowledge, habits, acquire behavior, sense of responsibility, life rhythms, eating habits, capacity to observe, to think and to act.

It is during this stage of life that the child develops hygiene habits, discovers his(her) body with its potentialities, its requirements and its limits, acquires behaviors propitious to the blossoming of health, carries out activities so that he(she) will develop his body and his(her) will.

It is equally during his(her) stage that he(she) will be confronted with puberty and sexual problems, and he(she) will discover social life with its advantages and dangers like unemployment, alcohol, cigarettes and drugs, which are potential hazards with regard to his(her) mental health.

Should school be the place where children could elaborate day after day appropriate health behaviors?

HEALTH OUTLINES

Statistics on childrens' health, children aged more than 5 years particularly, are more favorable compared with the under-five mortality and morbidity rates and with mothers' mortality rates, so governments do not pay attention to them.

We must say that school children and adolescents do not usually take medical advice and seem to be healthy. As a matter of fact, they are little consumers of medical care even for somatic pathologies or functional disorders. However, they do not represent a population free of problems.

School children and adolescents' health needs are very heterogeneous depending on their age group and their belonging to different social classes.

From 3 to 6 years, problems center on growth and development:

- Growth supervision in order to detect malnutrition or nutritional anemia whose consequences are severe on school performance;
- Observation in order to evaluate linguistic capacities, psychomotor skills – such as broad and fine motor ability, spatiotemporal organization and lateralization, emotional development. These multiple aspects of development must not hide any important

risks of infections, diarrheal diseases, dermatitis, malaria, parastic diseases in some regions and rheumatic cardiopathies elsewhere.

After age 7, children have grown and developed, but other risks and pathologies like visual and hearing problems, dental caries, and accidents can be noted.

Then it is puberty and the first steps in sexual and social life with their share of dangers and illnesses: early pregnancy, cigarettes, alcohol, sexually transmitted diseases, AIDS, drugs.

These rough outlines differ in a country from urban to rural or poor to rich regions and depend on socio-economic classes.

Few investigations take into consideration problems expressed by children like headaches, stomach aches, sleep or appetite disturbances.

Such investigations would allow people in charge of children/health to define some concrete objectives in the field of health care, prevention and health education.

SCHOOL HEALTH SERVICES

In many industrialized or developing countries, there is a department in charge of children's health.

These structures, when existing, are connected with the Ministry of Health or Education. Physicians, nurses sometimes helped by psychologists are responsible for them, but in many cases their action is limited to some periodic checkups during the school years or control of vaccination cards. We will not analyze the different systems but we will try to propose some solutions capable of meeting the specific children's needs depending on their age.

It is important to know the children's real needs so that health agents can help school children, teachers and parents to find the best solutions to improve health and healthy living conditions at school, in the families and in the milieu.

HEALTH MONITORING ACTIVITIES

PERSONAL EVALUATION OF HEALTH

There are many examples where the main activity of school health services is the individualized supervision of children, due to systematic checkup at the beginning of the school year or at any other period.

These checkups are done more or less carefully depending on countries. In some places they consist of mere vaccination supervision, in others they are clinical examinations concerning general condition, growth (height and weight measurements), detection of dental caries and visual or hearing disorders, and psychomotor skills.

In addition, children are sometimes administered psychological or intelligence tests. The use of tests is not always harmless and children are placed in different aptitude groups depending on their results, particularly their intellectual scores. But, the tests drawn up in Western countries are not adapted to the cultures of the different countries. Also, each child develops at his(her) own pace, each aspect of his(her) development has his(her) own rhythm; the evaluation of psychological development is described at a given time and may have no predictive value.

The advantage of such an evaluation is to observe the evolution of the different capabilities and to stimulate every child's deficiencies so he(she) may develop harmoniously.

All these activities carried out in order to detect pathologies, anomalies or developmental delays are useful if treatment or compensatory programs are joined, but it is far from being the case in every country.

Besides, children are submitted to these evaluations but they don't understand what they are used for, because of lack of information and communication.

Some experiences in which school children are responsible for some aspects of their own evaluation are developing. For example, children supervise their own staturo-ponderal growth; they measure periodically their height and weight at school, they draw their own weight and height curves and learn to read them.

Older school children are able to help with younger school children's supervision. This exercise can be repeated for many other aspects of evaluation such as the surveillance of visual acuity.

JOINT SURVEILLANCE OF HEALTH

In a given area, a district for example, it would be profitable to study the evolution of school children's health condition by means of appropriate indicators.

This joint diagnosis of school children's health would help to determine priorities and to start programs more adapted to the different children's needs.

All physicians and nurses' fields of activities cannot be approached so we have chosen to discuss five of them.

IMPROVEMENT OF SCHOOL LIVING CONDITIONS AND SCHOLASTIC ENVIRONMENT

School health teams have to intervene more and more frequently in order to analyze with teachers, school and municipal authorities, school living conditions: children's cleanliness, general hygiene, adequate and well maintained sanitation, water supply and waste water drainage, furniture, air and lighting of class-rooms, problems caused by insects, mosquitoes or other vector, animals transmitting diseases, playground equipment, prevention of accidents inside and outside school. These teams may have no competency to decide but they have to advise authorities and foster school children in participating in the analysis of needs and in helping to improve living conditions. It is during the early years that children develop health habits; it is necessary that the school helps them to carry out the different apprenticeships concerning health and stimulate them to improve their living conditions according to local possibilities. Needs and programs will be different in a small rural town and in a district of a large metropolis.

In many countries children have their lunch or at least a snack out of their home. Whatever may be the organization concerning food, whether children bring food from home or get it at school, it is necessary to conform with hygiene rules, well-balanced diet and family habits.

School restaurants may become training laboratories where children could experiment, day after day, how to get a well-balanced and hygienic diet and learn about managing a budget.

School teachers should be trained in the field of nutrition. They also should know a lot about food to help children discover food, their various origins and transformations, cooking. Children should know how food helps the body to grow and be healthy and eating habits.

Health teams have to take part in the establishment of well-balanced school rhythms. The alternation of scholastic activities and their balance (working, playing, moving, sitting, sleeping, waking) require health teams to look after the children's rhythms taken both individually or collectively. Children's fatigue is a normal reaction. Teachers should know how to recognize signs of fatigue in order to stop some activities before children are exhausted.

Attending school is not always easy and school pupils may have problems. Children's difficulties need to be analyzed in order to know what are the reasons for maladjustment to the constraints of school life: family and health problems, overcrowded classes, heterogeneous levels of development, inappropriate curricula, language difficulties, teachers' motivation and training, dull pedagogical methods.

Some attempts to make improvements must originate from this analysis.

HANDICAPPED CHILDREN

This is another field of interest to which health teams' attention should be drawn. More and more frequently (depending on the handicap) it is recommended to integrate handicapped children in the normal school system. This choice includes evaluating the handicapped and his(her) possibilities, to act in concert with parents, teachers and health teams and to adapt schooling.

HEALTH EDUCATION

School is not only commissioned to teach children. It has to play a great part in helping them become healthy adults, able to adapt to living conditions and to help in development. Consequently health education ought to be one of the most important actions concerning school structures.

At an early age children are interested in health themes. They are eager to understand how the different vital functions of their system are working and why they are disordered. They want to know about the influence of environment on their health.

There are many ways to realize health education: The first one is to transmit to children notions such as "you must not throw garbage on the ground" or "you must wash your hands."

This training consists of orders, prohibitions, advice directed at children by adults and helps to instill reflexes: children are not allowed to acquire some understanding, helping them to choose freely healthy habits of life. It does not explain the reasons for particular attitudes and the consequences when they are ignored. It does not allow children for any alternative.

Another approach consists of giving children information and knowledge. Unfortunately it is not always possible to put them into practice or they do not allow children to improve their own behavior. Should health education rather be a dynamic phenomenon consisting of transferring useful knowledge from the analysis by school children of a real situation they lived through and in putting scientific ideas in daily life through actions at school and in the family? Children are given possibilities to choose. In such an approach children are obliged to act, that is to participate in the improvement of their life surroundings and in altering their own behavior.

These actions accompany and extend the acquisition of knowledge; they are practices, certain ones of which are transformed into habits of life.

Thus the educator must include knowledge of the environment in health education activities.

Taking the environment of some events such as a birth in a family, an immunization campaign as starting point, educators and children must analyze it, identify needs, means, actions and express these as part of the children's instruction and as acts to be carried out. These activities should not constitute a separate program in themselves but be included in various activities undertaken with the children such as mathematics, geography, grammar. Children must be encouraged to act, to observe, to analyze but by proposing actions that are practical and consistent with their age, possibilities, religion and culture. Every health field can provide educational program opportunities.

In health education, the role of example is very important. Small children are great imitators, especially of those they love; there must be close correspondence between what children are told and taught and what the entourage practices.

Some of the above-mentioned activities, like checkups, involve school health teams (physicians, nurses) directly but have to be accompanied with information and answers to school children's questions. Other activities like health education activities will be lived through with school teachers who will have support and appropriate knowledge from the health staff.

Ideally, programs would be planned by pluridisciplinary teams.

In some countries, another duty assigned to health teams is health teachers' surveillance.

TEACHERS' HEALTH TRAINING

Daily attendance with children gives teachers a privileged place to observe their health condition, its evolution and the improvement of childrens' wellbeing.

That is why teaching staff must be given the required information during their initial training to be able to cope with health education.

Later on, regularly, during in-service training, teachers should have meetings with well-informed specialists in order to deal with new health problems.

In 1983, Dr. E. Berthet, convinced of the teachers' interest in school children's health problems, proposed 6 main themes which training programs should include:

- child growth and development
- childrens' needs: sanitary, nutritional, affective, psychosocial and cognitive needs
- major risks threatening childrens' health and preventive measures
- knowledge of the collectivity in which children are living
- practical problems for children to adapt to school
- principles and technics in school health education with the school health team and the parents.

In certain regions, the installation of primary health care teams gathering school teachers and school children has given very good results and has been an opportunity to initiate them into concrete preventive acts.

Teacher training in health education requires that health teams agree to share and transmit their knowledge, proficiencies and abilities by making use of an appropriate and concrete pedagogy and understandable language. As for teachers they have to work with a multidisciplinary team in close collaboration with parents.

REFERENCES

1. Deschamps, J.P., M. Manciaux, and R. Salbreux, et al. L'enfant handicape et l'ecole. Paris Flammarion Medecine-Sciences, 1981.

2. Berthet, E. Information et education sanitaires. Paris PUF n° 2069 1983 The state of the world's children. Oxford University Press, 1989.

3. International Children's Centre: the early childhood development centres in Benin. Notes, Comments n° 181, UNESCO-UNICEF-WFP cooperative programme. Paris, 1988.

4. d'Agostino, M., and A.M. Masse-Raimbault. Health habits: a learning experience. Children in the Tropics. International Children's Centre. Paris, 1980, no. 128.

5. d'Agostino, M., M. Chauliac, and A.M. Masse-Raimbault. Teaching nutrition to young Children. Children in the Tropics International Children Centre. Paris, 1987, no. 166.

6. d'Agostino, M., and A.M. Masse-Raimbault. Proceed with caution... Children under six. Children in the Tropics. International Children's Centre. Paris, 1987, no. 170-171.

7. International Children's Centre: One day you will grow up, children of Benin. Videotape (20 minutes).

8. Chiland, C. L'ecole maternelle, L'enfant et sa sante. Paris Doins Editeurs, 1987, pp. 551-560.

9. Levy, B., and M. Dubois. Le temps de l'ecole. pp. 561-573.

10. Pissaro,A. Ecole et sante. pp. 575-587.

11. Brasseur, A., and P. Hennart. La restauration en milieu scolaire. pp. 589-595.

12. Jolibois, R., and M. Manciaux. Activities physiques et sportives a l'ecole. pp. 597-606.

13. Vermeil, G., and M. Manciaux. Difficultes et echecs scolaires. pp. 1257-1265.

14. Levy, B., and A. Rancurel. Formation du personnel enseignant. pp. 1257-1265.

37

ACCIDENTS AND INJURY
IN CHILDHOOD

Narayan Bahadur Thapa, M.B.B.S., F.R.C.S.

IMPORTANCE

Children are a high vulnerability group in accident situations. They have little experience and awareness of danger with inadequate muscle coordination and speed to escape from it. They are less liable to know what to do when accidents do occur. The younger the child, the more these factors apply. In the developing countries special conditions prevail. Children are a group who are more likely to be left to their own devices while the parents work in the fields. An older child is usually the minder of smaller children and even babies. Children frequently play by the side of badly designed and poorly maintained roads. During winter, children are often sitting around open kitchen fires unsupervised. In many countries older children work in the fields, on construction sites and in some industries. Many houses have accident traps like steep stairs without any light (Graphic 1, next page), windows without any bars and flat roofs without any protecting railings or walls. Above all, there is poor awareness on the part of the parents that a child needs to be protected from hazards (Graphic 2, page 430). Indeed in many societies accidents are accepted as inevitable and, therefore, there is no conscious thought on the matter. In the developing countries there are only a few accident and injury prevention schemes. Problems like infectious diseases are traditionally given priority. But there are compelling reasons why injury control should be given increasing importance. In many developing countries it is found that:

- Injury is the number one cause of death among children and young adults.[1] In the world as a whole it ranks fifth among leading causes of death in the population (World Health Statistics Annual 1984) and one child in every five or ten sustains an accident each year.[2]

- As the incidence of infectious diseases comes down, mortality and morbidity from injuries become more important by comparison.
- Since treatment facilities are minimal or nonexistent, injuries are liable to lead to more severe and more permanent disabilities.

Graphic 1
Steep Stairs

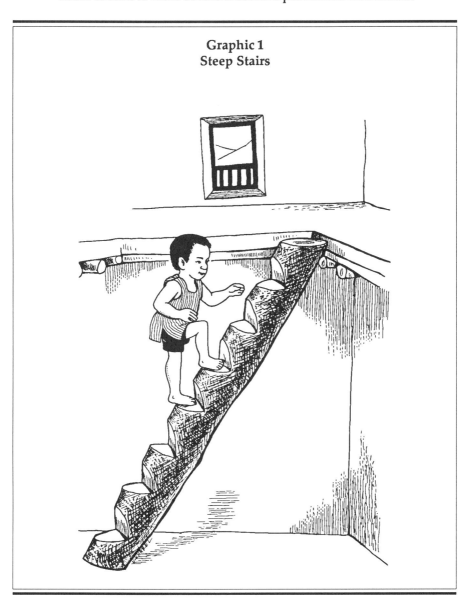

- Children form a much larger proportion of the population (more than 40%) than in developed countries, making this an important target group for any health promotion activities, particularly prevention of injuries.

COST OF INJURY

- When accidents lead to injury, the cost to the individual and community is great.
- Damages to the agent causing injury, e.g., motor vehicle
- Cost of treatment of injury
- Loss of productivity
- Human suffering.

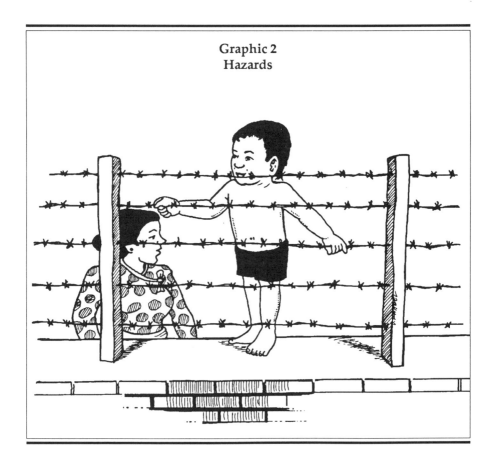

Graphic 2
Hazards

Disabilities tend to remain untreated. Rehabilitation programs are inadequate and ineffective to deal with the size of the problem. When children are the victims of injuries any uncorrected disabilities resulting from them are invariably longer lasting than in adults. The cost to the individual is tragic and to the community enormous.

CAUSES OF INJURY

Common types of accidents that lead to injuries among children are given in Table 1. Frequencies of particular types of accidents may differ in different countries but burns and fall injuries are universally common.

BURNS

Burns are among the most severe injuries that occur with great frequency in many countries. The main reason for this is that many villagers use firewood for cooking and this is done on open fire (Graphic 3, next page). In countries where kerosene stoves are used the fire hazard is less but even then the stoves are usually unstable, some are liable to explode and used mostly on floor level. To this kind of cooking area the children have ready access. In cold regions they spend most of the time around the cooking area for warmth. Burn injuries are seen more frequently in rural than urban areas.

<table>
<tr><td colspan="4">Table 1
Common Causes of Injury and Age Groups Involved</td></tr>
<tr><td></td><td colspan="3">Age Group</td></tr>
<tr><td>Common Causes</td><td>Under 1
year</td><td>1 to 5
year</td><td>6 - 15
year</td></tr>
<tr><td>Burns and Scalds</td><td>+</td><td>+</td><td>+</td></tr>
<tr><td>Falls</td><td>+</td><td>+</td><td>+</td></tr>
<tr><td>Poisoning</td><td>-</td><td>+</td><td>+</td></tr>
<tr><td>Animal Bites-Snake Bites</td><td>+</td><td>+</td><td>+</td></tr>
<tr><td>Drowning</td><td>-</td><td>+</td><td>+</td></tr>
<tr><td>Traffic Accidents</td><td>-</td><td>+</td><td>+</td></tr>
<tr><td>Agricultural Accidents</td><td>-</td><td>-</td><td>+</td></tr>
</table>

FALLS

In the rural areas falls are mainly from climbing trees. Boys climb trees to pluck fruit or gather fodder for cattle. In urban areas fall injuries are more frequent. This is due either to faulty design of houses, e.g., flat roofs without protective parapets, stairs without railings or to bad maintenance like missing bars from old windows. In India and Nepal, during kite-flying season in the winter many boys suffer severe head injuries caused by falls. Most of the kite flying is done from the roofs of the houses (Graphic 4, next page).

POISONING

In some countries accidental drinking of kerosene is very common. Kerosene is stored in beer bottles which are also used to keep water – a situation

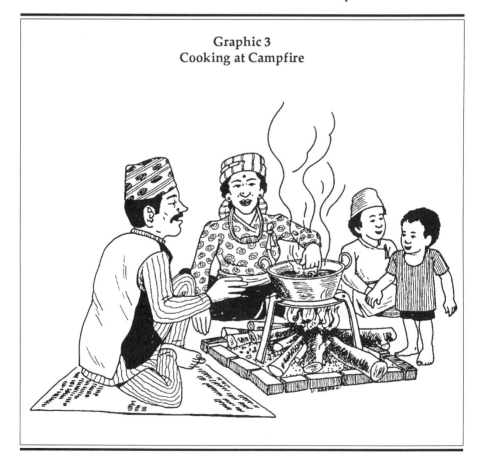

Graphic 3
Cooking at Campfire

fraught with danger. Medicines and other chemicals are kept where a curious child may easily reach and ingest. Poisoning from insecticide is a large problem in some countries; in Sri Lanka mortality from pesticide poisoning is greater than that from malaria, tetanus, diphtheria, whooping cough and polio combined.[3] The sales of drugs, poisonous chemicals and insecticides are not properly controlled and their storage may be haphazard.

ANIMAL BITES

Stray dogs are endemic in many poor countries. Bites themselves are usually not severe; the main danger is from rabid dogs. Poisonous snake bites may be fatal. Many African and Asian countries have large populations of poisonous snakes.

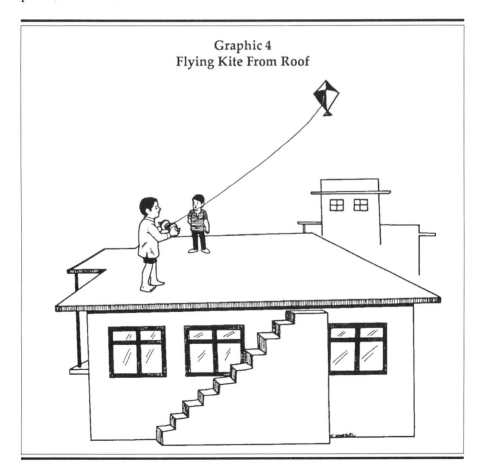

Graphic 4
Flying Kite From Roof

DROWNING

Rural areas have many ponds for the cattle to drink from. These ponds are always without any protective barriers and are a cause of many deaths from drowning. Swimming is not taught as a rule and adventurous children may approach rivers and lakes without appreciating the dangers.

TRAFFIC ACCIDENTS

Traffic accidents in developing countries are, so far, not a big problem in terms of absolute numbers. But the small number of vehicles in some of the countries cause many more deaths than an equivalent number in Western Europe and North America, very often twenty times more.[4,5] The reasons are bad design of roads, indifferent conditions of vehicles, unsafe number of riders (Graphic 5), inadequacy of traffic rules and lack of proper driver licensing. Thailand[6] and many Middle-East countries[7,8,9] where the road and vehicle conditions are better than many other countries, still show very large traffic accident rates.

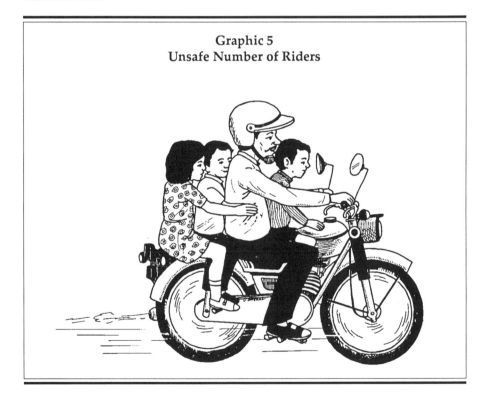

Graphic 5
Unsafe Number of Riders

AGRICULTURAL INJURIES

Some older children are liable to suffer injuries from farm implements as they are expected to work in the fields with their elders. Most of these injuries are minor in nature like cuts and punctures of hands and feet. Occasionally axes or large farm implements may cause deep cuts and mangling injuries. But even minor injuries may become fatal if tetanus is the result. Large sections of population are without the benefit of tetanus prophylaxis in many countries.

OTHER ACCIDENTS

Other accidents like electrocution, suicide, homicide, explosions, etc., form a small proportion of the total injury picture. Electrocution may be an increasing problem in rural areas when electrification is made possible without the necessary safety measures. Injuries like industrial and sport injuries will become a larger problem in the future. Lack of adequate legislation and faulty manufacturing are already responsible for many injuries from fireworks during festival seasons in many Third World countries. Natural disasters seem to affect a large number of people in countries like Bangladesh where every year many lives are lost due to floods. Earthquakes and landslides also take a yearly toll of many lives.

DEATH AND DISABILITY

Injury is a common day-to-day occurrence in many people's lives. Fortunately the majority of injuries are minor in nature. Perhaps this is the reason why most people are apathetic toward ideas about preventing accidents. However, the fact remains that some types of accidents are liable to lead to severe injuries with distinct possibilities of death or disability. Any fall from a significant height can cause severe head injury, internal or spinal injuries and fracture of limbs. Traffic accidents are well known for producing many fatalities. Poisons and drowning lead to deaths in many countries. Burn and scald injuries involving more than 15% of body surface in a child can lead to death, but it is the association of long-term morbidity and disability that increases the significance of this particular type of injury. In Nepal it is estimated that 3% of the population are disabled and that 25% of all disabilities are caused by injuries, one-fifth of which are due to burns and scalds (Thapa 1986, as yet unpublished).

TYPES OF ACCIDENTS BY AGE

When formulating strategies for prevention of accidents it is important to look at types of accidents in terms of their frequency in particular age groups. The groupings should be done in such a way that they reflect a child's natural activities and the environment in which children perform these activities (Table 1). Infants under one year are especially prone to foreign-body ingestion and inhalation. They frequently fall into open cooking fire in rural countries sustaining severe burn injuries. Young school children are at risk of being drowned as they are liable to approach open ponds. Adolescents are more likely to be involved in motorcycle accidents and suicides. Falls in this age group are particularly severe as they tend to be involved in activities like climbing trees and flying kites on flat roofs.

PREVENTION OF ACCIDENT AND INJURY

In considering the specific problem of children in a developing country it is important to state certain general principles. First, not all accidents are preventable. Second, the effects of many accidents can be minimized or sometimes be completely eliminated. For example, head injuries due to a crash among motorcyclists can be avoided if properly designed crash helmets are worn. In human terms it is important to consider preventing injuries when it may not be possible to prevent accidents that cause them.[12] Figure 1 illustrates some key issues related to injury control.

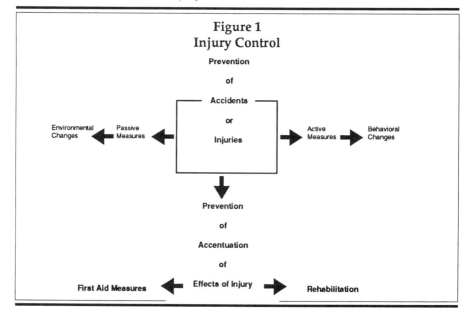

Figure 1
Injury Control

In considering the best way to keep people and particularly children from getting involved in accidents, one is aiming either at modifying the behavior of individuals or altering the environment they live in or the equipment they might use. Modification of behavior calls for ACTIVE MEASURES like preventing children from going into cooking areas or playing on the roads or flying kites from unprotected roofs. This means that first of all the parents and teachers have to be educated to recognize the dangers, who in turn must educate and supervise children to avoid risk-taking behavior and activities. This is particularly important as many accidents to children occur in and around their homes and schools. However, it has been found that a blitz of health education activity through mass media does not always bring a long-lasting change in the behavior of people.[13] What health education needs to do is to focus its attention on children through inclusion of information on prevention in the school curricula so that the exposure to this material is longer lasting and thorough. Another interesting and successful approach is a child-to-child program. This program is meant to teach school children to look after the health of their younger brothers and sisters or other younger children in the community. This is done through publication of a child-to-child book. The original book of these ideas about children helping each other was published in the International Year of the Child[14] and contains a chapter on accidents. This is an idea that can be adopted to many circumstances. Among the general population health education must promote dissemination of information about the actual possibility of prevention of accidents as this is a fact which is not always obvious to human thought. We must also supply information about what they can do to change their environment to make it safer. Above all education must include attempts to influence decision makers who can help to make the environment we live and travel in safer.

Changes in environment or the equipment people use provide examples of PASSIVE MEASURES where people do not have to take any action individually. If road design defects are subjected to low-cost remedial measures, accidents become less likely.[15,16] Similarly, in a vehicle designed with safety in mind even if accidents do occur injuries can be avoided or minimized. Provision of speed humps in certain areas keeps the speed of vehicles down, thereby increasing the safety of the area. In Nepal it was found that changing the cooking stove from the usual open fire to an improved closed type of stove brought down the incidence of burns by nearly 70% (Thapa, 1986, as yet unpublished). An important aspect of prevention is to minimize the accentuation of the effects and after-effects of injury. People who deal with the injured should know that proper handling is vital. For example, a child who has a part burned or scalded should have that part immersed in cold water immediately to reduce further damage by continuing high temperature of the burned area.

Programs of surgical correction of disabilities and rehabilitation program for handicaps resulting from injury should be developed on a priority basis. Aids for the handicapped should be simple, reliable, inexpensive and in designing them the needs of the user should be given due consideration.[17] Legislation has an important role to play in any injury-prevention effort. In many undeveloped countries potentially lethal situations are tolerated. For example, a motorcyclist may be required by law to wear a crash helmet. But his wife and children as pillion riders can travel without any protection. Legislation can help to stop this sort of situation. In making any plans for prevention of injuries it is useful to consider ten strategies.[18]

1. Prevent the creation of the hazard.
2. Reduce the amount of the hazard brought into being.
3. Prevent the release of the hazard that already exists.
4. Modify the rate or spatial distribution or release of the hazard from its source.
5. Separate, in time or in space, the hazard and that which is to be protected.
6. Separate the hazard and that which is to be protected by interposition of a material barrier.
7. Modify the relevant basic qualities of the hazard.
8. Make that to be protected more resistant to damage from the hazard.
9. Bring to counter damage already done by the hazard.
10. Stabilize, repair and rehabilitate the object of the damage.

In all underdeveloped countries where resources are scarce one has to make priorities. For it is essential to have reliable data on injury and its causation. After having established the priority areas it is also vital to consider what injuries are amenable to prevention. In agricultural countries it may not be very practical to try to prevent injury caused by farm implements, but burn injuries are amenable to preventive measures and should be tackled urgently.

Whenever possible National Injury Prevention Programs should be initiated. Efforts in this direction should be aimed mainly at the decision makers and groups that may be more aware of problems concerning themselves. For examples Youth Organizations and Mother's Groups may be particularly interested in any program to prevent accident/injuries to children. Other national and international non-governmental organizations (NGOs) may be willing to launch pilot projects to prevent injuries. When these pilot projects have demonstrated the efficacy of preventive measures the next step would be to influence the decision makers. For anyone particularly interested in promoting the idea of prevention of injuries a worthwhile initial step would be to co-ordinate the inputs from these national and international NGOs. This method has been used already with some success in Nepal where a momentum is gathering.

Lastly, any national program should be multi-sectoral as injuries occur in situations covered by a host of agencies. Unless these agencies sit together in the planning stage, chaos might prevail or worse still non-action might be the result. Therefore, an integrated approach by authorities dealing with health, education, legislation and law enforcement is essential to ensure success. Private agencies like construction companies, architectural consultants, manufacturers and media should also be made aware of possibilities of improvement in public safety. Injury is everyone's problem; if it is not their concern, it should be.

REFERENCES

1. Himan, A.R., et al., (eds). Health services in Shanghai County. Am J Public Health 72 Supp:1-95, 1982.

2. Manciaux, M. Accidental injuries in the young: From epidemiology to prevention. Effective Health Care 2(1): 21-28, 1984.

3. Jeyeratnam, J. Planning for the health of the worker. In D. Bull. Pesticides and the Third World poor: A growing problem. Oxford: Oxfam Public Affairs Unite, 1982.

4. Jacobs, G.D., and P.R. Fouracre. Further research on road accident rates in developing countries. Department of the Environment Department of Transport, TRRL Report, SR 270. Crowthorne: Transport and Road Research Laboratory, 1977.

5. Jacobs, G.D., and W.A. Hards. Further research on road accidents rates in developing countries (2d report). Department of Environment Department of Transport, TRRL Report, SR 434. Crowthorne: Transport and Road Research Laboratory, 1978.

6. Punyahotra, V. Epidemiology of road traffic accident in Thailand. National Accident Research Center, National Safety Council in Thailand, 1982.

7. Bayoumi, A. The epidemiology of fatal motor vehicle accidents in Kuwait. Accident Analysis and Prevention 13(4):339-48, 1981.

8. Weddell, J.M., and A. McDouglass. Road traffic injuries in Sharjah. Int J Epi 10(2):155-159, 1981.

9. Eid, A.M. Road traffic accidents in Qatar: the size of the problem. Accident Analysis and Prevention, 12:287-298, 1980.

10. Learmouth, A.M. Domestic child burn and scald accidents. J Ind Med Assoc 73(2):43-47, 1979.

11. Rao, B.S. Burns in childhood and early adolescence: An epidemiologic study of hospitalized cases. J Indian Med Assoc 46(1):23-27, 1966.

12. Baker, S.B. Injury control: Accident prevention and other approaches to reduction of injury. In Sartwell, P.E. (ed). Preventive Medicine and Public Health, 105th Ed. Englewood Cliffs, NJ: Appleton-Century-Crofts, 1972.

13. McLoughlin, E., et al. Project burn prevention: outcome and implications, Am J Public Health 72;241-247, 1982.

14. Aarons, A., H. Hawes, and J. Gayton, (eds). Child-to-child. The Macmillan Press Ltds, 1979.

15. Landies, J.R. The work of the GLC black-spot team: GLC Road Safety. London, 1979.

16. Wilson, J.L.S. Before and after accident studies at blacksites. Hertfordshire Country Council, Nov 1978.

17. Mohan, D. Amputees in India: Who they are, what they need and what they get. National Association for Equal Opportunities for the Handicapped News, XIII:4, Bombay, 1983.

18. Haddon, W., Jr. On the escape of tigers. Am J Public Health 60(12):2229-2234, 1970.

38

HANDICAPPED CHILDREN AND YOUTH IN DEVELOPING COUNTRIES

HELEN M. WALLACE, M.D., M.P.H.

GENERAL PICTURE

There is no uniform picture of handicapped children and youth in "developing" countries. Rather, the picture varies from country to country, depending on such factors as: (1) The stage of development of basic preventive programs and services, both general public health and more specific maternal and child health services; and (2) the stage of development of specific case finding; diagnostic, treatment, and rehabilitation; special education; and vocational programs and services for handicapped children and youth and their families.

Programs and services in "developed" countries by comparison on the whole are quite well developed. These include such countries as the United Kingdom, Australia, Western Europe, Scandinavia, and the United States.

COMMON TYPES OF HANDICAPPING CONDITIONS IN CHILDREN AND YOUTH IN DEVELOPING COUNTRIES

Data are lacking in regard to the incidence and prevalence of handicapping conditions in children and youth in most developing countries. This would require special surveys and/or special community studies.

One example of a recent national survey is that done in the People's Republic of China (which currently has a population of 1.2 billion) in 1987. (Table 1, next page). As seen in Table 1, from this survey, it was estimated that there was a total of 51,640,000 people (4.8% of total population). The largest single estimated groups are communication (both hearing and speech) –

441

11,700,000; intellectual handicap – 10,710,000; handicaps of extremities – 7,550,000; visual handicaps – 7,550,000; psychiatric handicap – 1,940,000; comprehensive handicap – 6,730,000. The criteria used to differentiate the various types of handicaps in this list are not known to this author; nor is it known how the survey was done. "Comprehensive handicap" probably refers to multiple handicaps.

MAJOR TYPES OF HANDICAPPING CONDITIONS IN CHILDREN AND YOUTH IN DEVELOPING COUNTRIES

Major types of handicapping conditions in children and youth in developing countries include the following:

- Post poliomyelitis
- Post trauma – fractures, burns
- Tuberculosis of bone and joint
- Cerebral palsy
- Mental retardation
- Epilepsy
- Hearing
- Vision - due to Vitamin A deficiency or to Ophthalmia neonatorum
- Cretinism due to iodine deficiency
- Other congenital malformations

Table 1 Sampling Investigation for Handicap (1987 - China)	
Total handicapped persons	51,640,000
% of handicapped persons in total population	4.8%
Communication Handicap	11,700,000
Intellectual Handicap	10,710,000
Extremites Handicap	7,550,000
Visual Handicap	7,550,000
Psychiatric Handicap	1,940,000
Comprehensive Handicap	6,730,000
Source: Reference 1	

The exact listing may vary from country to country, depending on the extent and effectiveness of the individual country's preventive efforts. Thus, one cornerstone of a community program and services for handicapped children and youth is prevention. Some of the basic preventive services and steps are as follows:

DEFINITION OF PREVENTION

Prevention services for persons at risk of parenting a handicapped child may be defined as those activities which may correct or avoid conditions or actions which result in handicap or disability for infants and children.

Prevention services have traditionally been classified into three types:

- **Primary Prevention** — Activities which attempt to eliminate causes of handicaps and thus reduce their prevalence in the community.
- **Secondary Prevention** — Procedures to cure or lessen the full development of a condition after it has been recognized.
- **Tertiary Prevention** — Services which minimize long-term disabilities or lessen some of their effects.

COMMUNITY EFFORTS TO PREVENT HANDICAPPING CONDITIONS IN CHILDREN AND YOUTH

Essentially, the most common types of community efforts to prevent handicapping conditions in children and youth in developing countries are those basic efforts which are carried on as part of general public health and maternal and child health services in the country. These include:

1. IMPROVED MATERNITY CARE

This includes such services as:

A. Making prenatal care accessible and available for all women who are pregnant.
B. Screening all pregnant women for high risk.
C. Arrangements for a referral system for special care of high risk pregnant women.
D. Provision of a safe labor and delivery service for all women, by a trained attendant.
E. Training of untrained traditional birth attendants, and incorporation of them into the "maternal health care" system.

2. IMPROVED NEONATAL AND INFANT CARE
   A. Prompt and safe resuscitation of the baby showing signs and symptoms of asphyxia.
   B. Use of a prophylactic solution of 1% silver nitrate in the eyes of all newborns.

3. SAFETY AND ACCIDENT PREVENTION
   Special care in conditions around the home, the school, roads, etc., to prevent falls and burns around the home and schools, and to prevent injury to children and youth on roads.

4. NUTRITION
   A. Prevention of blindness due to Vitamin A deficiency by providing adequate breast feeding and supplementary foods (including Vitamin A-containing foods) to infants, children, pregnant and lactating women.
   B. Prevention of thyroid deficiency and cretinism through the use of supplementary iodine in salt, bread or by injection, in those countries known to have a significant iodine deficiency (Nepal, mountainous areas of Latin America, etc.).

5. IMMUNIZATION
   This includes the use of the continuous mass application of all known safe effective immunizing agents available to all infants, children, and youth (BCG vaccine, DPT, measles, mumps, German measles); and of tetanus toxoid to all pregnant women to prevent such conditions as:

   Post-poliomyelitis paralysis
   Tuberculosis of bone and joint
   Encephalitis resulting from measles
   Congenital malformations from German measles

PRIMARY HEALTH CARE

One example of the PHC approach as a preventive device is to educate the mothers to recognize respiratory infections in their infants and children and to bring them immediately to the local health center for treatment and care. This is one example of a preventive approach to preventing the development of otitis media and a conductive type of hearing loss.

Still another example of the use of PHC approach as a preventive tool is education of the mother in the various aspects of safe maternal and child health care for herself and for her family, as a general approach to prevention of handicapping conditions in children and youth.

CARE OF HANDICAPPED CHILDREN, YOUTH AND THEIR FAMILIES

ASSESSMENT OF NEED

One of the early stages is to determine the needs of handicapped children, youth, and their families. This depends on the extent of the problems (i.e., number of known cases, incidence, prevalence, needs of children and families); and the extent to which such needs are being met. Discussions with providers of care (doctors, nurses, teachers, and other health providers), and parents are essential.

ASSESSMENT OF RESOURCES

A related question is the extent to which there are any resources for services and care – i.e.:

1. Case-finding and early identification

Finding the child who is handicapped represents the first step in assisting him (or her) and his family to receive care. Early case finding is essential in order that the child may receive the necessary care and services as soon after the onset of the condition as possible. The earlier the child is found, the earlier the diagnosis may be made, and the earlier treatment may be begun. If treatment and habilitation measures are to be provided at the time most appropriate for the child, early case finding is essential. Methods of early case finding include the following:

- Careful examination of all newborn infants;
- Continuous health supervision and observation of infants, preschool children and children of school age;
- Screening of infants and children for developmental and metabolic defects; and
- Especially close follow-up, observation, and study of infants and children at increased risk — those born of mothers with complications or of difficult labor and delivery; those of families with a known genetic condition.

2. Evaluation, diagnosis, treatment, and habilitation

All children having or suspected of having a handicapping condition should have a comprehensive evaluation promptly after the child is "found." The objectives include:

  a) to establish or rule out the diagnosis;
  b) to ascertain the etiology of the child's condition;
  c) to determine the extent of involvement, the degree of handicap, and the presence and extent of the child's abilities and potentialities for functioning;
  d) to appraise the effect of the condition upon the child and family;
  e) to estimate the short-term and long-term needs of the child and family, and to establish goals for the child and family;
  f) to interpret the child's condition to the family;
  g) to recommend, provide, and assist the family in carrying out the plan for treatment, habilitation, and management.

The approach needs to be a broad one, considering the social, psychological, educational, vocational, and recreational needs of the child and family. A team is usually necessary to provide this step.

An important aspect of this step is the appraisal of the child's abilities in certain functional areas of activities of daily living: feeding, dressing, toilet care, walking, and speech and communication. Training of the child (and of the child's family members) is an important part of habilitation of handicapped children.

3. Early intervention

Early intervention refers to any organized treatment that supports the developmental progress of young children and is aimed at ameliorating or eliminating a current or anticipated deficiency. Early intervention includes the entire family. Following the initial appraisal of the child, an individual plan needs to be developed for each child and family, which will promote and facilitate the child's physical, social, emotional, and developmental progress.

4. Education

Education, including special education, includes a wide range of services and programs designed to help handicapped students learn. In "developed" countries, special education programs begin with infants and very young children and extend throughout the periods of childhood and adolescence. The purpose may be to improve academic knowledge and skills for the mildly handicapped. Or it may be to teach life skills for students with more severe handicaps to live as independently as possible. The term "education" is used in its broadest sense to refer to traditional academic education as well as instruction in toilet training, dressing or communicating.

5. Vocational assistance

One of the objectives for handicapped children is that most of them as adults will become independent, self-supporting and productive members of society. This means the provision of services to make it possible to test, guide, train and place handicapped youth and adults in the appropriate vocational and employment setting. It includes consideration of the individual's physical, psychological, social, and educational status and interests.

6. Follow-up and case management

Handicapping conditions in children and youth usually require long-term care. Furthermore, as children and youth grow and develop, their needs for care and management may change appropriately. Thus, the plan of care includes a method of long-term follow-up, periodic appraisal of needs of the child and family, and modification of the plan for care as the needs of the child and family change. Case management through an interdisciplinary team is one method of providing individual follow-up care.

7. Respite care

Respite care is the provision of appropriate services on a short-term basis in a variety of settings to individuals unable to care for themselves, because of the absence, illness, emergency, or need for periodic relief of persons normally providing care. The severity of the child's handicap, the extent of related health or behavioral problems, and the drain on the family's physical and emotional health are the chief reasons for the family seeking respite care. Respite care services include the following: community in-home approach which offers respite providers, homemaker services, home health aide services, community out-of-home approach, placement in group homes, and short-term placement in residential facilities.

8. Transportation

The provision of transportation is an essential service for handicapped children. The ready availability of such service means that handicapped children will be able to attend regularly such activities as an evaluation and treatment program, a school program, a recreational program or a vocational program. The absence of transportation frequently means that handicapped children are either unable to attend or do so on a very irregular basis.

9. Recreation

Recreational activities are a necessary adjunct in services for handicapped children. They provide socializing experiences and are a means of enriching childrens' development. Group experiences are particularly desirable.

STEPS TO TAKE

The above is a list of some community services provided in communities in developed countries.

- An early step is to identify who and how many trained people are available to provide services and care, and to train others.
- An early step is to make a plan to train key personnel. One step might be to select a small number of key personnel for training who will return and establish new in-country training programs for long- and short-term training of other key personnel.
- Still another early step is to establish a community planning and advisory committee to:

1. Look at needs,
2. Determine unmet major needs,
3. Recommend plans for development of services and development of training programs,
4. Monitor progress,
5. Recommend legislation and funding.

Such a community planning and advisory committee would be composed of key professionals interested in the field of handicapped children and youth; major community political leaders; major representatives of parents and parents groups.

PRINCIPLES OF CARE AND MANAGEMENT

1. The care of many handicapped children is life-long. Therefore, for each child and family, an individual plan is needed which is both long term and short term. This plan should include continuity of care, monitoring of the child's growth and development, and the ability to modify the plan as the needs of the child and family change.

2. The family plays a central role in the care and life of the child in providing day-to-day care; in participating in all decisions about their child; in knowing the most information about their children and sharing this information with health professionals; in serving as advocate for their child and for other handicapped children. Care should be child- and family-centered.

3. The problems of handicapped children and youth and their families are many and varied. They include health, social, educational, vocational and housing. For this reason, a spectrum of community services is needed. Also, an interdisciplinary team is usually required, both in a diagnostic, treatment, and habilitation service, and in special educational and vocational services. Usually, the support of such interdisciplinary team services, which are required to provide comprehensive care, is expensive and beyond the reach of most families. Community support is essential.

4. Prevention of handicapping conditions in children and youth should be an important goal of all services and programs for handicapped children.

5. Training of personnel is an essential part of planning for the care of handicapped children and youth and their families.

6. Care of handicapped children and youth should take place in the least restrictive environment, wherever possible.

7. The long-term plan for community services for handicapped children, youth, and their families when fully developed should include a regionalized plan, with one or more central major centers for diagnosis, treatment, habilitation; training of personnel; and research. It should include district services providing diagnosis, treatment, habilitation, and follow-up continuing services; and

locally, where the child and family live, it should include therapy (physical, occupational, communicative), education, training of parents, training the child.

REFERENCES

1. Professor Yao Guo-Ying, Professor of Pediatrics, Chengdu Sixth People's Hospital, Chengdu, People's Republic of China. Personal communication. January 1989.

2. Wallace, H.M., R.F. Biehl, L. Taft, and A.C. Oglesby. Handicapped Children and Youth – A Comprehensive Community and Clinical Approach. New York: Human Sciences Press, 1987, p. 378.

3. Lypsky, D.K. Family Supports for Families with a Disabled Member. New York: World Rehabilitation Fund, 1987. 79 pages.

Section IV
ADOLESCENT HEALTH

39

ADOLESCENT HEALTH: PROMISE AND PARADOX

Herbert L. Friedman, M.D.; Mark A. Belsey, M.D.;
Jane Ferguson

INTRODUCTION

Health care for adolescents (those aged 10 through 19) presents something of a paradox. In terms of physical morbidity and mortality, young people are among the healthiest groups in all societies. They have survived illnesses of infancy and childhood which still take a high toll in many developing countries, and they are not yet suffering from the infirmities of old age, or, from damage arising from decades of hard labor at home or in the workplace, although many young people are still put at risk through too-early marriage and childbearing. As a result the health of young people has traditionally been given low priority in public health programs. Yet, in recent years, interest has grown in the health of young people for a number of disparate reasons:

1. Public health successes in regard to infectious diseases have made it possible to give more attention to health problems arising from behavior, an issue of particular relevance to the adolescent period;

2. Massive changes underway in sociocultural and demographic conditions including urbanization, the decline of the extended family, and the revolution in telecommunications have eroded traditional support and control systems for young people, eased social and sexual constraints and increased the exposure of adolescents to health-threatening situations and substances;

3. In developing countries both the absolute and relative size of the adolescent population has increased rapidly. More than half the world's population is currently under the age of 25;[1] and

4. As the adolescent period lengthens because of a generally earlier start to puberty and later age at marriage, there has been growing understanding that adolescence constitutes a series of choice-points which determine whether young people develop behavior patterns which promote their own health and that of their societies, or embark on life styles which are likely to do lasting harm to themselves and others.

In this chapter we will look first at health needs and problems of adolescents and then at some of the current approaches to the promotion of adolescent health.

ADOLESCENT HEALTH NEEDS

Adolescence is a period of transition between childhood and adulthood in which the body develops in size, strength and reproductive capability, the mind becomes capable of more abstract thinking, future orientation and ethical conviction, and social relationships move from a family base to a wider horizon in which peers and other adults come to play more significant roles. But while these changes are highly interrelated, development is usually uneven. While the adolescent is childlike in some spheres and continues to need strong material and psychosocial support, in others, it is important that the opportunity for independent experiment, adventure and accomplishment be encouraged. The health of adolescents is dependent on the people and conditions in the family, school, the community, places of recreation, work and worship, the mass media and the health and its many related sectors. Achieving an appropriate balance between support and opportunity to ensure healthy development in a rapidly changing world, is the challenge which faces societies in all regions of the world today.

ADOLESCENT HEALTH PROBLEMS

The health problems of young people fall broadly into those over which they have little or no control – particularly those which originate in childhood

– and those which are largely the result of voluntary behavior, although behavior itself is the product of many factors. Below we will look first at conditions which arise in childhood and adolescence, and secondly at those which can be traced to behavior during the adolescent years.

HEALTH PROBLEMS ORIGINATING IN CHILDHOOD

Poor health during infancy and childhood, a common problem for those living in impoverished conditions, is likely to have an adverse effect on the adolescent. The impact of perinatal anoxia, toxic exposure or a number of central nervous system infections in infancy and childhood may become apparent only after the child enters school. Minimal brain damage and visual, auditory or speech defects may cumulatively affect the child's ability to learn and consequent aspirations and self-esteem. Those who survive repeated cycles of diarrheal and respiratory disease or undernutrition are likely to fail to attain full adult growth and perhaps full psychosocial development. Physically underdeveloped girls are at greater risk of giving birth to low birthweight infants. Rheumatic heart disease is aggravated by pregnancy and will contribute to a higher mortality rate of those afflicted. Those disabled by poliomyelitis or indeed from any cause, will have special psychosocial as well as physical needs in adolescence and need assistance which will enable them to be integrated into the mainstream of society with their able peers to the extent possible. Insulin-dependent diabetes mellitus (juvenile diabetes) may be further complicated by adolescents' denial of the disease and resulting difficulties with therapeutic compliance. Owing to advances in treatment and care many children with genetic and metabolic diseases such as cystic fibrosis, hemophilia, and the hemoglobinopathies survive to adolescence and adulthood and pose new challenges to health care systems to facilitate their integration into society.[2]

HEALTH PROBLEMS ORIGINATING IN ADOLESCENCE

During adolescence normal physical development may be adversely affected by inadequate diet, excessive physical stress, or pregnancy before physiological maturity is attained. In the absence of immunity, harm arising from infectious diseases, such as paralysis from poliomyelitis and infertility from mumps, tends to be more frequent and more severe. Greater energy needs arising from the adolescent growth spurt combined with inadequate diet may contribute to tuberculosis. Adolescent girls require 10% more iron than boys to compensate for the loss of menstrual blood or they will suffer from anemia which is twice as common in women as in men. In sport, where competition is becoming increasingly fierce, and in recreation or work, excessive stress may be placed on bones before the epiphysis has fused and result in skeletal damage or impaired growth. The conditions of work are designed for adults rather than adolescents and put them at greater risk of accidental injury and death. The disabled adolescent – between 5% and 10% of the adolescent population – has special needs because of the increase of self-consciousness and the strong need for peer approval during this phase of life. The objective of health promotion should be to integrate the individual as fully as possible into the mainstream of life in his or her community.

ADOLESCENT BEHAVIOR AND HEALTH

While many of the health problems of young people arise from circumstances of impoverishment or disease beyond their control, perhaps many more originate through the behavior of young people – though behavior itself is determined by multiple factors.

As public health measures such as improved sanitation, a clean water supply and immunization have succeeded to some degree in controlling diseases, attention has been turned toward those health problems which arise more from voluntary acts than from involuntary infection. While most young people lead healthy and responsible lives, some, at least some of the time, put their health at risk. Many of the health problems which arise in adolescence – unwanted pregnancy and induced abortion arising from it, or unwanted childbirth and parenthood, sexually transmitted diseases, drug and alcohol abuse increasing risk for accidents and social disruption and illness in later life, infection with the human immunodeficiency virus (HIV) leading to AIDS, the use of tobacco with long-term damage to health, those accidents and injuries arising from excessive risk taking, and suicide – are direct consequences of behavior, although there are many factors which contribute to such acts.

There is evidence to suggest that problem behaviors cluster together.[3] Those who smoke cigarettes are more likely to progress to cannabis; the use of one drug is more likely to lead to multiple drug use; problem drinkers are more likely than others to use illicit drugs; heavy drinking and the use of certain other drugs are accompanied by antisocial behavior and implicated in traffic accidents. The use of tobacco, alcohol and other drugs is associated with poorer performance at school, at work and in sport. Sexual precocity is associated with substance abuse.

SEXUAL BEHAVIOR AND REPRODUCTIVE HEALTH

Puberty, in all societies, is a significant milestone in the transition from childhood to adulthood. It is often marked by religious rites, and changes in what is permitted and expected from girls and boys. Segregation between the sexes is often enforced to prevent illicit sexual relations and the possibility of conception outside of marriage. But sexual health and fulfillment is fundamental to human well-being. For adolescents the way in which sexuality is dealt with in their families, the degree and soundness of information which they are given about it, and the nature of the relationships they have with other people including their eventual sexual partners will determine whether their sexual behavior contributes positively or negatively to their overall health.[13]

One of the great health problems of adolescents worldwide is too-early pregnancy. In developing countries this frequently arises from early marriage, sometimes just after menarche, but in most countries an increasing proportion of young people are becoming sexually active at earlier ages and pregnant prior to marriage. Whether in or outside of marriage, however, the biomedical consequences of pregnancy in the young adolescent pose risks to mother and child, especially in the absence of adequate care. The unmarried adolescent is often reluctant to seek care early enough because of fears of negative reaction to her sexual activity. Similarly, contraception to prevent pregnancy is often absent or ineffective in this population whether because of pressure to conceive among the married girls in traditional societies, or the anxiety at their anticipated negative reaction of others to their sexual activity. In adolescent pregnancy girls who have not reached full physical and physiological maturity are as much as three times as likely to die from eclampsia, obstructed labor, hemorrhage, or infection as women in prime childbearing years. If they survive, they run a high risk of vesico-vaginal fistula or recto-vaginal fistula which, if not repaired, may leave them physically and emotionally disabled for the rest of their lives.[2]

An unwanted pregnancy often leads to an induced abortion which is likely to come later in a pregnancy for a girl who is frightened, ashamed and/or embarrassed to seek care, uncertain how to get appropriate help or too poor to pay for medically safe procedures. She is at greater risk of death and injury including infertility if the abortion is performed late in the pregnancy and in the hazardous conditions common to clandestine and/or illegal procedures.

The damaging consequences of childbearing too young are not merely biomedical, however. Even for the adolescent who marries young, it is likely

to bring an abrupt end to her education, and social and economic development. The adolescent's mother or mother-in-law, who, in an extended family,
would once have helped her to look after the baby, is increasingly likely to be
employed away from home. The adolescent who is not married is likely to
suffer even greater social and economic hardship as is her child. She may have
to bring up the child single-handed in poor economic conditions when she
herself is not sufficiently mature to provide necessary psychological and material support for her child who is also likely to be fatherless.

A second major hazard of unprotected sexuality in adolescence is the
possibility of contracting one of the many sexually transmitted diseases (STD)
including gonorrhea, chlamydial infection, syphilis, herpes and AIDS (also
transmitted by other means). The incidence of STD among adolescents has
increased markedly during the last twenty years.[5] As a consequence, in both
developed and developing countries, hospital admission for pelvic inflammatory disease is also rising, especially among those 15-24 years in age, as is
ectopic pregnancy. Young people are particularly vulnerable because they are
less likely than adults to be aware of the symptoms or the consequences of an
STD; some STDs, particularly in women, are asymptomatic, and young people
are often reluctant to present for help because, as with pregnancy in an
unmarried adolescent, they fear the reaction of the health provider and the
possibility of disclosure to others.

The new scourge of AIDS poses special problems for a number of reasons. It is not only at present incurable as is herpes, but, unlike herpes, is also
fatal. With respect to adolescent behavior, its transmission may come through
sexual contact – which in the West has been preponderantly of a homosexual
nature although it can also be transmitted heterosexually, or through the
sharing of a contaminated needle among drug users. As indicated earlier,
problem behavior is often clustered, and this makes drug users among adolescents particularly vulnerable. For an adolescent to seek help for suspected
infection may well mean facing the suspicion that he (or she) has been sexually active, possibly homosexual and/or using drugs – suspicions which might
be particularly difficult to tolerate. Furthermore, for an individual to learn
that he or she has an HIV infection (or AIDS) can have devastating personal
consequences since from that moment on responsible behavior will mean a
drastic permanent restriction on sexual habits and exclusion from future parenthood. Disclosure to others, despite many efforts to promote a supportive
attitude to those afflicted, may lead to varying degrees of social ostracism and
economic hardship. Despite vast publicity, many myths remain, perhaps particularly among the adolescent population who have limited access in most
societies to sound information about sexuality and sexual behavior.

SEXUAL DIFFICULTIES AND HEALTH

Awakening sexuality during adolescence can generate anxieties about sexual dysfunction, i.e., the inability to achieve sexual satisfaction, and sexual variation – sexual feelings and behavior which are uncommon. Dysfunction is most commonly experienced in the male as secondary impotence which itself is likely to stem from anxiety. Another problem which may appear is premature ejaculation in the quickly arousable sexual response system of the adolescent who also will have less expertise at controlling response. Both difficulties are relatively easy to deal with if the young person has access to a skilled and knowledgeable person in whom he has confidence.[6] Sexual variation, particularly homosexual feelings, are likely to cause considerable anxiety since in most societies the young person who acknowledges them is likely to meet with a negative reaction. Homosexual feelings are quite common in early adolescence and only a small percentage of young people will remain primarily homosexual in orientation. Sensitive handling of this issue is essential to the healthy development of young people and their future relationships with both sexes.

Sexual harassment or abuse of young people is another problem which is receiving increasing attention. Intercourse with a minor (other than a spouse), whether forced as in rape, or enticed as is sometimes the case in incest or pedophile relationships, is universally condemned. Incest is particularly difficult to deal with since the adolescent who experiences it, most commonly a girl with father or stepfather, is likely to face extreme hazards if she reports it. She may be condemned, punished, or the family broken up and is likely to retain feelings of guilt whatever the justice of the situation. Adolescent female and male prostitution is another problem which sometimes arises out of economic hardship, and sometimes from unresolved personal difficulties. As with all problems faced by adolescents, none should be neglected since at this time of life young people remain highly responsive to appropriate help.

THE USE OF ALCOHOL AND HEALTH

In the last three to four decades increasing percentages of children and adolescents have started to drink alcohol, the quantity and frequency of their alcohol consumption has increased, and the age at which drinking starts has declined.[4,7] Alcohol use has both short- and long-term effects on the adolescent. In the long term excessive consumption shortens the life span and puts the individual at greater risk of cancer, ulcers, heart disease, muscle wastage, malnutrition and cirrhosis of the liver. The pregnant woman who drinks exposes her unborn child to a greater risk of brain damage, growth deficiency and mental retardation. But alcohol use affects not only the body, it also affects behavior. In the longer term the alcohol abuser is more likely to suffer from marital instability, loss of friends, child abuse, failure at school, sport, and at work. Intoxication removes inhibitions that would otherwise prevent risky sexual behavior and is especially heavily implicated in aggression, crime, suicidal behavior and accidents on the road, at work and at home – a major cause of death and disability in adolescence.

The use of alcohol by adolescents is more likely to occur if family members drink, but young people are also highly susceptible to peer pressure, and examples set by popular idols. Accessibility plays a major role in the use of alcohol by young people. It may be reduced by enacting and implementing legislation which prohibits the sale of alcohol to minors and increases in cost.

Young people drink for a number of reasons – sometimes to gain peer approval particularly among males, sometimes as a way of behaving as adults appear to do, and sometimes for relief from anxiety (like adults). But the use of alcohol by adolescents can be compounded by a lack of knowledge of the consequences, and to some extent, the sense of immortality that characterizes youth.

THE USE OF DRUGS AND HEALTH

In recent years the mean age of illicit drug users has declined and multiple drug use has become more common.[4] While drug use by adults has been present in virtually all societies in one form or another, in recent decades it has become associated with youthful rebellion and the "counter-culture." But what was once restricted to small numbers has spread to many more and is becoming epidemic in some parts of the world. Opium has been used in parts of Asia for thousands of years, but its derivative heroin has more recently become a threat to the young. Mescaline and LSD are used for their hallucinogenic effects, coca and khat as stimulants and to produce feelings of euphoria. Solvents which can be found in everyday materials are being used by adolescents including those living in urban slums. Cannabis is used in all regions of the world, and there appears to be an increase in the use among young people of drugs prescribed for others such as amphetamines and barbiturates.

Drug use poses many hazards for young people including the possibility of psychotic reactions induced by amphetamines and hallucinogenic substances. Dangerous behavior including suicide and accidents arise from the use of drugs which alter perception and psychomotor reactions. There is now a new danger of infection of HIV leading to AIDS resulting from shared use of contaminated needles. And, of course, the effects of longer term use of drugs are likely to damage and limit every aspect of the young person's life including their relationships with people, and performance at work, school and recreation. Drug use is made more likely by a number of factors including families and peers who tolerate or encourage it, weak parental control and discipline, alienation, and ready access to drugs.[8]

THE USE OF TOBACCO AND HEALTH

One of the greatest threats to the health of adolescents is the use of tobacco. Unlike alcohol or other drugs, its immediate impact is relatively minor but its long-term effects are implicated in 90% of lung cancer deaths, 75% of cases of chronic bronchitis and emphysema, 25% of cardiovascular disease, and an increased risk to health if the oral contraceptive is used.[2] In the short term it increases the severity of influenza, reduces the immune response, adversely affects the fetus of pregnant women, and diminishes respiratory and athletic performance. The smoking of tobacco is increasing in developing countries and especially among girls, while it appears to be decreasing in some developed countries which have waged strong campaigns against its use. Unfortunately, for young people, it is seen as the first step toward "grown-up" behavior and is frequently seen as a symbol of liberation from constraints – a symbolism which has been exploited by the tobacco industry in encouraging women to smoke.

As with drinking, the onset of tobacco use is strongly influenced by its use in the home and by peer pressure. While it may begin to be used for symbolic or social reasons, its use is likely to continue for addictive reasons. Both the prevention of the onset of tobacco use, whether in the form of smoking or as smokeless tobacco, and its cessation, are essential for the health of all society, but the two objectives may require different tactics.

BEHAVIOR LEADING TO ACCIDENTS AND INJURIES

Accidents are a leading cause of adolescent disability and mortality accounting for as many as half of all deaths between the ages of 10 and 24 in many countries.[4] Accidents often occur because of a combination of excessive risk-taking, sometimes in association with alcohol or drug use, and dangerous contexts particularly on the road and sometimes in the workplace. But intentional injury is also a growing cause of concern. There appears to be an increase in crimes of violence by young people, though it is difficult to validate. In some situations it is a result of war in which the male adolescent is most at risk, and sometimes manifest by aggressive behavior toward self (suicide) or others. In places of work the adolescent is often vulnerable because conditions and tools are not designed for the youngster.

There appears to be a rise in suicide among adolescents, although it is consistently underreported because of feelings of shame and guilt, and legal and religious implications. The tragic loss of a young life usually leaves a trail of emotional devastation among the close survivors among family and friends. Young men complete suicides much more commonly than females, who, however, appear to be involved much more frequently in attempted suicide. The older adolescent is more vulnerable. In the Americas, for example, 4 to 5 times as many 15-19 year-olds commit suicide as those aged 10-14.[9] In many societies young people are facing increasing competition at school, in sports, and in seeking employment while at the same time the family support system has weakened. The transition from childhood to adulthood itself sometimes diminishes self-esteem as the individual begins to question his or her own identity, sexuality, appearance, and sense of self-efficacy. Perceived failure is acutely felt at this time of life, especially of new experiences, but the wish to be less dependent upon elders may reduce willingness to disclose difficulties. As suicide is frequently a taboo subject among adults, the adolescent may be left with a sense of growing despair and hopelessness and turn to suicide as a tragic solution.

EATING BEHAVIOR, ORAL HYGIENE, AND HEALTH

Undernutrition remains a serious problem particularly in developing countries, but malnutrition is sometimes the result of a poor choice of food.

Excessive consumption of sugar, fat and salt during childhood appears to engrain preference for those substances later. Inappropriate diet can increase the likelihood of developing cardiovascular disease, hypertension, obesity, and non-insulin-dependent diabetes. Obesity appears to be increasing among adolescents in both developed and developing countries, while at the same time being slim is publicized and valued. Unhealthy dieting is a common result, especially by girls. Inappropriate diet can also lead to acne (though not necessarily an exclusive cause) which is particularly upsetting to the self-conscious adolescent. Two eating disorders of psychopathological origin, anorexia nervosa entailing the virtual cessation of eating, and bulimia in which forced vomiting takes place after eating, require professional help. Oral hygiene is essential to avoid damage to teeth and gums, and to the appearance, a leading cause of anxiety among adolescents.

THE PROMOTION OF ADOLESCENT HEALTH

"If young people are helped to have positive and healthy relationships, to develop as individuals before they marry and have children, to exercise their minds and bodies in healthy ways – if they eat well, remain free of the abuse of tobacco, alcohol and other drugs, free of the risks of early pregnancy and parenthood, and free of infection, practice good hygiene, and are able to experiment and explore their worlds without excessive risk of injury and with an opportunity to care for others – their lives will be rich and productive and all will benefit."[10] This formula for physical, mental and social health calls for a combination of self care by young people themselves, in conjunction with the provision of the right conditions and services by others in the family, community, governmental and non-governmental organizations, and in all sectors relevant to health.

To achieve appropriate interventions, sound knowledge of what constitutes healthy development in diverse cultures is essential. It is important to have and assess indicators of biomedical and psychosocial health and acquire and maintain knowledge of the perceptions, beliefs and practices of young people themselves at all stages of adolescence and in all walks of life. Research is needed to assess the impact of policies and legislation, ways to promote effective intersectoral and interdisciplinary action, and the best approaches to the involvement of young people themselves in planning and implementing of programs for their health. Knowledge alone is insufficient; the skills with which knowledge can be communicated and applied is also essential. For this purpose training of all those who can effectively interact with the young is needed. Advocacy, too, is important, to achieve appropriate policies, legislation and public attitudes that support health needs. Whatever programs are developed require systematic evaluation which takes into account both objective and subjective measures of effectiveness and impact.

POLICIES AND LEGISLATION

The provision of services to promote health, or to prevent or correct problems, can be supported by policies and legislation which arise in many sectors including health, education, social services, criminal justice, youth sports and culture, religious affairs and others. But policies which impinge on adolescent health are rarely coordinated and often push in conflicting directions. Legislation is often inconsistent as, for example, minimum ages for marriage, legal age for military service, driving motor vehicles, drinking alcohol, leaving school and employment. Uncertainty about what laws exist, as well as failure to implement laws, compound the difficulties.

Legislation can be effective if it is implemented, however. As, for example, laws which reduce or eliminate advertising and availability and accessibility to adolescents of harmful substances such as tobacco, alcohol or drugs; adequate requirements for driving licenses; the use of seat belts in cars; safety measures at the workplace; raising the minimum age of marriage; and legislation which permits and encourages the provision of culturally acceptable sexual education and services to prevent too-early pregnancy. But policies and legislation need to be implemented not only formally, but through all those who influence the health of adolescents.

THE FAMILY AND ADOLESCENT HEALTH

Fundamental to the wellbeing of adolescents is the family which introduces the young person to life, and, at its best, provides them with basic support including unqualified love, adequate food, clean water, a place and time for rest, clothing, sanitary conditions, and a flexible system of constraints and opportunities which change as development takes place. The family exists in many forms – the extended family of multiple generations common to traditional rural societies, the nuclear family of two parents and children, more common in industrially developed societies, surrogate families in which the child's guardians are not necessarily blood relations, and increasingly, single-parent families, usually of mother and child where premarital adolescent childbearing is rising and the divorce rate increasing. Adult family members provide key role models to adolescents in their behavior and relationships. Despite the stresses which arise as adolescents become more autonomous, there is considerable evidence to show that most young people share the values of their parents and the differences tend to be about more ephemeral matters however intensely those battles may be fought.[11] For families to help adolescents, however, also requires knowledge and skills; a key challenge to the health and related sectors is how to help families obtain what they need.

THE HEALTH SECTOR

Many kinds of health services of potential usefulness to adolescents exist throughout the world from primary health care to teaching hospitals. But even where health services are available there are a number of reasons why they tend to be underutilized by the adolescent population. Health services are usually designed either for children or for adults. Adolescents are often reluctant to use them especially for sensitive subjects of special importance to them such as sexuality, their appearance, emotional difficulties and personal relationships. These topics frequently make health service providers (as well as teachers and parents) equally uneasy, especially when they are not adequately prepared to deal with them. Furthermore, both young people and adults may not think of these subjects as the legitimate domain of health services. Other health hazards such as the use of alcohol, tobacco or other drugs, or risk-taking on the road, are often not seen as health problems by young people, while adults frequently adopt a censorious attitude to the youngster who confesses to such behavior, thereby encouraging secrecy. A young person who drinks alcohol, smokes, uses drugs occasionally, and has premarital sex, may consider him or herself perfectly healthy while potentially sowing the seeds for a myriad of health problems as outlined above. These problem behaviors may not reach the health sector because they are often not labelled as "health" problems until it is too late.

People in the health and related sectors can be made more alert to warning signals. A young person who has poor relationships, low self-esteem, a low sense of self-efficacy, a poor body image, and is not succeeding in the eyes of his or her friends, may not be thought of as experiencing poor health by family or health providers if his or her physical health is good, despite the fact that the adolescent might be despairing and potentially suicidal, or turning to self-destructive or antisocial behaviors. While mental health services designed for adolescents are even less common in all countries and totally absent in some, other sources of help – the family and the school – could be strengthened in early detection and assistance.

A number of models for adolescent health services exist, including special services for young people embedded in a general service, free-standing services for adolescents only, which deal with all aspects of adolescent health, single-issue services such as those provided for alcohol or drug problems, and health services for young people which exist in other contexts, such as the school system or youth organizations. It is generally held that young people can be helped best with an integrated approach, rather than those that focus primarily on single issues. Many of the problems are interrelated, and share common roots. It is also likely that the promotion of healthy development in young adolescents will preclude the need for a curative response later. For the health sector to be effective in this way, however, requires intelligent policies with priority given to the promotion of health and prevention of problems coordinated across sectors, and trained staff who are knowledgeable and skilled in working with adolescents or in training others who influence their health.[12]

THE EDUCATION SECTOR

After the family, perhaps the most important influence on the health of young people for those who are or have been in school, are their teachers.

Learning to read, write, use mathematics, think and express oneself, are fundamental to healthy decision making. Knowledge acquired on the many subjects exposed in school including the physical and social sciences, and the stimulus of the arts, provides much of the raw material for healthy choices in life. School is usually the place where young people are introduced to sport, and can be provided with the conditions for healthy supervised physical as well as mental exercise. School health services can provide an invaluable basis for screening and care, especially when linked with community resources. Yet despite the potential for health presented by schools, many fail to achieve these objectives. Teaching is often didactic, and adolescent participation is low. Subjects of intense importance to adolescent development – sexuality, the prevention of pregnancy and sexually transmitted diseases, difficulties in relationships, personal anxieties natural to adolescence, for example – rarely find a place in school curricula, or people who are able to communicate well on these subjects.

The Youth Sector

Although enrollment in school and age at leaving have generally been increasing throughout the world, a significant number of adolescents are not in school and must be reached in other ways. There are many non-governmental youth organizations at international, regional, national and local levels which are active in the promotion of health throughout the world, not only for their own members, but in work which reaches other young people too, and frequently to meet wider needs. Given appropriate technical help, much more could be done. Behavioral research training in communication and counseling skills, advocacy, public information, and active interventions for health, are all variously within the capabilities of these organizations. There are also youth centers which cater to young people's needs, including health, which can provide the dual advantage of enabling an adolescent to seek help without publicly acknowledging the need, and bring health issues to the attention of young people who have been attracted to the center for other reasons.

The participation of young people in planning and providing services is important. Given the opportunity they can best articulate their needs and comment on the acceptability of approaches intended to promote their health. Peers have a powerful influence on the behavior of adolescents. With the appropriate skills and support by knowledgeable adults, they can provide effective counseling, information and social support for other young people. In addition, the involvement of adolescents in health promotion activities beneficial to their own health is attested by the success of many youth organizations. Being valued for meaningful contributions strengthens their self-esteem and confidence. Arousing the enthusiasm and energy of young people in improving their own and others' health can foster an approach to dealing with the problems and conflicts of life in a constructive manner. Adolescents and adults working as partners build foundations for joint action based on their respective strengths and competence.

THE MASS MEDIA

Young people are strongly influenced by popular culture which reaches them through the mass media channels of film, video, records and tapes, television, radio, magazines, comic books, etc., which have crossed cultural boundaries with unprecedented speed. Popular figures in entertainment and sports are influential and provide both positive and negative examples to the young. Much more could be done to promote health through such channels.

CONCLUSIONS

Adolescence is a period of life in which patterns are set with life-long consequences for health. Young people are highly sensitive to the influences in their cultures for good and ill. While adolescents have to accomplish their developmental tasks themselves, families, schools, the health and related sectors, and those who use or appear in the mass media, all have crucial roles to play, too. Adolescents need material and moral support, they need adult models of healthy behavior, they need services which will be sensitive to their needs, and they need opportunities to learn, work, play and contribute to their societies. Young people throughout the world are generally ready to contribute their energy and idealism to positive goals, given the chance. It is up to the adults in their cultures to provide them with this opportunity.

PRINCIPLES OF INTERVENTION FOR ADOLESCENT HEALTH

Experience to date suggests a number of principles that appear to be effective in promoting healthy development of adolescents:

- a prolonged supportive environment with graded steps toward autonomy enhancing self-esteem and promoting healthy life-styles;
- a positive interaction between adolescents and the key adults and peers in their lives;
- continual monitoring of the healthy development of adolescents within the sociocultural context;

- the development of the programs based on a sound understanding of adolescent's beliefs and behavior within any given culture;
- the use of people to implement programs who respect the young, have a sound knowledge of their needs, and are trained in communication skills;
- the use in programs of established principles of learning, behaviors, and development;
- the focusing of programs on groups of interrelated behavior rather than single forms;
- the use of an intersectoral approach in programs in which key groups interacting with the young are optimally involved, including the school, the family, the health system, religious and community leaders, and community organizations;
- a close linkage of community-based programs and complementary school-based programs with programs directed at those who have left or do not attend school, and the health care system; and
- the involvement of adolescents themselves in the planning and implementation of programs, to the greatest extent possible.

REFERENCES

1. World Population Trends and Policies: Monitoring Report. United Nations, 1987.

2. World Health Organization. The Health of Youth. Background Document, Technical Discussions. Geneva: WHO, 1989.

3. Jessor, R., and S.L. Jessor. Problem Behaviour and Psychological Development. New York: Academic Press, 1977.

4. World Health Organization. Young People's Health – A Challenge for Society. Report of a WHO Study Group on Young People and "Health for All by the Year 2000." Technical Report Series, 731. Geneva: WHO, 1986.

5. Silber, T. J., and K. Woodward. Sexually Transmitted Diseases in Adolescence. Health of Adolescents and Youths in the Americas. Washington, DC: PAHO, 1985, pp.. 87-94.

6. Kaplan, H.S. The New Sex Therapy. New York: Peregrine Books, 1978.

7. Moser, J. Alcohol problems in children and adolescents: A growing threat. Alcohol and Youth. O. Jeanneret, Karger, Basel, (eds), 1983, pp. 42-53.

8. Perry, C.L., and I.M. Murray. The prevention of adolescent drug abuse: Implications from etiological, developmental, behavioral and environmental models. J Prim Prev 6(1) Fall, 1985.

9. Cassorca, R.M.S., and M. Knobel. Depression and suicide in adolescence. Health of Adolescents and Youths in the Americas. Washington, DC: PAHO, 1985, pp. 158-168.

10. Nakajima, H. Opening Address by the Director General to the World Health Organization Technical Discussions on the Health of Youth, Geneva, May 1989.

11. Rutter, M. Changing Youth in a Changing Society: Patterns of Adolescent Development and Disorder. Abingdon: The Nuffield Provincial Hospitals Trust, 1979.

12. Report of the Technical Discussions on the Health of Youth, 42nd World Health Assembly, A42/Technical Discussions/13. Geneva: WHO,1989.

13. World Health Organization. The Reproductive Health of Adolescents – A Strategy for Action. A Joint WHO/UNFPA/UNICEF Statement. Geneva: WHO, 1989.

40

ADOLESCENT FERTILITY

PRAMILLA SENANAYAKE, M.B.B.S., D.T.P.H., PH.D.

WORLDWIDE OVERVIEW

Adolescence is a period of transition from childhood to adulthood, marked by interlocking changes in the mind, in the body, and in social relationships. However, adolescence is traditionally regarded as a period relatively free of health problems. Adolescents have survived the increased vulnerability to infection that endangers the early childhood period and have not as yet developed the chronic or degenerative diseases that afflict the elderly.

Definitions of the age range of adolescence vary according to cultures and also according to the purpose (legal, medical, psychological, or social) for which they are used. It has been suggested by the World Health Organization (WHO) that the period between the ages of 10 and 19 years, or the second decade of life, be designated as the period of adolescence.

Adolescents comprise a large part of the world's population; in many countries they form 20-25% of the population. Today there are just over one and a quarter billion people aged between 10 and 19. For many adolescents in developing countries the process of urbanization, industrialization and education have reshaped traditional relationships not only between themselves but in particular between the adolescent and the extended family. The competition for education, training, jobs and housing places great stress on young people.

PHYSICAL CHANGES DURING ADOLESCENCE

Breast development in girls begins at around 8-13 years and is usually the first sign of pubescence (thelarche). It is followed within a year or so with the development of pubic hair, height spurt and changes in general physique.

470

Menarche occurs quite late in puberty and is generally preceded by at least 2 years of breast development. The average age of menarche throughout the world is about 13 years but the range extends from 10-16.5 years. Over the past 4-5 decades or so it has been recognized that the age of onset of sexual maturation has been decreasing while growth and physical development have been proceeding at an accelerated pace. The age of menarche in Europe has become lower by 2-3 months per decade; evidence suggests that similar trends are occurring in developing countries, too. The reasons for these accelerations are not well established; however, factors such as better nutrition and improved social and economic conditions could be relevant.

The first sign of sexual maturity in boys is testicular enlargement. Growth of pubic hair is followed by spurts in height and penis growth. Axillary and facial hair appear on average 2 years after growth of pubic hair begins. Voice changes occur relatively late and can take 1-3 years to complete. "Spermarche," the first ejaculation, occurs during the final stages of puberty.[1]

It is important to realize that menarche and spermarche do not necessarily represent signs of fertility. Early menses are usually non-ovulatory and sperm released at spermarche are probably of low fertility potential.

While data on adolescent sexuality and fertility are still inadequate, particularly in developing countries, and while the situation in no two countries is the same, three patterns of sexual and reproductive behavior can be broadly distinguished.

The first category, which is found mainly in developed countries is characterized by onset of sexual experience in the mid to late teens, with a low use of contraceptives, a high incidence of unwanted non-marital pregnancy, a demonstrable tendency for recourse to abortion (largely legal and relatively safe), late marriage, low fertility and significant rates of sexually transmitted diseases.[2] The second type, which is almost the direct opposite of the first, is characterized principally by marriage at an age close to menarche, early and frequent childbearing. Premarital sexual activity is uncommon, as is premarital pregnancy and childbirth. Abortion usually is illicit and unsafe. In some areas, there is a high incidence of sexually transmitted diseases (STDs) with subsequent infertility because of inadequate health care. The third pattern, found particularly in urban settings in transitional societies occupies the stage between 1 and 2. Sexual as well as educational opportunities are expanding for youth, especially women. Patterns of sexuality and fertility are transitional and somewhat mixed. The traditional social restraints are still evident but less effective than in the past. The age of marriage is rising, premarital sex and pregnancy increasing among youngsters, as is recourse to abortion. There is increasing use of contraception.

Within the above-mentioned definitions there are a number of groups of adolescents which should be considered where appropriate. These groups include: Male-female; early adolescence-late adolescence; in school-out of school; married-unmarried; rural-transitional-urban-refugee; parents-nonparents; contraceptors-non-contraceptors; normal-handicapped.

IMPORTANCE AND CONSEQUENCES OF ADOLESCENT REPRODUCTIVE BEHAVIOR

Today it is becoming increasingly clear that sexually active young people face serious health risks. The young person who is physically and emotionally unprepared for sexual intercourse, pregnancy and child bearing faces life-long harm. The major reproductive and sexuality-related health hazards that face young people include sexually transmitted diseases (STDs), including acquired immunodeficiency syndrome (AIDS); carcinoma of the cervix; unwanted pregnancy, sometimes leading to illegal abortion and complications of abortion.[3]

The acquisition of STDs during adolescence can often have devastating effects on future fertility. The incidence of STDs among adolescents has increased markedly in the last 20 years. As a consequence the rates of admission to hospitals for pelvic inflammatory disease are also rising in the developed and the developing countries. As a further consequence the rate of ectopic pregnancy is rising sharply. Included among the major STDs are gonorrhea, chlamydial infection, syphilis, herpes and HIV/AIDS (also transmitted by other means). Three of the major obstacles to the control of these among adolescents are the ignorance of young people of the symptoms of STDs, the asymptomatic nature of some STDs particularly in women, and the reluctance of young people to present for help because they fear that they will be met with anger and hostility.[4]

Young people, like adults, sometimes have sexual problems that are especially frightening because they encounter them without a wider experience of the world. These problems include sexual dysfunction, sexual variation and sexual harassment and abuse (especially of young girls by older men).

It is now well established that early child bearing (pregnancy before the age of 18) can pose health hazards for both mother and child. The major cause of death in young women is childbirth. For women under the age of 18, there is a greater risk of maternal mortality and morbidity, when compared to women who have children when they are in the age range 20-29. This is true for both the developed as well as for the developing countries. Although social and economic factors such as nutrition and prenatal care may reduce mortality arising from obstetric complications to some extent, the maternal age factor has an independent influence on relative risks. There are two main risks for the pregnant young adolescent: pre-eclamptic toxemia and cephalopelvic disproportion. Both can present serious problems. A study carried out in Nigeria showed that 17% of 14 year-olds and 7% of 16 year-olds developed eclampsia but only 3% of the girls aged 20-24 suffered the same consequences. Cephalopelvic disproportion can lead to obstructed labor which in turn can give rise to fistulae which can be devastating to the young women. Fistulae can result in incontinence of urine and feces and the women can be made social outcasts.[5]

The children of the adolescent mother are also at a biological disadvantage. Retardation of fetal growth and premature birth are common. Low birth weight can be a major problem, resulting in high perinatal and infant mortality. It can also affect the subsequent mental development of the child. These children are also more likely to show neurological defects which may involve lifelong mental retardation. All of these problems seem to be more serious if the mother is 15 years or under.

STATUS OF WOMEN

In general the majority of women in developing countries have a lower social status than men. They have a much lower level of education and a higher rate of illiteracy. They also marry at an early age and start child bearing early mainly due to tradition and also lack of education. An estimated 40% of females aged 15-19 in Africa are married, and almost 30% in Asia compared with 15% in the Americas, 14% in Oceania, 9% in the Soviet Union, and 7% in Europe.[6]

Women in general are less likely to find jobs in countries where unemployment levels are high. Women are less skilled, and less educated and therefore have fewer employment opportunities. Inadequate attention is given to providing services and technology that would make women's tasks less burdensome.

Consideration should be given to empowering young women to achieve their educational, economic and social aspirations and to enhance their participation in their societies in partnership with young men.

PREVENTION

The necessity of providing adequate services for the fertility-related needs of the adolescent has recently received the international recognition it has long deserved. The United Nations International Conference on Population held in Mexico City in August 1984 sought to define the rights of adolescents in this area. Recommendation 29 of the report of the conference (adopted by consensus) stated, "Governments are urged to ensure that adolescents both boys and girls receive adequate education, including family life and sex education with due consideration given to the role, rights and obligations and changing individual and cultural values. Suitable family planning information and services should be made available to adolescents within the changing sociocultural framework of each country."[7]

In designing services for the adolescent, many important factors have to be kept in mind. These include social attitudes toward reproductive health services for young people, legal and policy issues, and staffing in relation to the provision of services, especially the involvement of young people as service providers. Family planning services should be able to respond specifically to the needs expressed by the adolescent. In addition factors such as whether, for example, the person to be served is a male or female, married or unmarried, or has mental or physical handicap should be borne in mind. Counseling is a very important aspect of service delivery. Wherever possible counseling should be designed especially for the adolescent and should cover a wide variety of subjects including sexuality, contraception and sexually transmitted diseases. The programs should provide contraception, obstetric care and treatment for sexually transmitted diseases.

An important factor in the success or failure of adolescent reproductive health programs will be the international communities efforts to improve the status of women. Dr. Nafis Sadik, Executive Director of the United Nations Population Fund, has so clearly identified, specific development goals involving the improvement of the status of women as follows:[8]

- Reduction in levels of illiteracy, especially female illiteracy which is almost 50% in the developing countries;
- Expansion of girls' enrollment in schools and their retention in the school system;
- Securing women's legal and social rights to free marriage, land and ownership, and paid employment; and
- Increasing income-generating programs for women.

Globally it would require the commitment of national governments, governmental and non-governmental organizations working at the village and district level empowering individuals, especially young people, to enable them to have control over their reproductive lives for their own benefit, for the benefit of their families and for the ultimate good of the communities in which they live.

REFERENCES

1. Senanayake, I.P. Adolescent Sexuality and Pregnancy, FIGO Manual of Human Reproduction, vol. 3. M. Fathalla et al. (ed). Carnforth: Parthenon, in press.

2. Hoffman, A. Contraception in adolescence: A review. I Psychosocial Aspects. Bull-WHO 62:151-162, 1984.

3. Senanayake, I.P. Contraception and the adolescent. Outlook 5(2):2-5, 1987.

4. World Health Organization. Background Document for the World Health Assembly Technical Discussions on the Health of Youth. Geneva: WHO, May 1989.

5. Harrison, K. Presentation at the International Safe Motherhood Conference, Nairobi, Kenya, Feb 1987.

6. International Planned Parenthood Federation: Statement on Adolescent Fertility. London:IPPF, 1977.

7. United Nations. Department of Technical Co-operation for Development: Report of the International Conference on Population. Mexico City, 6-14 Aug 1984. New York: UN, 1984, p. 24.

8. United Nations Population Fund. UN Population Fund calls for International Action to Balance Population Growth and Resources. UN Press Release POP/378,25 Jan, 1989.

41

ALCOHOL, DRUGS AND SMOKING IN YOUTH

Helmut L. Sell, M.D.

1. INTRODUCTION

During childhood, behavior is under the basically unchallenged control of parents and, to a lesser extent, of teachers and other adults in temporary contact with the child. Unsanctioned use (use not permitted by the environment) of mind-altering substances in children below the age of 12 years is therefore rare. It occurs mainly if a child is actively induced into use by an adult, for example, by a drug dealer who wants a child to become drug-dependent to serve him as a reliable and inconspicuous drug carrier, or into smoking by an older brother.

During adolescence two new determinants of behavior appear which are important in the context of drug use: One is the increasing importance of peers as role models in addition to the continuing role modeling by parents. The second is a tendency to take risks and to challenge established rules and values. In combination, these two sets of determinants of behavior can lead to groups of adolescents taking risks or challenging established rules by a behavior which none of the group would be likely to show alone or where none of the participants has had previous experience with the behavior concerned, for example, initiation into group violence, alcohol intoxication or into taking of illicit drugs.

These behaviors may exemplify the emotional and behavioral transitions accompanying puberty and the process of establishing one's individuality and individual personality. It has been observed in Western countries that personality traits (apart from psychopathology, which in many instances has been shown to have observable precursors) become measurable only towards the end of puberty, or, that personality measures taken before the age of about

14 years do not correlate with measurements of adult personality as it expresses itself before adulthood, or that important traits of adult personality are shaped during puberty (or, of course, a combination of both). It is surprising that this issue has only recently started to attract major research interest, although the latter possibility would appear to open a promising area for preventive and promotive interventions. If in fact major aspects of adult personality are formed during adolescence, then it would perhaps be possible to develop interventions to promote the establishment of protective personality traits like good social adaptational status and psychological well-being,[1] and prevent the formation of maladaptive behaviors like delinquency or drug dependence.

However, these observations relate to industrialized countries. Very little is known about puberty in developing countries although anecdotal evidence seems to suggest that puberty in developing countries or more traditional societies tends to be a considerably smoother transition, often times even only a ritualistic initiation, into adulthood. But the behavioral determinants of risk-taking and challenging of established rules do certainly exist in the urban and educated youth in developing countries also.

2. PATHWAYS TO DRUGS

It has been convincingly argued that people take drugs because they are offered to them.[2] It is very rare, at least for illicit drugs, that first drug contacts happen on the initiative of the user. As a rule, careers of drug-taking begin with an offer to take the drug. This offer, when successful, normally happens in circumstances where it is difficult to turn the offer down, in a situation which tends to be described – not very aptly – as social pressure or curiosity. More often it is in a situation which could probably best be described as conducive to impetuous or precipitous behavior: A mixture of peer modeling, risk taking and challenging prescribed rules of behavior. Or, "it will simply be an offer of the opportunity to join with others in what appears to be a method of extending pleasurable aspects of a conventional recreational situation. So, in spite of being 'anti-drug,' he or she evaluates the offer not in terms of the drug education/morality tale (which is still believed) but in terms of the current situation and the normal rules of behavior (sociability, enjoyment, reciprocity, keeping one's cool, presenting self, etc.) appropriate in such recreational situations. This is true both for early offers of legal drugs (cigarettes, alcohol) and for later offers of illegal drugs."[2]

Hardly any studies have been undertaken to elicit the circumstantial and emotional details of such situations of drug initiation. It is difficult to see how programs of "preventive education" can be effective if so little is known about the behavior which is to be prevented. "Just say no" is certainly not the full answer, especially when proposed by representatives of the very norms and rules which the behavior is challenging.

This lack of knowledge on the initiation into drugs has led to the generalization of the medical model of dependence to drug use in general. We are asking for "causes"of using drugs. There is evidence to suggest that dependence has a certain medical connotation in that there exists a genetic predisposition toward it. However, the behavior of taking a drug or accepting the offer of a drug does seem to resemble a medical condition about as closely as do other behaviors which imply a definite risk to health like skiing or mountaineering. All these behaviors are pleasurable. And in all of them risk-taking is one component of the pleasure. The fact that people do things which they enjoy doing does not seem to need further explanation. However, it is important to keep in mind that risk-taking can be fun, and especially so during adolescence. The physiological reactions to fear and fun are very similar. From observing only hormonal and some other physiological changes we are normally not able to say whether the person is living through a frightening experience, is enjoying a good joke or is experiencing an orgasm. The smooth and virtually timeless undulations between fright and fun can well be observed on the faces of people on a roller-coaster. It is therefore not surprising that the probability of an adolescent accepting the offer of a drug is not correlated to his knowledge about drugs. There is anecdotal evidence that drug initiation tends to be a highly emotional and exciting experience independent of the effect of the drug. The component of pleasure experienced in the process of drug initiation in many instances neutralizes the often unpleasant experience of the drug effect itself. This excitement permits, for example, adolescents to become smokers in spite of the initial unpleasant bitterness and cough provocation by cigarettes. They often times have to literally 'work' themselves into regular use. Like skiers, mountaineers or car drivers, drug users are convinced that they can control the risk. Some of each fail.

Whereas it is quite clear that in the beginning drugs are taken because they are offered, it is much less clear what makes certain people continue drug use and others to abandon it. A number of occasional users continue to be passive users, i.e., they take drugs only if they are offered. This is true even of highly addictive drugs like cigarettes and heroin. It is of course even more true of less addictive drugs like alcohol or cannabis. Unfortunately, nothing seems to be known about the protective mechanisms which permit certain people to use highly addictive substances occasionally without ever proceeding to the state of active use, i.e., use where the drug is actively sought and purchased. In contrast, some mechanisms have recently been described which permit regular users of heroin to maintain control over its use without moving on to compulsive use (controlled use meaning regular use with effective controls to make sure that the drug use does not substantially interfere with the user's social and professional life, compulsive use meaning that the drug use has taken such priority over other life concerns that it is continued in spite of adverse consequences for the professional or social life of the user.[3] Such controlled use is of course much easier to achieve with licit substances where unpredictable social (especially legal) sanctions are much less likely to occur, and where, therefore, the likelihood of consequences affecting the social and professional life of the users are easier to control. Furthermore, occasional users of highly criminalized drugs are much more likely to leave the mainstream of youth and proceed into the "drug scene" in a process of polarization between the establishment and a pro-drug-use counterculture.[4]

3. HEALTH EFFECTS OF DRUG USE

It is striking that the two drugs licitly used in most countries, viz., alcohol and tobacco, also appear to carry the highest risks when consumed at higher levels. A certain protective effect of alcohol against atherosclerosis has often been described. A recent study has confirmed previous findings that moderate users of alcohol tend to have fewer hospital admissions then teetotalers;[5] (also for references on alcohol and ischemic heart disease etc.). However, about one-third of all admissions to mental hospitals in Western countries are for reasons of alcohol dependence, and many more succumb to liver cirrhosis or are affected by other complications of heavy alcohol use like pancreatitis, stomach ulcers and neuropathies. The correlation between the amount of alcohol consumed and these alcohol-related health problems starts to rise steeply with a daily consumption of about 100 to 125g.

The causal relation of tobacco with oral cancer (especially when chewed) and with lung cancer (when smoked) is well established. Smoking can also increase considerably the seriousness of respiratory diseases. The relationship between tobacco smoking and atherosclerosis and ischemic heart disease is also well documented, but appears to be causally somewhat complex. However, large-scale interventions to reduce smoking (either within the context of general public health campaigns or as special anti-smoking campaigns) have, although sometimes decreasing morbidity, not normally affected mortality beyond trends observed in control groups or areas, and the usefulness of such campaigns has recently been seriously questioned.[6] It may well be that such campaigns generate a certain amount of shift in mortality patterns rather than a reduction in overall mortality.

For tobacco chewing a reduction in oral cancer and precancerous lesions following a vigorous campaign to stop tobacco chewing has recently been demonstrated in India.[7]

The effect of alcohol and tobacco smoking during pregnancy has been convincingly demonstrated. Both reduce birth weight, and alcohol increases the risk of certain malformations in the newborn. For alcohol use during pregnancy the risk for the intrauterine development of the baby may begin only from a certain level of heavy consumption about which, however, nothing is known. For cigarette smoking during pregnancy this risk appears to manifest itself already with very limited cigarette consumption. It is certainly highly advisable that female smokers adhere to strict tobacco abstinence during pregnancy.

Negative health effects of cannabis have so far not been established with certainty. A careful comparison of long-term heavy daily cannabis users with matched controls in North India has not found any significant cannabis-related difference between users and non-users on any of the many physiological and psychological parameters studied. Of course, in cannabis smokers the differences due to the concomitant cigarette smoking were observed (S.M. Das Gupta: Long-term Effects of Cannabis Use in Man. Banaras Hindu University, Varanasi, 1986, unpublished). However, this was a cross-sectional study. It would not have been possible to uncover differentials in mortality or, for example, differences in admissions to mental hospitals.

It is difficult to assess the specific substance-related health problems associated with chronic opiate use because of the frequency and often pervasiveness of the social, legal and economical problems normally accompanying the same, and their repercussions on health, including the special health risks related to the practice of intravenous injecting. The classical image of the emaciated and apathetic chronic opium smoker of China is very different from the heroin-dependent hustler of American slums or a heroin-using taxi driver in India. It is impossible to disentangle the impact of the various problems involved. Certainly, the various and often fatal consequences of alcohol and tobacco dependence like delirium tremens, cirrhosis of the liver and lung cancer are not paralleled by the health risks specifically related to the effects of opiates. Moreover, health considerations do not play a significant role in the prescription of methadone maintenance. In fact, there is no evidence that long-term methadone maintenance has adverse medical consequences.[9]

The serious health risks involved in intravenous drug use are well known. The yearly death rate of dependent IV heroin users has consistently been found to be in the order of 2% per year in Western countries. The bulk of this mortality are overdose deaths. The rate of overdose deaths is, therefore, often used as an indicator of trends in IV heroin use. This indicator is of course not usable in countries where heroin is mainly smoked or inhaled. The other main health risks in IV drug use are consequences of improper handling of needles and syringes, especially sharing of injection equipment. Previously mainly confined to hepatitis, the transmission of the HIV-infection or the AIDS virus has now become the main concern. We are still only at the beginning of understanding the mechanisms behind the continuation of needle sharing in spite of the risk of contracting AIDS. Risk-taking with a sort of denial "it will not happen to me" and peer modeling are certainly among them, the latter enforced by a ritualistic component of togetherness which itself is a consequence of the polarization mentioned above. Therefore, peer-to-peer programs are considered especially promising to reduce unsafe practices among IV drug users. A related argument of "mainstreaming" is used by proponents of the decriminalization of opiate use, assuming that by a decriminalization the strength of the social ties within the "drug subculture" would be reduced. This would make the users more amenable to interventions aimed at the reduction of the spread of AIDS and other health risks. Along the same line of argument, the component of pleasure from risk taking would decrease or disappear in drug initiation thereby enabling youths to make more rational decisions. It is of interest in this context that cannabis use in the Netherlands has been reported to have decreased since its decriminalization.

4. PROBLEMS IN DEVELOPING COUNTRIES

A major difficulty when discussing problems related to the use of mind-altering drugs in developing as well as industrialized countries lies in the definition of what may be considered a problem. A government may wish that its citizens refrain from using any addictive substance (except, normally, tobacco) and may therefore consider the occasional use of alcohol by some of its citizens as a problem. Other governments may consider any mind-altering drug except the traditionally sanctioned substances alcohol and tobacco as a problem. In some countries "once ever" use of certain illicit substances is considered a problem, whereas in others only compulsive use of the same drug leading to social and/or health problems (little difference normally being made between problems related to the substance and those related more to its criminalization).

WHO has made efforts to clarify the issues involved by proposing a set of definitions concerning drug use in a WHO memorandum. They are:

- **Unsanctioned use:** Use of a drug that is not approved by a society or a group within that society. When the term is used it should be made clear who is responsible for the disapproval. The term implies that we accept disapproval as a fact in its own right, without having to determine or justify the basis of the disapproval.

- **Hazardous use:** Use of a drug that will probably lead to harmful consequences for the user – either to dysfunction or to harm. This concept is similar to the idea of risky behavior. For instance, smoking twenty cigarettes each day may not be accompanied by any present or actual harm but we know it to be hazardous.

- **Dysfunctional use:** Use of a drug that is leading to impaired psychological or social functioning (e.g., loss of job or marital problems).

- **Harmful use:** Use of a drug that is known to have caused tissue damage or mental illness in the particular person.

In the same memorandum <u>drug dependence</u> is defined as a syndrome manifested by a behavioral pattern in which the use of a given psychoactive drug, or class of drugs, is given a much higher priority than other behaviors that once had higher value.

The term syndrome is taken to mean no more than a clustering of phenomena so that not all the components need always be present, or not always present with the same intensity. They will probably include some of the following:

- a subjective awareness of compulsion to use a drug or drugs, usually during attempts to stop or moderate drug use;
- a desire to stop drug use in the face of continued use;
- a relatively stereotyped drug-taking habit, i.e., a narrowing in the repertoire of drug-taking behavior;
- evidence of neuroadaptation (tolerance and withdrawal symptoms);
- use of the drug to relieve or avoid withdrawal symptoms;
- the salience of drug-seeking behavior relative to other important priorities; and/or
- rapid reinstatement of the syndrome after a period of abstinence.

Like the above classification into passive, active, controlled and compulsive use, this set of definitions is convincingly pragmatic and relatively free of value judgments except for a judgment on health risks or damage for the

WHO and a judgment on the effective containment of unspecified damage (health, social or professional) for the term "controlled use." This freedom from value judgments is probably one of the reasons why both have met with little acceptance worldwide. In an area where moral and otherwise emotional issues play such a strong role as the one of drugs, the preference for ill-defined but value-charged terms like "abuse" or "misuse" is understandable. After all, this is not the only area where the issue is "morality in the name of public health" (Washington Post, January 14-15, 1989).

In many developing countries the prevalence of regular tobacco use is very high indeed. But this is often limited to males. For example, in Sri Lanka, about 70% of males above 20 years are smokers, whereas less than 1% of women of this age group smoke. In such instances, tobacco use seems to represent a "cultural norm" to an extent that non-users are mainly those who, for example due to their special sensory sensitivity against bitter substances, simply "did not manage" to follow the general pattern. In such instances the earlier described role of risk-taking as a major motivator does of course not apply. Accordingly, in Sri Lanka the average age of smoking initiation is relatively high, viz., about 21 years as compared to 13 to 14 years in the USA.[10] The same is true of countries or societies with a very high rate and a high degree of social acceptability of beer consumption, as is the case in some parts of Europe and Africa. In such societies youth may even be initiated into this by their parents. But, in the absence of any polarization, the vast majority of users remain occasional or moderate users. In the case of smoking in Sri Lanka, for example, 50% of daily smokers smoke fewer than 8 cigarettes per day, and 10% of all smokers are occasional, not daily, smokers.[11]

Surveys on health problems related to the use of mind-altering drugs from developing countries are virtually non-existent. There are some fairly representative studies on drug use like the one cited above on smoking in Sri Lanka. But, unless one assumes the use itself to be a problem (if, for example, one considers a legal infraction like the use of an illicit drug a health problem), the extrapolation from such drug use figures to actual health problems remains problematic. This would require large, prohibitively expensive and difficult longitudinal studies. The author is not aware of any such study from a developing country. Furthermore, such survey data would not appear of a high priority unless they are linked to interventions. Figures from prisons and treatment facilities in India, Pakistan and Sri Lanka, for example, show that heroin use is highly prevalent in some parts of these countries. Although the seeking of treatment/detoxification is a fairly dynamic phenomenon (as is the use itself), these figures indicate high rates of heroin use. More detailed and exact information will not significantly change or improve the intervention responses, since there is no clear relationship between prevalence of heroin use and treatment needs or requests. In developing countries these are more often than not dictated by worried parents or a selectively vigilant police, whereas in industrialized countries they often reflect substantial fluctuations in price and/or availability of the drug. Yet, survey data do not appear normally to serve a particularly useful purpose apart from drawing attention to the fact that there is more or less widespread heroin use (which, as stated, can be inferred also from more easily available information). Furthermore, heroin and other illicit drug use may fluctuate in the form of epidemics. Survey data may then become obsolete in a matter of months.

5. PREVENTION

Since the 1960s it has become increasingly accepted to see drug abuse from a public health point of view: As a behavior which is transmitted from person to person. Terms like susceptibility and resistance therefore apply. The behavior is transmitted more often by "healthy carriers" (controlled users) than by persons afflicted by the illness, i.e., by compulsive or dependent users. Using this model, traditional preventive education in schools and via other means of information dissemination (e.g., by mass media campaigns) can only be based on the assumption that youngsters experiment with drugs (resistance is low) because they are unaware of the effects and risks involved. This has consistently been shown not to be true. The probability of a youngster accepting the offer of a drug is not correlated with his/her knowledge about the drug.[2] In fact, in view of the limited, if any, usefulness of media campaigns against drugs and of their potentially negative effects of polarization as mentioned earlier, a moratorium on media campaigns was imposed in 1973 and special guidelines established by the White House.[12]

Another approach to increase resistance against drug experimentation was based on the assumption that drug use is based on inadequate socialization and incomplete social development, i.e., that drug users are in some ways psychologically flawed. There is some evidence that youngsters who develop drug problems later in life are somewhat less conformist (less likely, for example, to be regular church goers in the USA), have a higher degree of alienation from their parents, and are more likely to have negative attitudes towards authority. This leads to the "generic approach" toward the prevention of drug use aiming at an improvement in their perception of authority, in their social interaction and their self-esteem. However, evaluation studies on this approach showed little, if any, impact on attitudes towards drugs or on actual patterns of drug use.[4]

Dorn[2] has summed up the results of the informational and generic approaches succinctly:

"All types of people take legal and illegal drugs. Some are knowledgeable about them and some ignorant. Some are psychologically unusual in some ways, but most are not. Most pupils believe that they would not take a drug if offered; but many, perhaps most, do."

Summing up, the Department of Health and Human Services reports to the US Congress:[13]

"Unfortunately, the inescapable conclusion to be drawn from the substance abuse prevention literature is that few of these programs have demonstrated any degree of success in terms of actual prevention of substance use or abuse."

However, in spite of this somewhat gloomy outlook, the DHHS review, as well as the review by Durell and Bukoski,[4] cites examples of successful prevention interventions. They are basically of three types:

A. The "macro" or "drug-free zone" approach. To use the terminology that is now used in the tobacco smoking reduction field, it is essentially an effort to create a climate of nondrug use. It depends on collaboration among parents who are concerned about their children's drug usage and who see that schools and other community agencies can be vehicles for change. It focuses on the entire environment in which a child is living. It has been remarkably successful in some countries and environments in reducing smoking in general and the beginning of smoking by youngsters in particular. It is not clear, however, to what extent this approach can be applied in regard to the use of other substances. For example, smokers can be accused of doing harm to their environment, by forcing passive smoking on them; they can easily be identified as an object of justified discrimination. This may not be true for other substances. Especially, it is not clear whether this approach is promising in regard to drugs which are already illicit, criminalized and socially disapproved.

B. Peer-to-peer programs. They involve youngsters as positive role models, often together with their training as peer counselors. Such programs aim at training youngsters, through using peers, to resist the subtle or explicitly persuasive seducements that emanate from their peers or the media. Such programs have been able to train youngsters effectively that saying no to a cigarette is socially acceptable and is, in fact, the desirable thing to do.

C. Programs for the prevention of drug initiation which are <u>situation-oriented</u>. Such programs tend to focus specifically on the offer situation. They are therefore relevant for passive users, i.e., drug users who have not yet proceeded to the state of actively purchasing the drug for consumption. They involve first a detailed descriptive study of the circumstances of offer situations a youngster is most likely to encounter. Descriptive material (visual or audio-visual) is then prepared aiming at a realistic portrayal of such situations. This material is presented to youngsters up to the point when a choice has to be made whether to accept the offer or not. This choice is then acted out in role-playing or in discussions. This approach, therefore, is a preparation for making a rational decision in a situation where the choice would otherwise be under strong situational control; i.e., this approach is basically a training in decision-making skills. It is a "think twice before you act" rather than a "just say no" approach.

These three promising approaches share a common feature: They require large numbers of dedicated and creative people for their implementation. Furthermore, especially the situation-oriented approach requires teachers (and parents) who accept the goal of decision-making skills rather than teachers insisting on merely moralistic and "anti-drug" goals.[2] All three approaches also contain a component of empowerment; empowerment of youngsters to make decisions for B. and C., and empowerment for community groups to take actions. This aspect is probably the main reason why large-scale official programs worldwide tend to continue along the more indoctrinational lines of traditional health education of little, if any, impact. (Except, as mentioned, anti-smoking campaigns which can thrive on the spirit of crusading against an identifiable wrong-doer and environment polluter. Furthermore, the thrust in these campaigns tends to be community action beyond what governments can plan. Equally vigorous anti-alcohol campaigns are more difficult to conceptualize in many countries.) When confronted with this issue of empowerment, it appears to be difficult to overcome the resistance of many professionals to give away power.

6. TREATMENT

A study group convened by the WHO in 1984 has, after a thorough review of the literature, prepared a check-list of factors which are, to the best of published knowledge, likely to improve treatment outcome. They are the following:

- returning to a drug-free environment
- living in a family or in another socially supportive environment
- employment or in school
- long-term follow-up
- supportive home visits
- education on drugs to the patient's family (not to the patient which does not seem to make any difference in outcome)
- continuing treatment after a relapse
- involvement of the patient in establishing a treatment plan
- development of marketable skills in patients where these are absent
- establishment of self-help groups of ex-addicts or relatives
- contingency contracting (detailed agreements on consequences following certain behaviors related to drug use)
- religious conversion
- early treatment
- methadone maintenance, especially if a reduction of crime is a major objective

It is obvious from this list that, in general, interventions aimed at the environment of the drug-dependent person hold more promise than interventions aimed at the dependent person alone.

Treatment efforts which follow the narrow medical model of treating only the addict himself and aiming at full abstinence are marred by a very high relapse rate. In general, such treatments when given alone make little difference, showing a yearly spontaneous abstinence rate of 2-5% in most follow-up studies of heroin- or alcohol-dependent persons. However, abstinence rates increase sharply with age.

In their 40s and 50s, most heroin users seem to "mature out" of their dependence. This is in marked contrast to the more sociable and less "juvenile" use of alcohol and opium. Where these are prevalent, the rate of spontaneous abstinence does not seem to follow this pattern of a sharp increase with older age, although moderate use tends to replace compulsive use in many dependent alcohol and opium users with older age.

A further observation corroborates the importance of social determinants of the dependence syndrome: Where opiates are used for pain relief over a longer period of time withdrawal symptoms appear at discontinuation. But they are not normally followed by craving.[14] Equally, anecdotal evidence from India and Sri Lanka suggests that persons who were made heroin dependent without their knowledge by, for example, adulterating cannabis products or ice cream with heroin, or by temporarily substituting heroin for cannabis in local markets, show a generally better prognosis than youngsters who were initiated into heroin use in the usual peer group manner. These anecdotal observations are in line with the finding that the first epidemic of heroin dependence which occurred in the USA in the early years of the 20th century following the free availability of heroin as a pain killer subsided with great speed once the dependence liability of heroin was publicized and it was banned from the market.[15]

As stated above, the large number of at least somewhat effective treatment modalities described in the literature show as a commonality their focus on the social environment of the dependent person. Especially the return after treatment into a drug-free environment has been shown to be a powerful predictor of success. From there evolve treatment responses which follow an explicit public health model: Drug use spreads through inter-human transmission like a contagious disease. Effective containment therefore requires early identification and treatment or otherwise elimination of foci of infection, and an increase in the effectiveness of treatment as well as prevention by maximizing community involvement under a sanitation-like perspective. Hughes, et al.[16] have described the management of a localized heroin epidemic along such lines. Similarly, Westermeyer[17] reports a very successful campaign to control opium dependence by an approach of "village-wise detoxification" highlighting the overall importance of a drug-free environment after whatever "treatment" has been given. Unpublished data from Myanmar, India and Sri Lanka suggest that this "camp approach" toward the establishment of "drug-free zones" may be equally effective in urban heroin-dependent youth.

As with prevention one may ask why large scale "treatment" programs to this day are still in so many instances oriented on traditional doctor-patient models thereby bringing their effectiveness to near insignificance. As with prevention, effective intervention seems to require a degree of dedication and creativity which large–scale programs may not be able to generate. Hughes' and Westermeyer's models, for example, require a "street corner epidemiology" and a "street corner involvement" which seem to be unacceptable to many professionals. Furthermore, they require considerable involvement of drug users, ex-users, relatives and volunteers. Such lay involvement is seen by many with suspicion and resentment against amateurish interventions. Certainly, their essentials of effective prevention and treatment programs are very difficult to generate in the context of large-scale government-sponsored programs.

CONCLUSIONS

Although little is known about the motivational pathways of youngsters into the use of licit and illicit drugs some approaches to primary and secondary prevention appear to emerge with some clarity. They are linked with the recognition that drug use and dependence are best considered in a public health or epidemiological context. They are transmitted from person to person. Environmental factors can enhance transmission or reduce its likelihood. However, unlike in many contagious diseases, environmental factors are also instrumental in the individual treatment outcome.

Large-scale changes in social norms will determine the spread or containment of the use of licit drugs. For illicit drugs, social changes for their containment seem to be effective only if effected on a smaller scale and in localized initiatives.

REFERENCES

1. Kellan, S.G., J.C. Anthony, and C.H. Brown, et al. Prevention research on early risk behaviors in cross-cultural studies, needs and prospects of child and adolescent psychiatry. Schmidt, M.H. and H. Remschmidt. Stuttgart: Hogrefe and Huber, 1989, pp. 241-254.

2. Dorn, N.Teaching decision-making skills about legal and illegal drugs. London: Institute for the Study of Drug Dependence, 1977.

3. Zinberg, N.E. Drug, set, and setting. The basis for controlled intoxicant use. New Haven and London: Yale University Press, 1984.

4. Durrell, J., and W. Bukoski. Preventing substance abuse: The state of the art. Public Health Reports, vol. 99, 23-31, 1984.

5. Longnecker, M.P., and B. Macmahon. Association between alcoholic beverage consumption and hospitalization, 1983 National Health Interview Survey. AJPH Feb 1988, vol. 78, 152-156, 1988.

6. McCormick, J., and P. Skrabanek. Coronary heart disease is not preventable by population interventions. Lancet, Oct 8, 839-841, 1988.

7. Gupta, P.C., J.J. Pindborg, and R.B. Bhonsle, et al. Intervention study for primary prevention of oral cancer among 36000 Indian tobacco users. Lancet, May 31, 1235-1239, 1986.

8. Arif, A., and J. Westermeyer. Manual of drug abuse. Guidelines for teaching in medical and health institutions. New York: Plenum Medical Book Co., 1988.

9. World Health Organization. Nomenclature and classification of drug- and alcohol-related problems: A WHO Memorandum. Bull WHO 59 (2), 225-242, 1981.

10. Johnston, L., P.M. O'Malley and J.G. Bachman. National trends in drug use and related factors among American high school students and young adults. Washington DC: U.S. Public Health Service, DHHS Publication no (ADM) 87-1535, 1987.

11. Sri Lanka, National Cancer Control Programme: Smoking patterns in Sri Lanka, 1989.

12. Special Action Office for Drug Abuse Prevention (SAODAP): The media and drug abuse messages. Washington, DC: The White House, 1974.

13. Department of Health and Human Services. Drug abuse and drug abuse research. National Institute on Drug Abuse. Rockville, MD: DHHS, 1984.

14. Mount, B.M., I. Ajemian, and J.F. Scott. Can Med Assoc J 115:122, 1976.

15. Krivanek, F. Addictions. Sydney: Allen & Unwin, 1988.

16. Hughes, P.H., E.C. Senay, and R.P. Parker. The medical management of a heroin epidemic. Arch Gen Psychiat 27, 585-591, 1972.

17. Westermeyer, J., and P. Bourne. Treatment outcome and the role of the community in narcotic addiction. J Nerv Ment Dis 166, 51-58, 1978.

42

ADOLESCENT REPRODUCTIVE HEALTH

SUPORN KOETSAWANG, M.D.

Adolescence is a transitional period from childhood to adulthood. Definitions of adolescence may vary, but in the context of reproductive health, adolescence begins at puberty and extends to 19 years of age. Adolescence has been defined by the World Health Organization as being between the ages of 10 and 19 years.[1] During this period, the adolescent has to cope with many difficult problems and needs understanding and help from parents and society.

PHYSICAL DEVELOPMENT

The adolescent experiences rapid physical growth during puberty. This growth spurt does not start at the same time in all parts of the body causing disproportionate body image. The development or delayed development of secondary sexual characteristics and the external genital organs may be extremely embarrassing to the adolescent. Also those who find themselves different from their peers may feel inferior. For instance, boys may be excessively worried about their penile size and girls may be unduly worried about the size of their breasts. These concerns are not particular to modern societies but are found throughout the developing world as well.

ADOLESCENT SEXUAL BEHAVIOR

There is a general impression that adolescent sexual activity is increasing considerably in developing countries leading to more reproductive health problems among adolescents.[2]

Increasing sexual activity is related to the following:

1. Early sexual maturation. This is an apparent trend to a lowering age of menarche resulting in more chance to have sexual problems.
2. No consensus on acceptable adolescent sexual behavior. Parents in developing countries seldom discuss sex-related problems, leaving the adolescents to interpret and experiment on their own. Increasingly, peers become the source of information on sex, often attendant with exaggerations and inaccuracies.
3. Lack of proper knowledge about sex and reproductive health. Despite exposure to a sex education course in the high school curriculum in Thailand, the standard and detail of instruction are known to be rather limited.
4. Declining cultural and religious influence. Aspects of adolescent life style are frequently counter to prevailing local cultural and religious values. In many developing societies, the influence of modernization is gaining dominance over traditional values. The pervasiveness and magnetic effect of the audio-visual electronic media combined with messages which often include an undercurrent of sexual independence and assertiveness, can contribute to an erosion of conventional behavior restraints designed to curb sexual behavior.
5. Urbanization. The number and variety of educational and employment opportunities that are available in growing urban centers lead many adolescents to migrate to cities. In the process, they are removed from the close parental and community supervision. The adolescent migrants may live independently or live with relatives who have less concern and control over the adolescent's behavior. Thus urbanization is a significant force in shaping the reproductive health or behavior of the adolescents in rapidly developing countries.
6. Late Marriage. The age of marriage rises substantially in developing countries. People delay marriage because of longer educational period and longer economic dependence.[3] The longer the young people delay their marriage, the higher they are at risk of premarital pregnancy.

PREMARITAL SEXUAL RELATIONS

A study in Bangkok[4] showed that 5.3 percent of female adolescents in schools had experienced premarital intercourse. The majority of them had sexual relations with their boyfriends.

A much higher proportion (45.2%) of male adolescent students had sexual intercourse with prostitutes and/or girlfriends.

REASONS FOR PREMARITAL INTERCOURSE

Reasons for premarital intercourse among male adolescents were rather unique. Most of them thought that men should have sexual experience before marriage. Physical pleasure was another important reason for premarital intercourse among them.

However, premarital intercourse among women is still culturally unacceptable. The reasons for premarital sexual relations among female adolescents are much more complicated. A study in Bangkok[5] reviewing 200 single pregnant adolescents found that most of them had combined reasons for becoming sexually active. Five major reasons were: physical pleasure, love affairs, to show maturity, to conform to peers and to search for new experience (Table 1).

Table 1 Reasons for Premarital Intercourse in 200 Female Adolescents (≤19 years) (Multiple responses allowed)		
Reasons	No.	% of Total (n=200)
Physical pleasure	179	89.5
Love affairs	177	88.5
To show maturity	118	59.0
To conform to peers	85	42.5
To search for new experience	51	25.5
To escape from parent's pressure	9	4.5
To get support	8	4.0
To challenge parents/teachers	3	1.5
Under alcoholic influence	3	1.5
Under drug influence	2	1.0
Being trapped in irresistable condition	14	7.0

(Adapted from "The study of women seeking abortion": Koetsawang S. et al., 1989).

Contraceptive Practice

Generally, among married couples, the wife takes responsibility for contraception and attending the family planning clinic. Because premarital sex is not acceptable in most developing countries, single women, especially adolescents, are not usually accepted or sympathetically served in family planning clinics. This cultural objection discourages the single girl from seeking contraceptive advice. The adolescents also tend to have limited knowledge on contraception. A study in Bangkok[4] showed that 57 percent of unmarried male adolescents had ever used contraception, though not regularly, when having sexual intercourse with their girlfriends. Similarly, 52 percent of unmarried female adolescents involved in sexual intercourse had ever used contraception. The condoms, oral contraceptive and natural family planning methods were the three most common methods used by both male and female adolescents. Over 40 percent of both male and female adolescents never used any contraceptive during intercourse. Among 200 female adolescents requesting abortion[5] only 18 girls (9%) used contraceptives in the month of conception. Most of the 182 adolescents who did not use contraception have a combination of reasons (Table 2). The five major reasons include:

Table 2
Reasons for not Using Contraception in 182 Adolescents
(Multiple response allowed)

Reasons	No.	% of Total (n=182)
Little concern for pregnancy	142	78.0
Poor or lack of contraceptive knowledge	76	41.8
Partner unwilling to use	45	24.7
Fear of contraceptive risk	23	12.6
Unprepared at time	21	11.5
Could not find any suitable method	18	9.9
Previous unsatisfied experience	11	6.0
Risking parent's discovery/devaluation	11	6.0
Contraceptive decrease sexual pleasure	7	3.8
Voluntary conception	5	2.7
No appropriate service	1	0.5

(Adapted from "The study of women seeking abortion": Koetsawang S. et al., 1989).

1. Little concern for pregnancy. The most common reason among all was that the girls were not concerned about the consequences of unprotected intercourse.
2. Poor contraceptive knowledge. Though many girls had heard about commonly used contraceptives, they did not know enough details to be able to seek for or to use contraception.
3. Lack of male cooperation. This reason is mainly related to the use of condoms as it was generally observed that the males felt that condoms decrease sexual satisfaction. Some of the girls had the same belief themselves.
4. Fear of contraceptive risks. News or rumors about contraceptive risks among adolescents could substantially discourage the contraceptive use.
5. Unplanned intercourse. Traditionally it seems immoral for any girl to have the contraceptives readily available for use as it implies that she is planning or expecting intercourse. This could be one reason why they had nothing available when they needed it.

It may be noticed that less than one percent of these girls mentioned problems related to contraceptive services. This is because most were not concerned about the negative consequences of unprotected sexual intercourse and therefore did not seek contraceptive services. Whenever this pattern is found in society, there is an urgent need for the expansion of effective sex education programs for adolescents.

The consequences of unprotected intercourse

The increasing incidence of unprotected sexual intercourse is invariably accompanied by the undesirable consequences of this behavior. Three major concerns are premarital pregnancy, sexually transmitted diseases and psychological consequences.

ADOLESCENT PREGNANCY

In certain developing countries, many girls marry at an early age. Without family planning and contraceptive knowledge, the girls tend to become pregnant when they are still in their adolescent period.

In many developing countries, however, there is a trend towards increased age of marriage because of urbanization, increasing years of education and economic status. These factors increase the chance of premarital intercourse and premarital pregnancy among adolescents.

In countries where abortion is not legalized, it is difficult to estimate the incidence of adolescent pregnancy as many of them end the pregnancies as unrecorded illegally induced abortions. A nation-wide study[4] in Thailand reported 636 adolescent pregnancies (17.2%) among 3700 illegally induced abortions. Of 466 female clients visiting the Adolescent Counseling Clinic at Siriraj Hospital, Bangkok, there were 67 (14.4%) adolescent pregnancies.[6]

Obstetric risk

Obstetric risks associated with adolescent pregnancy include the following:

1. pregnancy-induced hypertension,
2. anemia and malnutrition,
3. cephalopelvic disproportion,
4. difficult delivery, and
5. perinatal mortality.

With the exception of the pregnant girls under 15 years old, most problems related to adolescent pregnancy could be eliminated by proper antenatal care, early recognition of complications, psychological and social support. A study[8] of 16-19 year-old patients delivering in Siriraj Hospital, Bangkok, showed similar obstetric outcome to those of the adults. However, this study did not include adolescent pregnancies which terminated by illegally induced abortion.

Psychological and socio-economic consequences

Though most of the adolescent obstetric problems can be managed effectively, psychological and socio-economic consequences of adolescent pregnancy tend to be serious in the developing world where social welfare services are still inadequate and premarital sexual intercourse in female adolescents is considered highly shameful.

Psychological and socio-economic consequences include:

1. psychological stress, poor self-esteem with social stigma,
2. disrupted education, poor academic achievement,
3. poor socio-economic future, poor earning capacity,
4. poor parental job,
5. unstable marriage, and
6. unwanted child.

The condition is usually more serious if the pregnant adolescents are from a poor or broken family.

The father of adolescent pregnancy

A study[6] of pregnant adolescents in Bangkok showed that only 26 percent of the fathers of the adolescent pregnancies were adolescents themselves. The majority of fathers were between 20-24 years old. Most of them had little responsibility of the pregnancies.

Approach to reducing the negative consequences of adolescent pregnancy

The adverse consequences of adolescent child bearing could be ameliorated by the following plans:

1. provide continuing education,
2. provide childbirth and parenthood classes,
3. increase the adolescent's self-esteem, confidence and sense of responsibility and counseling for both the adolescents and their parents, and
4. provide contraceptive advice to delay further adolescent pregnancy.

Induced abortion in adolescents

It is obvious that continuing pregnancy in adolescents will severely disrupt their future lives and cause many difficult problems. Most unmarried pregnant adolescents risk their lives in the hands of crude abortionists. A nation-wide study on health hazard of illegally induced abortion in Thailand showed that illegally induced abortion is associated with high maternal mortality and morbidity due primarily to infection, hemorrhage and trauma to the pelvic organs. Deadly infections such as tetanus and gas gangrene infection and serious complications such as renal failure and disseminated intravascular clotting were still found.[6]

Access to illegal, but medically skilled abortion service through private organizations and clinics also exists in many developing countries. Such services, however, are inaccessible to poor adolescents because of the high service fees. The majority of abortion-seeking adolescents are still economically forced to choose low-cost services from unqualified abortionists.

Contraceptive Choices for Adolescents

Contraceptive use in the adolescent is a complex issue. In countries where early marriage is still widely practiced, it is agreeable that these young couples should be motivated to use contraception until they pass the adolescent period.

In cases of unmarried adolescents, contraceptive use is still controversial. It has been repeatedly stated that contraceptive services may promote pre-marital promiscuous behavior though there has been no definite evidence to prove this belief.

Generally, there is an agreement that a society should try to preserve its traditional culture. However, there is also concern about the discrepancy between these ideals and present situation such as increasing unwanted pregnancy and maternal mortality from illegally induced abortion.

Contraceptive services for the unmarried adolescent seem well tolerated by developing communities provided that the intervention is not too obvious and is combined with other services (e.g., counseling to reduce adolescent sexual problems).

Another problem is the low contraceptive acceptability among adolescents because of various reasons already mentioned. Sex education, the better communication program and adolescent-oriented clinics may help to overcome this problem.

Suitable contraceptive for adolescents

Contraceptive use in married adolescents may be similar to the use of temporary contraceptive methods in the adult population. In unmarried adolescents, however, their sexual relations are usually irregular and unpredictable. Contraceptive use in this group should be well-fitted to each situation. Recommended methods are briefly reviewed below.

Condoms Condoms are one of the highly recommended methods for adolescents whose sexual activity is irregular. They have several advantages as follows:

1. effective,
2. simple; easy to carry; do not require prescription or medical supervision,
3. no systemic effects,
4. delay premature ejaculation, and
5. protect against sexually transmitted diseases.

However, the condoms are not well accepted by the male adolescents because they tend to believe that condoms decrease penile sensation during intercourse.

Vaginal Contraceptive Sponge The Collatex sponge is a disposable polyurethane sponge impregnated with one gram of nonoxynol-9. The sponge has three contraceptive mechanisms:

1. mechanically blocks the external os,
2. trapping and immobilization of sperm, and
3. nonoxynol-9 in the sponge kills the sperm.

Immediately before sponge insertion, the sponge should be wet thoroughly with clean water and squeezed several times until foamy. With the dimple facing upward; the sponge is inserted into the vagina as far as it will go. Once the sponge is inserted, intercourse can occur immediately. One sponge contains enough spermicide for repeated intercourse during 24 hours. It must be left in place at least 6 hours after the last intercourse. It should be removed no later than 30 hours from original insertion.

The contraceptive efficacy of the sponge is lower than those of systemic contraceptives and IUDs. However, it may be convenient for the adolescent with irregular sexual activity. One additional advantage is that nonoxynol-9 contained in the contraceptive sponge can substantially reduce the risk of acquiring chlamydia infection and gonorrhea.

Oral Contraceptives The oral contraceptive is the most popular temporary contraceptive method in many adult populations. In prescribing oral contraceptives for adolescents, the same contraindications as for the adults should be followed. The low-dose combined pill containing ethinyl estradiol 30 μg or less is recommended.

In addition, the following points should be considered regarding the pill and adolescents:

1. Menstrual Irregularity – It is usually recommended that adolescents should not use the oral contraceptives until they have regular menstrual cycles, as it has been found that the adolescent with irregular menstruation tends to develop post-pill amenorrhea. However, it has been demonstrated that oral contraception does not alter the maturation of the endocrine system of the young girls.[10] Therefore, if they are not able to use other effective methods and are at high risk of pregnancy, the pill can be prescribed.

2. Acne Vulgaris – Acne vulgaris which is common in adolescents may be aggravated by the oral contraceptive. Oral pill formula-

tion containing cyproterone acetate* (which possesses an anti-androgenic property) can be used to improve acne.

The oral contraceptives may be suitable for the adolescents who have regular sexual activity. It may not suit those whose sexual intercourse is irregular and often unanticipated.

Post-coital Oral Contraceptive Pill If a highly effective post-coital pill is ever developed, it should be one of the ideal methods for the unmarried adolescent with irregular sexual activity. Unfortunately, the efficacy of the post-coital pills available at present is still not satisfactory. If failure occurs, there is a theoretical risk of teratogenicity.

Both estrogen and progestogen compounds have been used for post-coital contraception. Many regimens have been tried.

Two regimens presently used will be given as examples:

1. Levonorgestrel 750 mcg given orally within one hour after sexual intercourse, and

2. two tablets of the combined pills containing ethinyl estradiol 50 mcg and levonorgestrel 250 mcg taken immediately after intercourse and another two tablets 12 hours later.[11]

Injectables: Two available long-acting injectable contraceptives are:

1. Depot medroxy-progesterone acetate 150 mg given intramuscularly every 90 days, and

2. norethisterone enanthate 200 mg given intramusculary every two months.

Both preparations are not commonly used in adolescents because of their common side effects: prolonged irregular bleeding and amenorrhea. These preparations are not usually recommended for adolescents because of the high incidence of delayed return to fertility after discontinuing medication.

Subdermal Implants At present, the only commercially available contraceptive implant is Norplant®6. This implant system consists of six silastic tubings, each containing 36 mg of levonorgestrel. The six implants are placed in a fanlike manner subdermally in the inner upper left arm. Norplant constantly releases levonorgestrel to prevent pregnancy up to 5 years after insertion. The six capsules will be removed 5 years after insertion or earlier if required. Similar to the 3-monthly injectable, Norplant®-6 may cause irregular

---

*Formulation containing ethinyl estradiol 50 mcg and cyproterone acetate 2 mg per tablet.

bleeding or amenorrhea but there is no delayed return to fertility after removal. A study of Norplant in different parts of Thailand showed high efficacy, high acceptability and high continuation rates of use.[12]

Intrauterine Contraceptive Devices An IUD is not generally recommended for nulliparous patients because its use is associated with more pelvic pain and a higher expulsion rate[13] and higher incidence of pelvic infection[14] which may not relate directly with the IUD but with sexual promiscuity.

The IUD may be a good alternative for some adolescents because once it is inserted, it does not require user compliance. It may be particularly suitable for the adolescent who is not willing to use or cannot tolerate other contraceptives. The small size copper IUD should be selected as it will cause fewer side effects while still retaining high contraceptive efficacy. Though this method is not currently used among adolescents it may later prove to be well accepted by married and sexually active adolescents.

ACTION PLAN ON ADOLESCENT FERTILITY

The IPPF's Bellagio Consultation held in 1983[15] has given a very useful general program guideline for an action plan on adolescent fertility as follows:

1. In dealing with issues related to adolescent fertility, it is important to respect different cultural and social norms.
2. The community, including local organizations, should be encouraged to support and participate in programs for adolescents.
3. Programs should encourage responsible behavior by adolescents of both sexes.
4. Adolescents of both sexes should take an active role in designing and implementing projects which concern them.
5. Research should be fostered both to uncover and understand the issues in each country as well as to assess programs already under way so that the most suitable policies and programs can be formulated and replicated if feasible.
6. Programs for adolescents should endeavour to include information, education, counseling and health services.
7. Personnel should be given appropriate training to develop their skills and attitudes.
8. Every effort should be made to develop financial resources to support adolescent programs.
9. The exchange of experience between countries with similar problems and similar sociocultural norms should be encouraged.

REFERENCES

1. World Health Organization. The Health of Youth. Background Document/Technical Discussion. Geneva: WHO, 1983, p. 5.

2. Friedman, H.O.L., and K.G. Edstrom. Adolescent Reproductive Health: An Approach to Planning Health Service Research. WHO Offset Publication, no. 77. Geneva: WHO, 1983, p. 7.

3. ESCAP: Urbanization in Thailand and its Implications for the Family Planning Programme. Population Research Leads no. 17. Population Division. Bangkok: ESCAP,1984, pp. 9-10.

4. Koetsawang, S. Siriraj Adolescent Counseling Program: 1983-1985 Report. Theera Press, 1987, pp. 19-22.

5. Koetsawang, S. The study of women seeking abortion. (in prep, 1989).

6. Koetsawang, A., and S. Koetsawang. Nation-Wide Study on Health Hazard of Illegally Induced Abortion. Bangkok: Theera Press, 1987, p. 15.

7. Annual Statistics, Siriraj Family Planning Research Center, 1988.

8. Swadimongkol, S., and S. Toongsuwan. Teenage pregnancy. Siriraj Hosp Gaz 29: 961, 1977.

9. Rosenberg, M.J., J. Feldblum, and W. Rojanapithayakorn, et al. The contraceptive sponge's protection against Chlamydia trachomatis and Neisseria gonorrhoea Sexually Transmitted Disease 14: 147, 1987.

10. Wyss, R.H., I. Rey-Stocker, and M.M. Zufferey, et al. Influence of Hormonal Contraception in the Maturation Process of the Hypothalamic-Pituitary-Ovarian Axis. The Processings of an International Symposium, Amsterdam, March 1982. A.A. Haspels and A. Rolland (ed). MTP Press, 1982, pp. 156-167.

11. Haspels, A.A. Post-coital contraception. Female Contraception. B. Runnebaum, T Rabe, and L Kiesel (ed). Berlin: Springer-Verlag, 1988, pp. 371-380.

12. Koetsawang, S., O. Kiriwat, and M. Piya-Anant, et al. Clinical techniques and comparative performance with Norplant-6 and Norplant-2: Experience in Thai women. Recent Advances in Hormonal Contraception. M. Mizuno,(ed) Tokyo: Keidanren Kaikan, 1988, pp. 88-94.

13. Goldstruck, N.D.The use of IUCD in nulliparous women. Brit J Fam Plan 5:5, 1979.

14. Westrom, L., L.P. Bengtsson, and P.A. Mardh. The risk of pelvic inflammatory disease in women using intrauterine contraceptive devices as compared to non-users. Lancet 2:221, 1976.

15. McKay, J., (ed). Adolescent Fertility: Report of an International Consultation, Bellagio, 1983. London: IPPF, 1984. p. 41.

Section V
DELIVERY OF
CARE TO WOMEN
AND CHILDREN

43

A GLOBAL OVERVIEW OF THE HEALTH OF WOMEN AND CHILDREN*

MARK A. BELSEY, M.D., AND ERICA ROYSTON

INTRODUCTION

The health of women and children forms a continuum from one genera-tion to another. It reflects not only the vulnerabilities inherent in the biological and behavioral aspects of reproduction, growth, development, and matura-tion, but also the social, ecological, and historical situation of societies. The successful and healthy transition from one critical stage of life to the next is enhanced in societies that have made a commitment to social justice, and provide a minimum level and appropriate distribution of resources for health and social development. The health of women and children is threatened by imbalances in the distribution and access to resources by discrimination against women and illiteracy. Social changes, such as urbanization, economic crises, and natural and man-made disasters, all leave an imprint on the health of women and children.

Women's life-long health can be compromised by discriminatory treat-ment in childhood. Traditionally, many cultures prefer male children. Sons are perceived as an economic asset to the family, contributing productive labor. Girls, on the other hand, are seen as a burden, who often have to be provided with a costly dowry and whose economic productivity will benefit their husband's family rather than that of their parents. Sons usually have the main responsibility for the care of their parents in old age. Girls may get less food, be sicker before they are taken for curative health care, and receive less preventive health care. Evidence of such practices includes poorer nutritional

*Reprinted from *Maternal and Child Health Practices, Third Edition*. Helen M. Wallace, M.D., M.P.H., George M. Ryan, Jr., M.D., M.P.H., and Allan C. Oglesby, M.D., M.P.H. Oakland, CA: Third Party Publishing Company, 1988.

status of girls than boys, fewer girls than boys immunized, higher case fatality among girls brought to hospital, and higher mortality overall (Table 1). Significantly, where women's economic productivity is high the preference for sons is less pronounced.

Table 1			
Infant, Toddler and Child Mortality Rates, Ratios (M/F)			
and Preference for Sex of Children			
Country	Infant	Toddler	Child	Index of Son Preference
Senegal	1.16	0.99	1.00	1.5
Nepal	1.03	0.89	0.95	4.0
Bangladesh	1.03	0.73	0.84	3.3
Pakistan	1.05	0.63	0.68	4.9
Cameroon	1.07	1.04	0.99	1.2
Egypt	1.01	0.71	0.94	1.5
Turkey	1.10	0.62	0.94	1.4
Ivory Coast	1.24	1.19	1.11	1.2
Indonesia	1.30	1.15	1.31	1.1
Morocco	1.06	0.88	1.11	1.2
Kenya	1.10	1.17	1.02	1.1
Ghana	1.22	1.15	0.95	1.0
Colombia	1.19	0.75	0.83	1.0
Tunisia	1.02	1.05	1.25	1.3
Mexico	1.25	0.86	0.88	1.2
Thailand	1.08	1.42	0.65	1.4
Syria	0.92	1.05	0.64	2.3
Sri Lanka	1.24	0.68	0.87	1.5
Jordan	0.85	0.81	0.99	1.9
Venezuela	1.27	1.14	0.90	0.8
Fiji	1.19	0.92	1.04	1.3
Jamaica	1.36	1.07	1.17	0.7
Malaysia	1.31	1.41	1.19	1.2
Portugal	1.49	1.52	0.59	1.0

SOURCE: World Health Organization. Evaluation of the Strategy for Health for All. Seventh
  Report of the World Health Situation. Geneva, WHO, 1987, and World Fertility Survey. Notes: a) Countries are ordered by level of under five mortality

b) Index of son preference (from the World Fertility Survey) - Ratio of the number of mothers who prefer the next child to be male to the number of mothers who prefer the next child to be female

Women's education is also an important determinant of their own health and that of their children. In every economic setting, the children of literate women have a better chance of survival than those of illiterate women. Educated women tend to marry later, delay the onset of childbearing, and are more likely to practice family planning. They generally have fewer children with a wider spacing between births. Women with no schooling, on average, have almost twice as many children as those with seven or more years schooling.[1]

MATERNAL MORTALITY

Each year at least half a million women die from causes related to pregnancy and childbirth.[2] All but about 6,000 of these deaths occur in developing countries (Table 2). Maternal mortality rates are highest in Africa, with community rates of up to 1000 per 100,000 live births reported in several rural areas. The risk of dying from maternal causes is somewhat lower in the urban areas of Africa, but rates of over 500 have been reported in several cities. High maternal mortality rates are compounded by high fertility.

Table 2
Estimates of Maternal Mortality

Region	Live births (millions)	Maternal Mortality Rate (per 100,000 live births)	Maternal deaths (thousands)
Africa	23.4	640	150
Asia	73.9	420	308
Latin America	12.6	270	34
Oceania	0.2		2
Developing Countries	110.1	450	494
Developed Countries	18.2	30	6
World	128.3	390	500

SOURCE: World Health Organization. Evaluation of the Strategy for Health for All. Seventh Report of the World Health Situation. Geneva, WHO, 1987, and World Fertility Survey.

Very young age is an added risk in childbearing the world over. Teenage marriage is widespread in the (developing world, with the highest recorded incidence in Bangladesh, where 90 percent of women are married before they are 18 years old. By the age of 17, almost half of all women in Bangladesh are mothers and by the age of 19, one-third have at least two children.[3] In Bangladesh, girls aged ten-to-14 had a maternal mortality rate five times higher, and women aged 15-to-19 two times higher, than women aged 20-to-24.[4] Even in the U.S., girls under 15 have a maternal mortality rate three times that of women aged 20-to-24.

Maternal mortality rates have declined significantly in almost all developed countries in recent years. Table 3 shows such trends for selected countries.

Sri Lanka is an interesting success story. From a level of 522 in 1950-1955, the maternal mortality rate, excluding abortions, fell to 260 ten years later, and to 87 in 1980.[4] No doubt the fact that 85 percent of the births in Sri Lanka are attended by trained attendants, and 76 percent take place in institutions, provides at least part of the explanation. Over the same period, the total fertility rate fell from 5.3 in 1953 to 3.8 in 1977; and contraceptive prevalence rose from 32 percent in 1975 to 48 percent in 1981-1982.[5]

As overall maternal mortality has fallen, it has usually been deaths from sepsis that have declined first. In Sri Lanka, in 1950-1955 one-quarter of the

Table 3
Changes in Maternal Mortality in Selected Countries

Country	1965	1975	Change	Latest
USA	32	13	-59%	9 (1980)
France	23	20	-13%	13 (1980)
Fed. Rep. Germany	69	40	-42%	11 (1983)
Czechoslovakia	35	18	-49%	8 (1982)
Greece	46	19	-59%	12 (1982)
Portugal	85	43	-48%	5 (1984)
Japan	88	29	-67%	15 (1983)
Romania	86	121	+41%	149 (1984)
Romania excl. abortion	65	31	-52%	21 (1984)

SOURCE: World Health Organization. Maternal Mortality data bank.

maternal deaths were due to sepsis. By 1977, the proportion had fallen to ten percent.[4] In China, where overall rates have fallen to 49 in 1984, deaths from sepsis now account for only some six percent of all maternal deaths. Such declines reflect both improvements in the standard of delivery care, such as, for example, the emphasis on the three *cleans* (*clean* hands, *clean* delivery surface, and *clean* cord care) and the lower case fatality resulting from the availability of antibiotics.[6] Deaths from hemorrhage are usually slower to decline. The short-time between the onset of serious bleeding and death means that access to lifesaving interventions is crucial.

Hypertensive disorders of pregnancy (HDP) remain one of the more common morbid conditions of pregnancy. The death rate due to HDP seems to fall more slowly than that from sepsis. The prevalence of HDP and eclampsia varies widely, as seen in the results from the WHO collaborative study. (Table 4) It is noteworthy that the fall of mortality from HDP in such countries as Sweden was not a function of a decline in the incidence of eclampsia but was the result of the decline in the case fatality rate.[7]

Severe anemia in pregnancy contributes greatly to maternal morbidity and mortality. In rural India, in 1981, anemia was given as the second most important cause of maternal mortality, after hemorrhage, where it is usually a contributing factor.[8] Together, these two causes accounted for 41 percent of maternal deaths. In one study from India, the risk of a maternal death was increased 14-fold when the woman had a hemoglobin level of less than 8 gm percent.[9]

On the basis of a review of all information available in 1979, it was estimated that, in 1975, there were some 230 million anemic women in the

---

Table 4
Proportion of Mothers with Pre-Eclampsia and Eclampsia

	Pre-Eclampsia (per cent)	Eclampsia (per cent)
Viet Nam	1.5	0.34
Burma	4.4	0.40
Thailand	7.5	0.93
China	8.3	0.17

SOURCE: World Health Organization, Hypertensive Disorders of Pregnancy, Technical Report Series No. 758, WHO, Geneva, 1987.

world; about half the nonpregnant women live in developing countries, and two-thirds of those pregnant. The highest proportion of women with hemoglobin concentrations below the WHO norm is in Asia, followed by Oceania and Africa.[10]

MALARIA AND PREGNANCY

In addition to the nutritional anemia of pregnant women, in many areas of the developing world malaria will lower the hemoglobin level by 1.5 g percent[11] and result in a 150 to 250 gram lowering of birthweight.[12] Malaria during pregnancy, among primagravida women, greatly increases the risk of cerebral malaria and death. The risks of chloroquine to the fetus are exceedingly low, and more than offset by the dangers that untreated malaria has for both mother and infant. However, with increasing prevalence and higher levels of resistance of the malaria parasites to chloroquine, the management of malaria during pregnancy becomes increasingly complex. The safety of the newer anti-malarial drugs has not been established with respect to effects on the fetus.[11]

UNWANTED PREGNANCY AND ABORTION

A considerable proportion of the very high fertility observed, particularly in developing countries, is unwanted. If all women who said they wanted no more children were actually able to stop childbearing, the number of births would be reduced by an average of 35 percent in Latin America, 33 percent in Asia, and 17 percent in Africa.[13]

The incidence of abortion and its consequences and complications represents a public health problem of major dimensions in a large number of countries, regardless of whether the procedure is legally available and accessible. In all settings, its occurrence and persistence reflect the failure to satisfy the fertility regulating desires and needs of women. That failure may represent a combination of societal actions or inaction (policies, access to information, and services, etc.), personal health behavior and choice, and contraceptive failure.

Even an estimate of the incidence of legally induced abortion is difficult to obtain, while estimates of illegally induced abortion are generally unreliable. However, estimates based on either official reporting or secondary data sources suggest that there are some 33 million illegally induced abortions performed annually (with a low of 30 million and a high of 40 million). The Soviet Union and China account for fully 25 million of these cases.[14] The estimates of illegally induced abortion are highly speculative. The total number of abortions is estimated to be between 40 and 60 million. On a global basis, that level of abortion would suggest there are from 24 to 32 induced abortions for every 100 known pregnancies.[13]

The effect on maternal mortality of a change in the legal status of abortion has been well documented in several countries. In Romania, where abortion had been widely available and practiced after it was made illegal, both the birth rate and the maternal mortality rate rose sharply. The maternal mortality rate has stayed high, with 80 percent of maternal deaths being abortion-related, while the birth rate has gradually returned to the low levels of the early 1960s. (Table 3) In Cuba, between 1968 (when abortions were first permitted in hospitals) and 1976, about half of the decline in maternal mortality, from 85 to 46, was attributed to the decline in abortion-associated deaths.[15]

BREAST FEEDING AND FERTILITY

Breast feeding has been recognized as a unique and critical factor in the health and wellbeing of both the mother and the infant. Although much maligned as a means of fertility regulation, the weight of demographic and epidemiologic data supports the conclusion that any changes in breast feeding practices that reduce the present high incidence and long duration of breast-feeding, and the high frequency of suckling, will have a profound effect on fertility. Thus, if in Bangladesh, for example, the breast feeding patterns were to change to those typical of industrialized countries, the already high fertility rates could be expected to rise by over 50 percent. To maintain fertility at current levels, contraceptive use would have to increase from nine percent to about 52 percent.[16] When feeding is provided on demand, particularly without any supplementation before four-to-six months, breast feeding prolongs the period of postpartum amenorrhea.[17]

LONG TERM REPRODUCTIVE MORBIDITY

Long term morbidity and disability are many women's legacy from inadequate or unskilled maternity care, unregulated fertility, and sexually transmitted diseases. If, singly or in combination, these conditions do not lead to a maternal death, they frequently result in serious physical suffering and social consequences for the woman. In physical terms, the consequences are measured in terms of pelvic inflammatory disease (PID), ectopic pregnancy, infertility, vesico-vaginal and recto-vaginal fistula, and uterine prolapse. The social and personal consequences are very much a reflection of the responsiveness, sensitivity, and supportiveness provided by the husband, the family, and the community. The long-term morbidity contributes to family disruption, divorce, and the ostracism and stigmatization of the women concerned.

Although information on long term reproductive morbidity is difficult to obtain, in many circumstances information on ectopic pregnancy serves as a useful indicator of the combination of conditions, i.e., sexually transmitted disease, post-abortal, and puerperal sepsis.[18] Both in developed and developing countries the incidence of ectopic pregnancy is increasing dramatically. Over a 17-year period, the rate has tripled in Finland.[19] Whereas in 1967, one in 142 pregnancies was ectopic; in 1983, one in 50 was ectopic. Ectopic pregnancies place a burden on hospital services, in terms of the capacity for emergency operative facilities, skilled staff, and blood transfusion services, the latter being greatly complicated by the problem of AIDS in many parts of the world.

The health and health service implications of infertility are emerging more clearly. In several countries, and in many subgroups, primary and secondary infertility may be as high as 15 percent to 20 percent, with consequently heavy demands placed on health services and unjustifiably heavy burdens placed on women, who account for only a portion of the infertility.[20] Care for the infertile couple in many countries is ad hoc, both expensive and frustrating for all concerned. Sexually transmitted diseases, and inadequate access to diagnostic and therapeutic services for the control of infections, are major factors in excessive levels of infertility in many countries.

LOW BIRTHWEIGHT AND PRETERM DELIVERY

The birthweight of an infant is the single most important determinant of its chances of survival, healthy growth, and development. Because birthweight is conditioned by the health and nutritional status of the mother, the proportion of low birthweight (LBW) infants closely reflects the health status of the communities into which they are born.

Low birthweight can be caused by short gestation and/or by retarded intrauterine growth. Although etiologically distinct, both have an important effect on fetal and neonatal mortality. A review carried out in 1984 led to an estimate of 20 million LBW infants, or 16 percent of those born in 1982. This constitutes a fall, in both relative and absolute terms, when compared to estimates for 1979 of 21 million LBW infants, making up 16.8 percent of the 122 million born that year.[21]

The incidence of LBW, by region, ranges from 31.1 percent in South Asia and 19.7 percent in Asia as a whole, to 14.0 percent in Africa, 10.1 percent in Latin America, 6.8 percent in North America, and 6.5 percent in Europe. There is no evidence of any improvement in South Asia, the region where the problem is most acute. Rates in that region remain between 20 percent and 50 percent.[19]

The major factors associated with low birthweight in developing countries include the pre-pregnancy weight and height of the mother; weight gain during pregnancy; infections, particularly malaria, anemia, parity, and sex of the infant, and racial factors. (Table 5) In the industrialized countries, infection plays a less important role and cigarette smoking a much more important role, accounting for one-third of the low birthweight.[22]

Table 5
Factors Associated with Intra-Uterine Growth Retardation
and Pre-Term Delivery

	Relative Risk of Intra-uterine Growth Retardation	Relative Risk of Pre-term Delivery
Maternal height		
157.5 - 158 cm	1.27	1.0
Pregnancy weight		
< 49.5 kg	1.84	
< 54.0 kg		1.25
Primiparity	1.23	?
Previous LBW infant	2.75	
Previous pre-term infant		3.08
Pregnancy weight gain		
< 7 kg (well nourished)	1.98	?
100 kcal/day supplement		
undernourished women	0.47	
well-nourished women	0.82	
Smoking	2.42	1.41
Alcohol -> 2 drinks/day	1.78	?

SOURCE: Belsey MA: The epidemiology of infertility. Bulletin of the World Health Organization, 54:319-341, 1976.

PERINATAL MORBIDITY AND MORTALITY

Information on perinatal mortality is often unreliable and difficult to obtain because of incompleteness of reporting and variations in the definitions used. Under-reporting of perinatal, or even neonatal mortality, is far more common than the under-reporting of infant mortality, and may have contributed to the failure of health authorities to recognize both the importance of the problem and the possible options for action.

High perinatal mortality rates of 80 to 100 per 1,000 live births are found among the least developed and most disadvantaged countries; and, moderately high rates, i.e., 40 to 60/1,000 live births are found in most developing countries. In most developed countries, and a number of developing countries with strong programs of maternal health care, the perinatal mortality rate is in the low 20s; and, in a few instances, such as Japan, the Nordic countries, and the Federal Republic of Germany, the rate is below ten. Because birthweight itself is such a major determinant of perinatal mortality, comparisons of perinatal mortality must make an adjustment for differences in birthweight distributions.[23] Even in many of the least developed countries as much as 40 percent to 50 percent of the infant mortality occurs during the first month of life, largely in the first week.

Decline in perinatal mortality is in large part a function of the health of the mother and the quality of pregnancy, delivery, and newborn care. Perinatal mortality rates within a country, therefore, are a very sensitive indicator of program interventions and are useful as an indicator of the quality of care in different populations and areas of a country. The timing of a perinatal death, i.e., antepartum, intrapartum, and postpartum, also provides a good measure of the quality of the maternal health care services. In European countries with perinatal mortality rates around 10/1000 live births, the ratio of fresh stillbirths to macerated stillbirths is 0.2. In two developing countries where special studies were carried out, the ratios were 1.5 and 1.7, suggesting inadequate referral and management of pregnancies at risk of complications.[21]

In a number of developed countries, and a few small developing countries, perinatal mortality has decreased by half over the period from 1965 through 1980. (Table 6, next page) Investment in high technology is not the only way such declines have come about. Regionalization of perinatal care, the application of a risk approach, and a greater understanding of the pathophysiological basis of perinatal morbidity and mortality, with better management of pregnancy and delivery, have, in many instances, contributed to this decline without major investments in facilities and equipment. Even within a four year period of time, with no increase in medical or maternity expenditures, over a 50 percent reduction of perinatal mortality and stillbirth rates was accomplished through a primary health care program among plantation workers and their families in South India. (Table 7)[24] In contrast to postneonatal infant mortality, social, economic, and environmental improvements have far less of an impact during this period, except insofar as they affect maternal health and low birthweight.

Table 6
Perinatal Mortality Rates (Per 1,000 Live Births)
for Selected Countries, 1965-1984

Year	Sweden	Singapore	England & Wales	France	Japan	Mauritius
1965	19.9	25.8	27.3	28.2	30.1	82.0
1970	16.5	21.7	23.8	23.7	21.7	60.9
1975	11.3	16.7	19.9	18.3	16.0	61.6
1980	8.7	13.5	13.4	13.0	-	39.5
1984	6.8	10.4	10.1	11.3	8.0	32.1

SOURCE: Edouard L: The epidemiology of perinatal mortality, World Health Statistics Quarterly, 383:289-301, 1985.

Table 7
Comprehensive Labor - Welfare Scheme Estates: Data on Stillbirth
and Perinatal Mortality Rates* (Per 1,000 Live Births)

Year	Still birth rate	Perinatal mortality rate
1979	69.8	109.7
1980	44.3	82.5
1981	36.6	73.2
1982	27.9	47.7

SOURCE: Kramer MS: Determinants of Low Birth Weight: A methodologic and meta-analysis Bulletin of the World Health Organization, 1987.

* Total population covered by the CLWS was over 250,000

INFANT AND CHILD MORTALITY

While not as great as the differentials in maternal mortality, the differences between the infant and child mortality in the poorest countries and the most privileged are up to 30-fold. On average, one in 12 infants in the developing countries dies before reaching the age of one, compared to one in 71 in the industrialized countries. For children under five, the ratios are one in eight compared to one in 56.

Differentials are not confined to comparisons between countries, for even within developed countries there are two to threefold differences in infant, neonatal and, postneonatal mortality rates between the most- and least-socially advantaged groups.

In 1986, WHO reported over 14 million children died before reaching their fifth birthday, two-thirds of them aged less than one year. Ninety-nine percent of all infant and child deaths in the world are in the developing countries, although these countries account for only 85 percent of all children under the age of five.

Nevertheless, considerable progress has been made over the last 30 years. Despite the fact that the annual number of births has increased from 86 million in 1950 to 130 million in 1986, the annual number of infant deaths has fallen from 16 million in 1950 to some 14 million in 1986. The infant mortality rate for developing countries, as a whole, fell from 188 in 1950 to 92 in 1980, and 81 in 1986; the under-five mortality rate fell from 295 in 1950 to 142 in 1980, and 124 in 1986. The UN Population Division projects a further reduction of some 30 percent in the infant mortality rate of developing countries between 1985 and 2000, to a level of 61. A similar fall is projected for the developed countries, to a level of 11 in 2000.

The main killers of young children in high mortality countries are the infectious diseases (Table 8).

Table 8 Causes of Death of Children Under Five	
Cause	Million p.a.
Acute diarrhea and related causes	5.0
Malaria	3.0
Measles	2.1
Neonatal tetanus	0.8
Pertussis	0.6
Acute respiratory infections	4.0
Typhoid fever	0.5
SOURCE: World Health Organization.	

INFANT AND CHILD DISEASE MORBIDITY

In many developing country societies, the common pattern is that of repeated infectious diseases during childhood, with as much as 30 percent to 40 percent of a child's life spent suffering gastrointestinal, respiratory, or other infections.

In 1974, when the Expanded Programme on Immunization (EPI) was established by the WHO, less than five percent of infants in the developing world were fully immunized. In 1987, 45 percent of the infants in the developing world now receive the third dose of DPT or polio, and more than 60 percent receive at least the first dose. However, vaccine coverage in the developing world is the lowest for the two EPI diseases which cause the highest number of deaths – measles and neonatal tetanus. These two diseases account for over 80 percent of the 3.4 million deaths annually attributable to the EPI target diseases. Measles immunization is at the level of 35 percent, while immunization of pregnant women against tetanus is at the level of 16 percent.[25]

Measles affects 70 million children yearly in the developing countries. About two million of these cases end fatally. Protein-energy malnutrition commonly increases the risk of death and is often an important factor in growth retardation. Although the case-mortality rate in developed countries is not high, complications are not infrequent. About one percent of cases are hospitalized, and encephalitis affects one case in 2000, with frequent sequelae of permanent brain damage and mental retardation. Case-fatality rates are often over one percent in the developing world.

Mortality from neonatal tetanus in some areas of the world has been as high as from 100 to 260/1,000 live births. In Haiti, the introduction and improvements in the training of traditional birth attendants had reduced those rates by as much as half that in 1962. The subsequent introduction of immunization of pregnant women, and later of all women, in an outreach program eliminated the disease as a public health problem.[26] Similar marked reduction in neonatal tetanus was found in China with the simple adherence to the principles of the "three cleans" in the training of the traditional birth attendants: clean hands, clean delivery surface, and clean cutting and care of the umbilical cord. (WHO 1985)

Of an expected 850,000 deaths from pertussis, approximately 30 percent have been prevented through immunization. Of an expected 365,000 cases of poliomyelitis, nearly 40 percent have been prevented. In a follow-up of the EPI program in Indonesia, the decline in the morbidity rate of diphtheria corresponded to the level of coverage achieved with two doses of DPT.[27]

DIARRHEAL DISEASE MORTALITY AND MORBIDITY

The incidence and case-mortality rates for diarrheal disease have been difficult to obtain, and difficult to compare over time and between different countries. Nevertheless, the Diarrheal Control Programme of WHO has summarized the results of 193 surveys in 49 countries, in which the standardized WHO/CDD methodology was used. (Table 9) The median number of diarrheal episodes per year for children, globally, is estimated to be 3.6, with the Americas-region surveys showing a median of 6.2 and the Western Pacific surveys having a median of 2.2. Globally, it is estimated that one-third of the child deaths are associated with diarrhea.[28]

NUTRITIONAL PATTERNS OF CHILDREN

It is estimated that 40 million preschool children in developing countries are living in conditions of acute malnutrition, and more than three times that number in a chronic state of insufficient nutrition and associated illness that is hampering their growth.[29] Growth patterns of children and their trends over

Table 9
Summary of Results of 193 Diarrhea Mortality, Morbidity and Treatment Surveys of Children Aged 0-4 Years, 1981 - 1986

WHO Region	Number of Surveys (countries)		Mortality rates/1,000 children (median)		Percentage of deaths Diarrhea Associated	Annual Incidence (episodes/ child/year)
			All Causes	Diarrhea-Associated		
AFR	40	(17)	32.0	11.5	41.1	4.7
AMR	6	(06)	11.0	3.9	34.9	6.2
EMR	32	(09)	15.7	6.7	43.2	3.8
SEA	67	(09)	13.7	3.6	28.3	3.2
WPR	48	(08)	8.4	2.2	22.4	2.2
Total	193	(49)	18.0	5.6	36.0	3.6

SOURCE: World Health Organization. Programme for Control of Diarrheal Diseases. Interim programme report 1986. WHO document No. WHO/CDD/87.26.

time have frequently been used as indicators of health and nutrition status. The most-widely used indicator, weight-for-age, has been used as a measure of protein-energy malnutrition. Interpretations of trends in nutritional status, based on weight-for-age, are complicated by the fact that weight-for-age is a composite of both stunting and wasting.

Anthropometric indicators for stunting (height-for-age) and for wasting (weight-for-height) provide a much clearer picture of the health status of children. *Wasting*, a highly sensitive indicator, varies widely by season and quickly reflects the impact of acute illnesses such as measles and diarrheal diseases. *Stunting* reflects more the accumulated health and nutritional legacy of a child.

Trends in stunting have been analyzed from nine countries in different parts of the world.[30] In seven, there was an improvement and in two a deterioration (Table 10). For all regions except Asia, the prevalence of protein–energy malnutrition among children under five appears to be decreasing over the last few decades. (Table 11, next page)

Table 10
Average Annual Change in Prevalence of Stunting

Country	Year 1	Year 2	Per cent change
Egypt	1978	1980	-2.95
Nicaragua	1965 - 7	1980 - 2	-1.69
Thailand	1975	1984	-1.41
El Salvador	1965	1975	-1.05
Lesotho	1976	1981	-1.04
Colombia	1965 - 6	1977 - 80	-0.47
Sri Lanka	1975 - 6	1978	-0.50
Sierra Leone	1974 - 5	1977 - 8	+0.92
Kenya	1978 - 9	1982	+1.03

For all regions except Asia, the prevalence of protein-energy malnutrition among children under five appears to be decreasing over the last few decades.

SOURCE: Filmore, C, 1986.

BREAST-FEEDING TRENDS AND CHILD HEALTH

The nutritional and infection protecting properties of breast milk have been amply demonstrated. The decline of breast-feeding has been associated with an increase in infant morbidity and mortality, especially among the more disadvantaged communities of both the developed and developing world. Among the direct results are an increase in diarrheal diseases in infants fed breast-milk substitutes.[31]

In developed countries, changing lifestyles, particularly involvement of women in the work force, changes in family structure, and developments in food technology, appear to have been important contributors to the decline in breast-feeding, which took place between the 1940s and the early 1970s. In developed countries, many of the potentially adverse effects on child health of the decline have been countered by improved sanitation, clean water, communicable disease control, family planning services, and general socio–economic improvements. However, a similar erosion of breast-feeding in the developing world could have a disastrous impact on health and family planning.

Early initiation of breast-feeding consistently appears as a key factor in the establishment and duration of breast-feeding.[32] While there is strong evidence that early mother-to-child, skin-to-skin contact, and demand feeding are important factors in enhancing breast-feeding[33] many of the maternity and health care routines limit, rather than facilitate, these practices.

Table 11 Estimated Protein-Energy Malnutrition Prevalence by Region, Determined as a Percentage of Children with Low Weight for Age		
Country	1963-1973	1973 -1983
Africa	31.1%	25.5%
Americas	25.9%	17.7%
Asia	50.6%	54.0%
Oceania	22.0%	11.5%
SOURCE: Filmore, C. 1986		

In reviewing the worldwide patterns of breast-feeding, WHO described a typology that appeared to conform to the dynamic changes in patterns according to stage of development and population subgroups within a country. Time-trend analysis from a few countries has confirmed the sequential nature of that pattern, with a sharp decline in breast-feeding in the urban higher-income groups first, followed by other groups, and then a resurgence of breast-feeding again initiated among the higher–income urban groups.

COVERAGE OF MCH, INCLUDING FAMILY PLANNING

Almost everywhere, there is a dearth of systematic, comprehensive, and critical reviews and evaluations of program coverage, performance, and effectiveness. Wide variations in the proportion of women receiving prenatal care exist both between and within geographic areas. In Africa, the proportions range from 33 percent to 90 percent; in Latin America, from 20 percent to 81 percent; and, in Asia, from five percent to 98 percent.[34]

MATERNAL CARE

In a significant number of cases, and especially in rural areas, the percentage of women receiving prenatal care (by a trained attendant) exceeds the percentage receiving skilled intrapartum care. This discrepancy between high levels of prenatal care coverage and somewhat lower levels of supervised delivery care coverage, in some instances, may be related to the geographic inaccessibility due to lack of transport, and the distances and time necessary to travel once a woman goes into labor. But, in many settings, cultural preference and distances may play an equal, if not greater, role. Hassouna has described how even the majority of nonprofessional health workers are delivered by a traditional birth attendant in Cairo, despite the availability and their knowledge of the delivery care facilities.[35] A similar preference for traditional birth attendants, who are more like family birth attendants, has been noted in Zimbabwe.

On the basis of available information, it is possible to build up estimates for the coverage of maternity care in the various regions of the world. These estimates show that only some 55 percent of the births in the world are attended by trained personnel. Even fewer take place in an institution. This means that some 58 million of the 128 million infants born in 1983 were delivered with the help of untrained traditional birth attendants, family members, or by the mother alone.

In the developed world, nearly all births are attended by trained personnel, but in the developing world, where 85 percent of the world's births take place, fewer than half were so attended. The coverage of child health care is extremely difficult to quantify. If one uses immunization protection as a measure, many countries have shown spectacular progress. However, the use of immunization coverage, as a surrogate for overall infant and child health care coverage, is only possible in situations where immunizations are provided almost exclusively by the organized health services. Social mobilization and mass campaigns, while admirably raising the level of protection in a relatively short period of time, and intended to lead to sustainability through the health system, do not really reflect overall care for children. Thus, for example, a recent evaluation of MCH services in Tanzania suggested that, apart from immunization coverage, which ranged from 70 percent for BCG to 30 percent for measles, the programs were having limited, if any, impact on the main problems of mothers and children.[37]

FAMILY PLANNING

From only a few countries with family planning programs in the beginning of the 1960s, currently 120 governments now support such programs either directly or indirectly. About 95 percent of people in the developing world live in countries which provide some form of public support for family planning programs, generally as part of MCH programs. Contraceptive prevalence, as a measure of family-planning program effectiveness, has increased. In over 75 countries, with 60 percent of the world's women, contraceptive prevalence rates of 30 percent or above prevail. However, in over 50 countries, with 20 percent of the world's women, prevalence rates are below ten percent.[38]

Despite the apparently high contraceptive prevalence rates in some countries, there does not appear to be a commensurate change in fertility. This somewhat paradoxical observation has been attributed to high discontinuation and failure rates of certain contraceptive methods and, at times, to over-reporting of acceptor rates in some programs. Another contributing factor to an apparent lack of effect on birth rates, despite an increased rate of contraceptive prevalence, is the use of such methods by older couples who are already at a low risk of pregnancy.[39] The World Fertility Survey has shown a marked discrepancy in many countries between current fertility, numbers of unwanted births per woman, and contraceptive prevalence. In Africa, only 23 percent of women not wanting any more births are practicing contraception; in Asia it is 43 percent; and in Latin America, 57 percent. Evidently, in many circumstances and in many countries, either the methods and/or the services are not accessible and/or acceptable in physical, cultural, or personal terms. As a consequence, deaths from illegally induced abortion continue to constitute from 25 percent to 50 percent of maternal mortality in many countries.

The pattern of use of different methods of contraception, often a consequence of availability, varies widely. (Table 12) For example, in Thailand, of the 65 percent of women practicing family planning, fully 90 percent are protected from unwanted pregnancies by such methods as sterilization, oral or injectable hormonal contraceptives, or IUDs. On the other hand, in Bulgaria, although 76 percent practice family planning, these effective methods are being used by less than ten percent of contracepting women. Globally, about 325 million couples, out of 800 million of reproductive age, are using an effective method of contraception, namely:

135 million – sterilization
70 million – IUD
55 million – oral hormonal contraceptives
37 million – condoms
30 million – injectable hormonal contraceptives, barrier methods, and
        other modern methods

Table 12
Contraception: Estimated Percentage of Married Women of Reproductive Age Practicing Contraception, 1980-1981

	Percent
World total	45
Total excluding China	38
Developing regions:	
Total	38
Total excluding China	24
Africa	11
Asia	42
East Asia	69
South Asia	24
Latin America	43
Developed regions:	
Total	68

SOURCE: United Nations_ Recent levels and trends of contraceptive use as assessed in 1983 New York, UN, 1984.

Another 20 million to 40 million use traditional methods, such as periodic abstinence or withdrawal.[40]

PRIMARY HEALTH CARE AND MCH, INCLUDING FAMILY PLANNING (FP)

Primary health care (PHC) has inherent to it the concept of placing the appropriate technologies at the most appropriate level of the system. Over the last several years, both research and experience have shown that many of the appropriate technologies in MCH/FP can be transferred successfully to families and communities. Such successful transfers have included: community-based distribution of contraceptives and of oral rehydration salts; home preparation of ORT; growth monitoring and follow-up action by women's organizations, teachers, and others; homebased monitoring of pregnancy, and of child health and growth through the use of home based records; and the identification and referral by traditional birth attendants of pregnancies at potential risk of complications.

Since some of the essential technologies for MCH/FP cannot be made available at the PHC level, they must be available and accessible at the level of first referral. Thus, for example, without the availability of the skills, supplies, and equipment for an assisted delivery, cesarean section, the provision of blood, etc, little progress will be made in significantly lowering the very high maternal mortality rates found in many countries.

If the different levels of care are not integrated and mutually supportive – although all the technologies may be appropriately placed – there will be only a limited impact, particularly in such areas as maternal health.

The field of MCH/FP experienced the debate, for many years, as to whether and how to integrate the MCH and FP components. In most countries, that debate has been resolved, although functional integration continues to elude many countries, in large part due to the legacy of discrepancies in policies, resource allocation (including external resources), management support, training, etc. More recently, major advances in the development and adaptation of other appropriate MCH/FP technologies have come about, such as those related to immunization and oral rehydration therapy. However, many countries have failed to learn the lessons of the MCH and FP debate, once again developing vertical structures for the delivery of these services.

Does the emphasis on one technology or program area have a beneficial spillover effect, a detrimental, or no effect on other aspects of MCH/FP? A recent evaluation of MCH services in Tanzania suggested that, apart from immunization coverage, which ranged from 70 percent for BCG to 30 percent for measles, the programs were having limited, if any, impact on the main problems of mothers and children.[37] There was no "spillover" effect.

The needs for the future in maternal and child health, including family planning, have been aptly summarized in the WHO Expert Committee report on MCH/FP.[41] "If the focus of health care is to shift from the hospital to the community, and from selected coverage to total coverage, community and family health, particularly MCH care, must be made the central objective of basic and continuing education for all members of the health team. Moreover, to ensure the integration of MCH care into the general community health services, the MCH content should be incorporated into the curricula for the basic and postgraduate preparation of health personnel in universities and professional or vocational schools. This calls for a vast expansion and reorientation of the educational system for health personnel, and for basic changes in the philosophies of medicine, nursing, and allied health professions, coupled with the reformulation and reshaping of curricula and methods of teaching."

REFERENCES

1. World Health Statistics Annual, 1985. Based on the findings of the World Fertility Survey.

2 Maternal Mortality. A tabulation of available information. 2d ed. WHO document No. FHE/86.3, 1986.

3. World Fertility Survey, Bangladesh. Geveva: WHO, 1987.

4. Chen, L.C., et a. Maternal mortality in rural Bangladesh. Studies in Family Planning, 5(11):334-341, 1974.

5. Sri Lanka. Ministry of Health, Family Health Bureau. Medium Term Plan. Family Health Program, 1985-1989. Colombo:The Ministry, 1984.

6. Zhang, L., and H. Ding. China: Analysis of cause and rate of regional maternal death in 21 provinces, municipalities and autonomous regions. Chinese J Obst and Gyn, 21(4):195-197, 1986.

7. Hobert, U. Maternal mortality in Sweden. Umea, Sweden: Umea University, 1985.

8. Registrar General, India, 1981 quoted in: Bhasker Rao, A: Maternal mortality in India. A Review. Paper presented to the Interregional Meeting on

the Prevention of Maternal Mortality, Geneva, 11-15 Nov 1985. WHO document no. FHE/PMM/85.9.4, 1985.

9. Shotri, A. Risk Approach Studies in Maternal and Child Health in Pune, India (in press).

10. Royston, E. The prevalence of nutritional anaemia in women in developing countries: A critical review of available information. World Health Statistics Quarterly, 35:52-91,1982.

11. Buck, A.A. quoted in Royston, E. The prevalence of nutritional anaemia in women in developing countries: A critical review of available information. World Health Statistics Quarterly, 35:52-91, 1982.

12. WHO Expert Committee on Malaria, Eighteenth report. Technical Report Series no. 735, Geneva: WHO, 1986.

13. Maine, D., et al. Prevention of maternal deaths in developing countries: Programme options and practical considerations. Paper prepared for the International Safe Motherhood Conference, Nairobi, Feb 10-13, 1987 (1986).

14. Tietze, C., and S.W. Henshaw. Induced abortion. A world review 1986. 6th ed. New York: Alan Guttmacher Institute, 1986.

15. Rodriguez Castro, R. Complicaciones del aborto a Corto Plazo. In: Reproduction Humana y Regulacion de la fertilidad. Simposio Cuba-OMS, Havana, 1978.

16. World Health Organization and U.S. National Research Council, Breast-feeding and fertility regulation: Current knowledge and programme policy implications. Bull WHO, 61(3):371-382,1983.

17. De Chateau, P., et al. A study of factors promoting and inhibiting lactation. Developmental Medicine and Child Neurology, 19:575, 1977.

18. Muir, D.C., and M.A. Belsey. Pelvic inflammatory disease and its consequences in the developing world. Am J Obstet Gynecol 138(7)part 2, 913-928,1980.

19. Makunen, J.I. Ectopic pregnancy in Finland 1976-83: A massive increase, Brit Med J, 294, 240-241, 1987.

20. Belsey, M.A. The epidemiology of infertility. Bull WHO, 54:319-341, 1976.

21. The incidence of low birth weight: an update.Weekly Epidemiological Record,59(27) 205-211, 1984.

22. Kramer, M.S. Determinants of low birth weight: A methodologic and meta-analysis. Bull WHO, 1987.

23. Edouard, L. The epidemiology of perinatal mortality. World Health Statistics Quarterly, 383:289-301, 1985.

24. Laing, R. Health and health services for plantation workers: Four case studies. London: Evaluation and Planning Centre for Health Care, London School of Hygiene and Tropical Medicine, p. 39, 1986.

25. World Health Organization. Expanded Programme of Immunization, 1987.

26. Berggren, W. A tetanus control program in Haiti. Am Journal Trop Med, 1974.

27. Kim-Farley, R., et al. Assessing the impact of the expanded programme on immunization: The example of Indonesia. Bull WHO, 65(2):203-206, 1987.

28. World Health Organization. Programme for Control of Diarrheal Diseases. Interim programme report 1986. WHO document No. WHO/CDD/87.26.

29. World Health Organization. Global nutritional status. Anthropometric indicators. WHO document no. NUT/AUTREF/87.3,1987.

30. Filmore, C. Protein-energy malnutrition trends in nine countries (unpublished document),1986.

31. Victoria, C.G., et al. Evidence for the protection by breast-feeding against infant deaths from infectious diseases in Brazil. Lancet ii(Aug 8):319-322,1987.

32. Slopar, K.S., et al. Increasing breastfeeding in a community. Archives of Diseases in Childhood, 52:700, 1977.

33. The dynamics of breastfeeding. WHO Chronicle 37(1):6-10, 1983.

34. Royston, E., and J. Ferguson. The coverage of maternity care: A critical review of available information. World Health Statistics Quarterly, 38:267-288,1985.

35. Hassouna, W.A. Health sector assessment study. Health Services Researcher, S1:4, 1982.

36. Mutambirwa, J. The role of traditional medicine in Zimbabwe. Presentation at Zimbabwe National MCH Workshop, June, 1983.

37. Shears, P., and R. Mkercnga. Evaluating the impact of mother and child health services at village level: A survey in Tanzania, and lessons for elsewhere. Annals of Trop Peds 5:55-59, 1985.

38. United Nations. Recent levels and trends of contraceptive use as assessed in 1983. New York: UN, 1984.

39. Amin, R., et al. Fertility, contraceptive use and socioeconomic context in Bangladesh. Paper prepared for the annual meeting of the Population Association of America, Boston, Mar 28-30, 1985.

40. Mauldin, W.P., and S.J. Segal. Prevalence of contraceptive use in developing countries. A chart book. New York: Rockefeller Foundation, 1986.

41. New trends and approaches in the delivery of maternal and child care in health services. Sixth report of the WHO Expert Committee on Maternal and Child Health. Technical Report Series no 600. Geneva: WHO, 1976.

44

UNICEF AND THE HEALTH OF MOTHERS AND CHILDREN

James P. Grant

INTRODUCTION

The United Nations Children's Fund (UNICEF) was founded on December 11, 1946, at a time when there was immediate need to deal with the urgent needs of children and mothers in Europe after the ravages of World War II. It later enlarged its scope of cooperation with all the developing countries.[1]

Since then, UNICEF has been concerned with all factors affecting child life and family health, particularly MCH, early childhood development, education, food and nutrition, urban poor, water and sanitation, women in development, the effects of economic crises, of war and conflict, and other situations that endanger the survival and development of children and the health of mothers. It has programs of cooperation with 121 developing countries, at peace or at war, and during emergencies.

UNICEF is governed by an Executive Board comprising 41 member countries, and is led by an Executive Director with his staff in Headquarters, New York, 6 regional offices and country offices in 121 developing countries. Contributions to UNICEF are entirely voluntary but have increased steadily over the years. In 1988 UNICEF income totalled over $700 million with virtually all governments in both industrialized and developing countries contributing. Seventy percent of income is from governmental and intergovernmental sources and the rest from private donations and sale of UNICEF Greeting Cards. Thirty percent of UNICEF income is raised by the national Committees for UNICEF in 34 industrialized countries.[2]

In 1984, 47% of UNICEF expenditures were for maternal and child health and nutrition programs, 29% for water and sanitation projects, and the rest for emergency relief, education, community and family welfare. UNICEF apportions resources to developing countries according to the level of infant mortality, the child population and the gross national product per capita.

BASIC SERVICES

During the 1950s and 1960s the assistance of UNICEF was extended rapidly to almost all the developing countries. UNICEF helped to strengthen training and provide support in pediatrics (social pediatrics and preventive medicine) in many developing countries, in applied nutrition programs and environmental sanitation. From 1962 UNICEF encouraged national governments to establish priorities for children and plan child-related projects as an integral part of an overall national development effort. The concepts of the "basic services" strategy to encompass the broad range of actions urgently needed for improving the quality of life for poor families, with their active involvement in developing countries, were developed in 1975.[3,4] Further to this approach, UNICEF and WHO organized the epochal conference at Alma Ata, USSR in 1978, where it adopted Primary Health Care as the appropriate strategy for achieving Health For All by the Year 2000.[5]

PRIMARY HEALTH CARE APPROACH

The Alma Ata Conference was a significant milestone for both WHO and UNICEF, and has profoundly affected their programs and working relationships. It was agreed that Primary Health Care was "essential health care based on practical, scientifically sound and socially acceptable methods and technology made universally accessible to individuals and families in the community through their full participation and at a cost that the community and country can afford to maintain at every stage of their development in the spirit of self-reliance and self-determination."[5] The Declaration called for an urgent social revolution, necessitating the creation of a world movement for the rapid attainment of health for all. UNICEF has placed its efforts in health work for children and mothers completely behind this call for action.

THE BASIS FOR CURRENT PROGRAMS
OF ASSISTANCE THROUGH UNICEF

The global economic recession starting in the late 1970s threatened the gains achieved in health services delivery and infant and child mortality reduction of the previous thirty years. UNICEF-commissioned studies clearly indicated that the economic recession was impacting negatively on children and mothers, especially among the poor communities and least developed nations, as well as among the poorer segments of some developed countries.[6] Each year, mainly in developing countries, there are 14 million deaths of children under five years of age and 500,000 maternal deaths, of causes largely preventable or curable with available and low-cost technologies. This situation was regarded as unconscionable especially in view of the availability of low-cost measures to save lives, and the UNICEF Executive Board directed in 1983 that the lowering of infant and child mortality should be a major priority of UNICEF's work.

CHILD SURVIVAL AND DEVELOPMENT STRATEGY

UNICEF's response has been to pursue the goal of accelerating PHC through a strategy which focused closely on the priorities of child health and survival, and which offered a rallying point for many organizations in national and international health programs. This was the UNICEF advocacy for a global child survival and development revolution, seizing the opportunity to synergistically combine effective low-cost measures in primary health care to social mobilization of the communities and the society.[7,8]

UNICEF stressed seven main health interventions; namely, growth monitoring and promotion, oral rehydration therapy, breastfeeding and better weaning practices, immunization against the six communicable diseases, food supplementation, family (child) spacing of children, and the promotion of female literacy and the enhancement of the role of women (GOBI-FFF).[9]

These seven interventions (GOBI–FFF) were put forward not as an exclusive, never-to-be-varied package of actions – but as a check-list of low-cost, high effectiveness measures which should be of high priority in many country situations because they can prevent the majority of infant and child deaths in most developing countries. To these, obviously, should be added disease interventions of local relevance.

This emphasis on child health and survival does not mean abandonment of UNICEF's other concerns with education, water, or the broader aspects of child development and women's advancement. Action in these other areas is important in their own right, and, in fact, contributes synergistically to child survival and development.

UNICEF PROGRAMMING

UNICEF supports these child survival and development measures by increased advocacy of these high priority cost-effective actions by countries as part of strengthening Primary Health Care (PHC) and other basic services, as envisaged at Alma Ata. UNICEF increased its own <u>financial and technical support</u> towards the priority actions advocated, and special support in the context of economic recession and financial constraints to help governments and NGOs to maintain and, if possible, expand their basic services for mothers (Adjustment with a Human Face).[10]

UNICEF cooperation with countries is based on a long tradition of country-specific programming. The cycle of program development starts with the Situation Analysis. This is a comprehensive study of the situation of women and children with the assistance of national specialists. It embraces all factors influencing the lives of children, the situation of women, their social, reproductive and productive roles, their education and health status. The analysis delves into the underlying causes, i.e., the environment, nutrition and food production, the health care system, educational and social communication sectors; and with structural causes such as the incidence, seasonality and the roots of poverty.

This document becomes a powerful informational and advocacy tool and forms the basis for the determination of strategies for actions to be taken in each country, linking these with current global concerns for women and children. Together with national authorities, plans of action and operation, including systems for monitoring and evaluation, are agreed to. UNICEF then seeks external resources additional to those allocated from UNICEF's general resources for the plan after approval by the Executive Board.

The implementation of the plan is the responsibility of the national authorities, e.g., the Ministry of Health, non-governmental organizations, as government may decide. Reviews of the program are carried out periodically and the evaluation at the end becomes part of the study of the situation for the next cycle of UNICEF collaboration.

SPECIFIC PROGRAM SUPPORT

In health care UNICEF's interest is on the needs of children and women, focusing particularly on actions that would lower mortality, and contribute to sustainable development. Health is interpreted in the broadest sense. Actions that significantly and rapidly reduce mortality give hope to communities, and mobilize them for development in general.

UNICEF supports <u>maternal health</u>* programs as it is very much aware that half a million women die each year because of the problems of unsafe

---

*UNICEF and WHO issued a joined statement on Maternal and Neonatal Care, 1986.

motherhood, and that 99% of these deaths occur in developing countries. The range of concerns for intervention include maternal nutrition, infection, child spacing, low birth weight and the care of the newborn which can be vigorously addressed, under the growing global initiative for safe motherhood.

For nearly forty years UNICEF has supported the training of midwives, traditional birth attendants and provided midwifery kits, and other related supplies to practically every developing country. It plays an important role in mobilizing communities for responsible parenthood. UNICEF emphasizes the close relationship between mortality reduction and fertility reduction; and the potential contribution of an improvement in child survival to slowing population growth, and it works in complementarity to WHO and UNFPA in family health without duplicating their specialized technical tasks.

Growth monitoring and promotion (GM/P) is the operational strategy for enabling the mother to visualize growth or lack of it, and to receive specific, relevant and practical guidance in ways that she, her family and community can act to ensure health and continued regular growth of the child. The growth chart therefore should be an outward and visible indicator of an established system of care for children in the community, a health passport. UNICEF therefore supports growth monitoring and promotion programs in all developing countries.

The Control of Diarrheal Diseases is a major program focus of UNICEF, since diarrhea is one of the most important causes of death in children under five years of age in developing countries and interacts adversely with nutrition. Apart from support for programs in the management of diarrhea with oral rehydration therapy, in water and sanitation, health education to improve personal and food hygiene, promotion of breastfeeding and good weaning practices, UNICEF in concert with WHO, USAID and other agencies has (through international conferences such as ICORT I, II and III, and regional and world congresses and seminars arranged with the International Pediatrics Association) significantly changed the climate of opinion of the leaders of the medical profession in the use of ORT and the management of diarrhea. It also supports applied research at the International Center for Diarrhoeal Disease Research, Bangladesh. By 1988, over half the under-five year-olds in developing countries had access to ORS, and with the use of home-available solutions, some one million child deaths from dehydration were averted.[11]

The Nutrition of Infants and Young Children in wide context has been an enduring UNICEF concern. The work of UNICEF, WHO and of many NGOs in the 1970s, culminated in the World Health Assembly Resolution in 1981 on the Code of Marketing of Breastmilk Substitutes.[12] UNICEF has assisted programs in many countries in the promotion of breastfeeding, working with numerous international and national agencies. It has also engaged in programs for frequent feeding using energy-dense and balanced food, the production of local weaning foods based on local recipes, and support for women as an essential component of programs to assure better infant and young child nutrition. This is linked to the roles and opportunities available to women, in terms of credit and other inputs. Family food security is another dimension to the problem.

Immunization - "Toward universal childhood immunization"[13] is one of the elements of the Child Survival Initiatives to which UNICEF has paid particular attention in the past few years, in an effort with WHO and other agencies to achieve the 1990 goal of universal childhood immunization set by the World Health Assembly in 1977 using the six vaccines, BCG, DPT, measles and polio, in an Expanded Programme on Immunization (EPI). UNICEF activities have been in advocacy at global, regional and national levels, in vaccine supplies, cold chain and immunization equipment, training, monitoring and evaluation in almost all developing countries.

It is of great public health significance that the aim of achieving universal childhood immunization with the six antigens, is now within sight. In 1974 immunization services were hardly existent in many countries. Now over 60% of all children under one year of age in the world have been immunized against measles, tuberculosis, tetanus, whooping cough, diphtheria and poliomyelitis. It is estimated that this was, by 1989, preventing some 1.9 million deaths from these diseases, and about 240,000 cases of poliomyelitis each year.[13]

ESSENTIAL DRUGS PROGRAM

Among the major developments of UNICEF over the past years has been the utilization of an efficient system of international tendering to purchase supplies on the world market at prices that have declined steadily in real terms and to pass on to governments in the developing world the information concerning these benchmark prices and of potential suppliers, so that governments can avail themselves of low price, assured quality and if required, consolidated setpacking of supplies for primary level health facilities.

The UNICEF Supply Division Warehouse in Copenhagen, UNIPAC, holds about $10 million of essential drugs in stock and in 1985 supplied, both as regular programs and on a reimbursable procurement basis, essential drugs and vaccines to the value of $60 million, to more than 100 developing countries.

BAMAKO INITIATIVE

In view of the African economic crises, UNICEF, together with WHO, is currently supporting the proposed African Health Ministers' plan (the Bamako Initiative of 1987) for improving the health of women and children in Africa. Provision of basic essential drugs will form the basis for community financing and the establishment of a revolving fund for drugs and for some of the local operating costs of the PHC system.

OTHER INTERVENTIONS

The range of possibilities for reducing infant, child and maternal mortality through low-cost and effective interventions, that lend themselves to accelerated coverage is increasing. Among the key problems identified are acute respiratory infections, malaria, especially in Africa, neonatal mortality and low birth weight. Attention also continues to be focused on micronutrient deficiencies such as vitamin A, iodine and iron deficiencies. In AIDS, UNICEF collaborated with WHO in programs for women and children in health education; communication and social mobilization; training of MCH/PHC workers; supporting studies of the socio-economic impact of the disease on children and works in the EPI field to assure the safety of immunizations.

Early Childhood Development is an important corollary to child survival efforts. Linkages have been established between survival and developmental programming, and to increase program coverage, which is currently biased towards children in the three- to six-year-old age group, to include the child from birth to age six. UNICEF, collaborating with Rehabilitation International, plays a significant role in the prevention, early detection and rehabilitation program for disabled children.

INFRASTRUCTURAL DEVELOPMENT AND CAPACITY BUILDING

UNICEF has a forty-year tradition of assistance in training of health workers, community leaders and workers in child development, as well as in equipment and supplies for clinics, health centers and other mother-and child-related institutions. This started in the European countries after World War II and has since been a major feature of collaboration with all developing countries. In 1986, UNICEF cooperated in maternal and child health programs in 113 countries.

- It provided grants for training, orientation and refresher courses for 410,900 health workers: doctors, nurses, public health workers, medical assistants, midwives and traditional birth attendants; and provided technical supplies and equipment for 61,500 health centers of various kinds – especially rural health centers and subcenters.

- In the same year it supplied medicines and vaccines against tuberculosis, diphtheria, tetanus, typhoid, measles, polio and other diseases.
- It helped to expand applied nutrition programs in 18,300 villages, equipping nutrition centers and demonstration areas, community and school orchards and gardens, fish and poultry hatcheries.
- UNICEF provided stipends to train 9,000 village-level nutrition workers.
- Delivered some 15,460 metric tons of donated foods and supplements;
- It cooperated in programs to supply safe water and improved sanitation in 93 countries.
- Helped to complete approximately 83,468 water supply systems including 71,341 open/dug wells with handpumps, 1,203 piped systems, with 567 motor-driven pumps and 10,357 other systems such as spring protection, rain water collection and water treatment plants.
- Benefited some 18.7 million persons with rural water supply systems.
- Completed 293,404 excreta–disposal installations benefiting some 2,483,100 people.[14]

INTERAGENCY COOPERATION

UNICEF has had the closest collaboration with WHO since the latter's establishment in 1947. The two organizations have regular mechanisms of consultation, development of new initiatives in health and review collaborative actions in health. UNICEF also cooperates extensively with UNFPA, the World Bank, UNESCO, FAO, World Food Programme and UNDP and with many governmental multilateral and bilateral agencies, as well as with international and national non-governmental agencies.

FUTURE DIRECTIONS

Among the many issues of concern to UNICEF is the raising of global consciousness even further to the needs of mothers and children, and to the empowerment of families with knowledge for healthy living. Together with WHO and UNESCO it is launching a "Facts for Life" program to involve all communicators to focus on 10 specific areas of health as part of their contribution to improving the quality of life. It is also working with many other agencies to ensure the adoption by the United Nations Convention for the Rights of the Child.

Another concern is to ensure that health and social indicators* are clearly specified in the goals for the Fourth Development Decade of the United Nations. There is a need to improve the quality and timeliness of vital social information and UNICEF is cooperating with WHO and FAO in an inter-agency food and nutrition program to establish surveillance programs in 60 countries in the next five years. The actual beneficial results of the Child Survival and Development Revolution in advancing primary health care are already notable. It is heartening to see that children's lives <u>are</u> being saved and that their chances for a healthy life are vastly increasing. As more and more countries take on the responsibility for mobilizing social forces at all strata of society to increase the health and wellbeing of their children, the world is moving toward a monumental effort to enact truly major changes at a level where it counts – among those most in need, the women and children of the poor people of the world. This is the mission of UNICEF.

---

* See Declaration of Talloires. 12 March 1988 Talloires France - Task Force for Child Survival (WHO, UNICEF, UNDP, World Bank and Rockefeller Foundation), reproduced in the front of this book.

REFERENCES

1. Black, M. The Children and the Nations: The story of UNICEF. P.I.C. Sydney, Australia, 1986.

2. Executive Director's Reports for 1986, 1987, 1988, 1989.

3. Planning for the Needs of Children in developing countries. UNICEF. 1964.

4. Assignment Children - Children, Youth, Women and development plans: The Lome Conference. UNICEF, 1972.

5. WHO/UNICEF: Primary Health Care - Report of the International Conference on P.H.C. Alma-Ata, 1978.

6. Jolly, R., and G.A. Cornia, (ed). The Impact of World recession on Children. Pergamon, 1984.

7. Assignment Children – A Child Survival and Development Revolution. 61/62, 1983.

8. Assignment Children – Going to Scale for Child Survival and Development. UNICEF, 1984.

9. Cash, R., G.T. Kensch, and J. Laamstein, (ed). Child Health and Survival – The UNICEF GOBI-FFF Program. Croom/Helm, 1987.

10. Cornia, G.A., R. Jolly, and R. Stewart. Adjustment with a Human Face. 2 vol. Oxford, 1988.

11. Executive Director's Report. 1988.

12. WHO International Code of Marketing of Breast-milk Substitutes. Geneva,1981.

13. Assignment Children: Universal Childhood Immunization by 1990. 69/72.UNICEF, 1986.

14. Executive Director's Report, 1986-1988.

Other Key UNICEF Publications on Women and Children's Issues

A. 1. State of the World's Children Reports: annual - over 300,000 copies in over 40 languages.

2. The Executive Director's Reports - annual reports on the work of UNICEF.

3. Mandl, P.E, (ed).. Assignment Children Series (other titles) editor: P.E. Mandl

   a) Vitamin A (5. Eastman) UNICEF. 1987-88

   b) Breastfeeding and Health 55/56. 1981.

   c) The Condition of Women and Children's Well Being 49/50. 1980.

B. Joint WHO/UNICEF Statements (Selection)

1. The management of diarrhoea and the use of oral rehydration therapy. 2nd edition, 1985.

2. Planning principles for accelerating immunization activities, 1985

3. Maternal care for the reduction of perinatal and neonatal mortality, 1986

4. Basic principles for control of acute respiratory infections in children in developing countries, 1987.

45

UNITED NATIONS POPULATION FUND (UNFPA)

NAFIS SADIK, M.D.

INTRODUCTION

The United Nations Population Fund (UNFPA) is the world's largest source of multilateral assistance to population programs in developing countries. Established twenty years ago in 1969, UNFPA has contributed to the significant expansion of maternal and child health care and family planning (MCH/FP) services worldwide. The Fund's policies and activities in maternal and child health and family planning have been developed in accordance with the recommendations of the 1974 World Population Plan of Action (WPPA)[1] and the International Conference on Population held in 1984 in Mexico City.[2]

This chapter starts with a brief description of UNFPA's mandate and program, followed by a discussion of the Fund's support to MCH/FP. It then highlights selected topics of particular concern for the future.

BRIEF HISTORY OF UNFPA

UNFPA became operational in 1969. The United Nations had addressed population issues long before this, but mainly by way of demographic work, statistical analyses of demographic conditions and trends. The Population Commission, established within the United Nations in 1946, was given responsibility for undertaking studies and making technical knowledge available to interested countries. During the 1960s however, demographic work within the United Nations progressed significantly, bringing population issues more to the fore. An emerging consensus among UN Member States on the importance of population issues led to the creation by the United Nations

541

Secretary-General of a Special Trust Fund for Population Activities in 1967. In 1969, the Special Trust Fund was renamed the United Nations Fund for Population Activities. Three years later, in 1972 UNFPA became a subsidiary organ of the General Assembly, with the Governing Council of the United Nations Development Programme (UNDP) as its governing body.

UNFPA's mandate, laid down by the Economic and Social Council of the United Nations in May 1973, is:

- to build up the knowledge and capacity to respond to needs in population and family planning;
- to promote awareness of population problems in both developed and developing countries and of possible strategies to deal with these problems;
- to assist developing countries at their request in dealing with their population problems, in the forms and means best suited to individual country's needs; and
- to play a leading role in the United Nations system in promoting population programs, and to coordinate projects supported by the Fund.

UNFPA provides assistance for a broad range of activities in the following areas in order of priority:

(a) maternal and child health and family planning;
(b) population education, communication and motivation, and dissemination of information;
(c) basic data collection and analysis;
(d) population dynamics (demographic research; training of national staff in demography, etc.); and
(e) formulation, implementation and evaluation of population policy.

Virtually all of the Fund's resources come in the form of voluntary contributions from governments. Most are made in terms of annual pledges at the United Nations Pledging Conference for Development Activities.

Since 1969, a total of 144 countries have contributed over $1.8 billion to UNFPA's work, the majority of it coming from the industrialized countries.

Despite a stable and expanding resource base, requests for assistance continue to exceed UNFPA's ability to meet them. A supplementary system has therefore been developed for matching the needs of countries with potential donors through a multi-bilateral arrangement. In a typical case, UNFPA administers funds on behalf of a donor government which are earmarked for a specific project or group of projects, usually in a country or region specified by the donor.

USE OF FUNDS FOR MCH/FP

The majority of UNFPA program funds are channelled in support of MCH/FP activities, be they at the national, regional or interregional level. On average, UNFPA expenditures for MCH/FP activities during the 1982–1988 period have accounted for 50 percent of the Fund's program. In dollar terms UNFPA assistance to MCH/FP between 1969 and 1988 has amounted to about $760 million. In 1988 alone, the Fund allocated some $74.4 million to support nearly 500 MCH/FP projects at the country and intercountry level.

MAJOR FUNCTIONS IN MCH/FP

UNFPA assistance for MCH/FP is oriented toward both the individual and the family. It may be provided in the form of programs which seek to integrate family planning with maternal and child health services, in the context of primary health care or in a variety of other programs, as appropriate to social and cultural conditions. These include: (I) delivery of services at the community level, including improvements in the logistical systems through which such services can be provided; (II) training of personnel; (III) strengthening of management; (IV) provision of logistical support, including provision of contraceptives, if required; (V) encouragement, where appropriate, of local production of contraceptives; and (VI) research into traditional and new contraceptive methods and development of safer, more efficient measures, including natural family planning methods.

Since abortion is not an acceptable method of contraception,[3] according to the consensus of the International Conference on Population, UNFPA does not extend assistance for supplies or services used for this purpose. Moreover, because abortion is an extremely sensitive issue in many developing and developed countries, the Fund takes particular care to ensure that none of its assistance is used for this purpose.

UNFPA has recently formulated policy guidelines governing its support for the prevention and control of acquired immunodeficiency syndrome (AIDS). These guidelines emphasize the importance of incorporating information and education activities into currently supported programs.

PROGRAMS IN MCH/FP

UNFPA has always been guided by two major principles in providing assistance for population activities, both of which are particularly important in the area of MCH/FP. The first is that every nation has the sovereign right to determine its own population policies and programs; the second is that all couples and individuals have the basic right to decide freely and responsibly the number and spacing of their children.

The policies and programs of UNFPA aim at encouraging appropriate information and education concerning responsible parenthood and at making available to persons who so desire the means of achieving their goals in terms of family size. Bearing this in mind, UNFPA support for family planning activities recognizes and respects any or all of the following rationales for family planning:

1. as a human right;
2. for improvement in family health;
3. for demographic change; and
4. as an adjunct to socio-economic development.

The great majority of UNFPA assistance in the area of MCH/FP goes to the delivery of MCH/FP services, to action programs and to informational and communication support. UNFPA supports all modes of delivery of MCH/FP services as long as such modes are feasible and effective. In the same vein, the Fund supports all methods of fertility regulation technically approved by WHO and in consonance with the policies of the requesting governments.

In providing assistance to this sector, the Fund has placed special emphasis on reaching underserved and difficult-to-reach groups. UNFPA thus encourages the provision of information and services to the disadvantaged, particularly to the rural inhabitants in remote areas and to the rural and urban poor, in forms which are both socioculturally acceptable and accessible with regard to distance and cost. UNFPA also emphasizes support to activities directed toward specific population groups, such as adolescents, newlyweds, men and low-parity women, which have often been overlooked in traditional service programs.

Recognizing the important role of the community in the success of a national family planning program, UNFPA encourages activities, as appropriate, to strengthen community participation in family planning and related programs. In this connection, UNFPA support may be used to train national staff in various techniques to generate community involvement or to help develop community-based motivation and contraceptive distribution systems.

In the last few years, the Fund has paid special attention to sub-Saharan Africa, where pervasive high maternal and infant mortality requires urgent attention and assistance. With the renewed emphases on maternal health arising out of recent international conferences,[4] UNFPA's support has concentrated on integrating family planning services with maternal health care, and expanding access to such services, especially in remote rural areas and urban slums.

The Fund has always given high priority to training in MCH/FP. Through the years, by assisting countries in building up their institutional strength in the training field and by financing in-country courses, fellowships and study tours abroad, as well as in-service training for health professionals, traditional midwives and paramedicals, UNFPA has helped countries build up a corps of trained staff.

In recent years UNFPA has focused considerable attention on the quality of training and on special topics, such as management training and adolescent health. Responding to the growing demand for training in MCH/FP in the Africa region, during 1988 UNFPA conducted a review and assessment of needs in the MCH/FP area and identified training facilities, courses, resources and programs for both French- and English-speaking countries.

Another major category of UNFPA assistance for MCH/FP is research. In family planning research, UNFPA supports the study of socio-economic and cultural factors that influence fertility and the practice of FP, as well as program-related operational questions and biomedical work in connection with methods of fertility regulation.

Most of the family planning research supported by the Fund is undertaken in conjunction with WHO, particularly in the context of the Special Programme of Research, Development and Research Training in Human Reproduction (WHO/HRP). In the face of shrinking commercial interest in development and marketing of contraceptives, UNFPA has initiated discussions with WHO on alternative options for developing countries. One such option would be a joint UNFPA/WHO undertaking to devise and fund a mechanism by which new contraceptives like monthly injections and vaginal rings could be marketed, distributed and introduced in the developing countries. Moreover, UNFPA is assisting in collaboration with The Population Council, in the introduction of NORPLANT contraceptive subdermal implants.

PRESENT AND FUTURE MAJOR NEEDS

One of the major challenges of the immediate future will be just to maintain existing levels of contraceptive prevalence in developing countries.

The fact that the number of new protected couples must be increased by some 94 million between now and the year 2000 conveys a sense of the magnitude of this challenge. Much greater support will also be needed to help save women's lives; an estimated half-million women die each year of pregnancy-related causes. In most developing countries this means a re-doubling of efforts to make MCH/FP services much more widely available.

There is also a strong need for more widespread and accessible provision of safe, effective and acceptable contraceptives, and for continued research leading to development of new contraceptives.

Improvement in program quality and in the motivation and skills of personnel remains crucial. Further efforts should be made to better identify concerns and needs of target populations and more carefully tailor MCH/FP information and services to the particular characteristics of users.

The issues of adolescent health and fertility will require special attention. To meet the needs of adolescents, various avenues for information and services have to be explored as alternatives or complements to MCH/FP clinics.

In all countries, and particularly for countries which have made only modest progress so far in MCH/FP, special care will have to be given to the role and status of women in family, community and society. Strong evidence shows that the success of population policies and programs is directly linked to improvements in the status and role of women—female education, women's rights in marriage, access and control of resources and other indicators of women's status. Countries will therefore have to take decisive steps to improve conditions of women if they wish to make significant advances in population and health matters and in socio-economic development in general.

Finally, program interventions have to be better planned using a broad-based and comprehensive strategy which links MCH/FP interventions to all other sectors such as agriculture, education, legal rights of women, and so on. Activities need to draw more on research findings and evaluations of past performance and take a longer-term perspective. Such a more strategic approach to MCH/FP and all other programs in developing countries, it is hoped, will prepare a firmer ground for institutionalization.

REFERENCES

1. Report of the United Nations World Population Conference, Bucharest, 19-30 August 1974. (United Nations publications, Sales no. E.75. X111.3), Chap 1.

2. Report of the International Conference on Population, 1984, Mexico City, 6-14 August 1984.(United Nations publications, Sales no.E.84. X.111.8).

3. Ibid.

4. For example, the International Safe Motherhood Conference, Nairobi, Kenya, February 1987; and International Conference on Better Health for Women and Children through Family Planning, Nairobi, Kenya, October 1987.

46

FAMILY PLANNING AND MATERNAL AND CHILD HEALTH IN THE WORLD BANK'S POPULATION, HEALTH AND NUTRITION PROGRAM*

JANET NASSIM, M.A. AND FRED T. SAI, M.B.B.S., M.P.H., F.R.C.P.

INTRODUCTION

The World Bank, which consists of the International Bank for Reconstruction and Development (IBRD) and the International Development Association (IDA), was established to promote economic and social progress in developing countries. To this end the IBRD and IDA help governments undertake policy reforms designed to establish economic growth and support a wide variety of projects. The IBRD was established in 1945 to help finance reconstruction and development in its member countries; IDA was established in 1960 to provide assistance to the poorest developing countries on terms that would bear less heavily on their balance of payments than IBRD loans. Most of IDA's assistance is concentrated on the very poor countries with per capita incomes of less than $400 a year. The IBRD is now owned by the governments of the more than 150 countries that have subscribed to its capital, and these subscriptions are in relation to their economic strength. Most governments that have joined the IBRD have also joined IDA. Although IDA is legally and financially distinct from the IBRD, it shares the same management and staff, and the projects it assists have to meet the same criteria.

The Bank's involvement in the Population, Health and Nutrition (PHN) sector began in 1969, with its decision to begin lending for population, and has grown steadily since. Although the proportion of total World Bank lend-

---

*Although the authors are employed by the World Bank, this article reflects the views of the authors alone and should not be taken to reflect the official policy of the Bank.

ing that goes to population, health and nutrition may seem relatively small, about 2% of the total lending program, this reflects mainly the magnitude of the Bank's involvement in economic development in general.

The Bank is, in fact, the largest provider of assistance in the health field,[**] and is one of the three largest in the field of population.[***] The size and nature of the Bank's activities as an International Development Bank help to define its characteristics vis-a-vis other donor agencies in the field. It provides loans or credits, not grant assistance, which often influences project design since countries are more willing to borrow for some components than others – for buildings, for example, rather than for costs incurred in running programs. It provides this assistance to governments, in support of their national programs. Bank personnel are not, therefore, directly involved in service provision to the client. Lending is only one feature of the Bank's activities: Lending is founded upon detailed analysis of the sector, and this sector work also informs policy dialogue with the government. In fact, the Bank's involvement in many aspects of a country's development program makes it possible for policy dialogue to be part of a process of formulating coherent country strategies, with population, health and nutrition data informing economic and social policy, and vice versa. This chapter reviews the Bank's activities in the PHN sector, among which family planning and maternal and child health activities are a major priority. Learning to meet the family planning, health and nutrition needs of the client in a variety of developing country settings, given the Bank's structure and modus operandi, is a continuing challenge. The evolution of the Bank's PHN program reflects its response to this challenge.

HISTORY OF THE WORLD BANK'S INVOLVEMENT IN PHN

The Bank entered the field of population as a result of growing awareness, shared by other development agencies, that since World War II the world was experiencing unprecedently high rates of population growth, and from concern that this growth, concentrated mainly in the developing world was seriously undermining attempts to raise living standards in many countries. The new initiative was announced by Robert McNamara in his first address as President of the World Bank at its 1968 Annual meeting: "The World Bank is concerned above all with economic development, and the rapid growth of population is one of the greatest barriers to the economic

---

[**] Japan and the United States are the two other major donors in the health field, providing assistance mainly by way of grants.
[***] In 1986, the Bank's assistance to population was about the same as the UNFPA budget and about half the size as the USAID budget for population activities at that time.

growth and social well-being of our member states."[1] The first Bank review of the sector written in 1972 gave two other reasons for Bank involvement: concern over the ultimate size of world population and the ability of the earth to support it, and concern for human welfare, particularly health. Since then the Bank has also recognized freedom of access to family planning information and services as a basic human right.

ADMINISTRATIVE STRUCTURE

Robert McNamara proposed that the Bank follow three courses of action in the population field and these have remained the foundation for the PHN program. First, dialogue with governments; second, financing of projects; and third, programs of research. The administrative structure for these activities was provided in 1969 with the establishment of the Population Projects Department. Lending began in 1970 with a $2 million dollar loan to Jamaica. In 1979 the Bank decided to lend directly for health projects, rationalizing and complementing a trend which began in 1975 when health components were introduced into several population projects. Support for nutrition projects had been the responsibility of the Nutrition Division of the Agriculture and Rural Development Department in the 1970s and in 1979 all these activities were brought together in a new Population, Health and Nutrition Department. The Department consisted of four divisions: three regional divisions responsible for lending operations, and one division whose work was devoted to research and policy formulation.

In 1987 as part of a major reorganization of the administrative structure of the whole Bank, the Population, Health and Nutrition Department was disbanded. Its functions are now carried out by Population and Human Resource (PHR) Divisions in Country Departments. The change reflects the growing trend toward "policy-based" lending and the adjustment of whole economies or sectors in the 1980s, as part of the process of developing overall country strategies. There are now 16 country PHR divisions, supported by 4 regional technical departments with PHN expertise. Policy and research are undertaken by a Population, Health and Nutrition Division within a new administrative unit (PPR) responsible for Policy, Planning and Research for the whole Bank.

THE BANK'S COMMITMENT TO PHN

Bank President McNamara's commitment to population activities was reaffirmed by his successor, A.W. Clausen, at the World Population Conference in Mexico in 1984. In his speech, which reflected the widening of the Bank's activities to include health-related activities, he pledged a doubling of Bank lending in the sector, to $500 million by 1990.[2] This pledge was endorsed by the present Bank President, Barber Conable, in his speech to the Safe Motherhood Conference in Nairobi in 1987: "By 1990 we expect to have projects in about 50 countries with approximately 12 to 14 new operations a year. Lending for population, health and nutrition could reach $500 million a year, about twice our level in 1984–5"[3] In fact, current indications are that commitments will exceed these levels by 1990.

The importance of the PHN sector at a time when the Bank is assisting many countries in programs of structural adjustment of their economies was stressed by Mr. Conable in his 1988 Annual Address. The curbing of population growth was identified as one of five critical fronts on which the war on poverty would be carried out. Population growth was seen not only as a cause of underdevelopment, but also as a consequence: "A vital part of the Bank's work involves development activities that have a strong impact on population. Many projects improve economic opportunity and education for poor people, particularly women and girls. We are financing health and safe motherhood programs, and we will expand our direct support for family-related activities. Population issues will be prominent in our dialogue with governments."[4]

THE LENDING PROGRAM

The pace of lending in the sector began fairly slowly, but by 1979 just under $350 million had been committed to 21 projects in 14 countries. After the formation of the Population, Health and Nutrition Department, the volume of lending increased. Lending in 1980 (four projects totalling $143 million) reflected commitments to projects developed under the old structure, but during the period 1981 to 1986 loans of over $1000 million were made to 34 projects. 1987, the year of the administrative reorganization, saw a temporary down-turn in the lending program, but in all, 14 projects were approved, and over $350 million committed in that and the following year. Preliminary estimates for the current financial year, 1989, indicate that the momentum of lending continues to increase, and that about $500 million will be provided to 10 projects.

POLICY AND PROGRAM DEVELOPMENT

While the lending program is the most visible evidence of the Bank's presence in the PHN field, a great deal of effort goes into another of the areas outlined by President McNamara: policy dialogue. As the largest economic development agency, the Bank has the status and the opportunities to discuss development policies across the board, and has often used its position to draw attention to population issues. One external review concluded: "Perhaps the single most effective element in the Bank's work on population and development is the policy dialogue that links population issues with other aspects of development."[5] This policy dialogue has firm foundations in the Bank's economic and sector work which also paves the way for project identification and development. The new structure of the Bank is designed to promote further the integration of demographic issues into country development planning and to ensure that the social sectors are not only protected but strengthened in the programs of structural adjustment currently underway.

The Bank's activities in sub-Saharan Africa are a good example of its work in policy and program development. Demographic and health issues have been an important area of concern. Sub-Saharan Africa has the highest population growth rates in the world, and these are not expected to peak until after the year 2000, twenty or thirty years later than in other major developing world regions. The average growth rate for the region as a whole is just over 3% per annum, at which rate a population doubles every 23 years. In addition the region has the highest rates of infant and child mortality and maternal mortality in the world. The links between high unregulated fertility and the health of mothers and children are increasingly well documented. Population has been and still remains a sensitive issue in many countries in Africa, for many reasons related to its colonial history, to economic relations between North and South, and other cultural factors.

Yet as time has elapsed since independence, many African governments have come to accept that control over their own destinies involves slowing their rates of population growth. The Bank's work has played a part in this process of change. It has put considerable effort into raising population and health issues in dialogue at all levels of government, into organizing high–level conferences and workshops in the region, and into dissemination and discussion of its research and sector work. With the advent of health lending the Bank has also been in a better position to add financial support to countries willing to address the problem. The Bank has contributed to policy breakthroughs in several countries that previously opposed or took a laissez-faire approach to intervention—notably Burundi, Malawi, Nigeria and Senegal, and its sectoral analyses have assisted even more in introducing family planning into their health system. Eleven of the 24 PHN sector reports completed in 1987 and 1988 were for African countries, and all but two included attention to population. And financial assistance to projects is increasing substantially, as documented below (see Tables 1, next page and Appendix Table, page 561). (For a fuller account of policy development see Fred T. Sai and Lauren A. Chester.[6])

Policy dialogue and program development do not necessarily result in a large role in project lending. The Bank is often the "lender of last resort – governments may be unwilling to borrow from the Bank, especially if they are

Table 1
Lending For Population and Health by Region: FY86-88[a]
Commitment in US$ million

Fiscal year	Region	No. of projects	No. with population component[b]	Total PHN lending	Total lending to population	Lending to population as % of total PHN lending
1986	Africa	5	5	81.1	9.7	12.0
	Asia	4	2	242.4	129.0	53.0
	EMENA	0	-	-	-	-
	LAC	2	1	96.0	0.3	0
	Subtotal	11	8	419.5	139.0	33.0
1987	Africa	4	4	30.8	7.9	26.0
	Asia	0	-	-	-	-
	EMENA	1	0	13.3	-	-
	LAC	1	1	10.0	6.8	68.0
	Subtotal	6	5	54.1	14.7	27.0
1988	Africa	5	3	121.4	19.9	16.0
	Asia	2	2	74.5	62.3	84.0
	EMENA	0	-	-	-	-
	LAC	1	0	109.0	-	-
	Subtotal	8	5	304.9	82.2	27.0
	Total	25	18	778.5	235.9	30.0

[a] The Bank's Fiscal Year runs from July 1 to June 30
[b] "Free-standing" population projects and projects with population components.

ineligible for IDA credits, and if grant assistance from another donor is available. Or governments may wish to borrow for "hard" components such as construction of physical facilities, and will turn to other agencies for assistance with the "soft" components – IEC, training and so on. Donor coordination in providing support to national programs is becoming increasingly common: In Algeria the Bank will provide family planning through support to the health program; UNFPA will support broader population activities through the Ministry of Social Affairs. In Sri Lanka the Bank's project supports a major UNFPA initiative. In Bangladesh, where the Bank does play a major role in financing the national program, it is the lead agency coordinating assistance from the many international co-financiers involved. The Bank's strength, therefore, lies not so much in its lending program, as in the opportunities it has to create the environment in which there will be project demand. Nonetheless, its lending program is substantial and varied, as the following section illustrates.

CHARACTERISTICS OF THE LENDING PROGRAM

One of the major reasons for the Bank's decision in 1979 to begin lending for health was the opportunity this would afford for dialogue on population and for supporting family planning through the health care system. The impetus given to lending in Africa is well illustrated by the figures in Table 1. Over the past three years, 14 projects have been approved in Africa. In the 1980 to 1985 period, 9 were approved. In contrast, there was only one project (in Kenya) in the 1970s. All but 2 represent the first borrowing in the sector in the 21 countries concerned. While the number of projects is greatest in Africa, the volume of lending in dollar terms is greatest in Asia, where the Bank has provided long-term support in the sector to national programs. These programs, for example in India, Pakistan, Indonesia, and Bangladesh were largely vertical programs in the 1970s but are now increasingly integrated with health.

Table 1 also indicates that lending for health predominates—for many of the reasons indicated in the preceding section. However, the great majority contain population components. All but two of the health projects in Africa have population components, strongly validating the approach to family planning through health. In fact, most health projects make some provision for family planning as part of basic health services (Appendix Table), and to this extent the figures in Table 1 understate lending for population-related activities. This table reveals that projects in Middle Eastern and Latin American countries also make provision for family planning services. In these countries, as in Africa, while discussion of family planning for reasons of fertility reduction is a sensitive issue, there is no such controversy over its use to improve maternal and child health through birth spacing.

Activities to improve family planning and maternal and child health (MCH) services are included in the vast majority of PHN projects. Indeed a Health Sector Policy paper, written in 1980 to guide the Bank as it entered the health field, identified the support and improvement of FP/MCH as one of the seven critical areas for action. Thirty-four of the 40 projects approved from 1981 to 1987 contained FP/MCH provisions, or family planning and other basic health service activities, typically a few key interventions such as antenatal and well-baby care, immunization, and diarrheal and respiratory disease control. In 1988 the 3 projects without a sizable population component included a project in Brazil to eradicate endemic tropical diseases, and two projects – in Guinea and Uganda – to build and renovate basic health infrastructure. While it is not possible to talk about a World Bank FP/MCH program in terms of finite projects, family planning and MCH are an integral part of the Bank's PHN work. The Bank's efforts to improve service delivery are therefore critical to FP/MCH objectives, and the following discussion relates to activities that include these objectives.

IMPROVING SERVICE DELIVERY

The main focus of the first generation of PHN projects was extending the coverage of basic health services. Attention was paid to improving the structure of health systems – to construction, equipment, training, facilities, management systems, staffing, and defining the roles and duties of different health workers. In subsequent projects increasing attention is being paid not only to increasing coverage, but to increasing the effectiveness and efficiency of projects.

Two important emerging themes in recent Bank research have been the development of cost-effective models of health delivery systems, and the problems of managing health delivery systems at the periphery, i.e., providing services to those whose poverty and geographic location make them least likely to have access to services, but who are often those most in need. One recent Bank study is of particular interest with respect to FP/MCH on both these topics. Using aggregate data from Indonesia it first confirms the frequently posited synergistic relationship between fertility and mortality. It demonstrates that the advantages of integrating family planning and health programs in the form of lower program costs and more effective service promotion are enhanced by the mutually reinforcing effects of fertility and mortality reduction. Second, it documents the substantially greater cost effectiveness of non-hospital, or community, health expenditures compared to hospital expenditures in reducing mortality.[7]

The question increasingly being addressed by Bank research is how to improve these community services, not only their availability, but their acceptance by the people they are intended to serve. Ninety-five percent of the Bank's PHN projects have included in their objectives extension of the coverage and/or quality of services, with emphasis on the provision of primary health care. A review of the Bank's record in reaching people at the periphery[8] documented a consistent effort to include outreach activities in the Bank's PHN projects – 70% use community health workers, 85% include IEC activities, over 50% involve the mobilization of community support groups. However, it concluded that there was a need for much more attention to be paid to client/provider interactions in project design and implementation. It suggested that innovative approaches already introduced in some Bank projects should be tried more widely. These approaches include targeting of population groups, and interventions; increased use of rapid anthropological surveys to learn more about client and provider attitudes and practices in the course of project preparation; more flexibility in the course of project implementation based on feedback from clients; investigation of incentives – both monetary and in the form of feedback on performance; and increasing mobilization of community resources outside the public sector – non-governmental organizations (NGOs) and community support organizations such as women's groups. Some indication of the move away from the heavy emphasis on physical capacity in current Bank projects is to be found in the fact that whereas past PHN projects committed from 40 to 80 percent of project resources to civil works, in projects approved in FY88 the range is 10 to 40 percent.

SPECIAL INITIATIVES

An important complement to operational activities are the programs sponsored by the Bank, or by the Bank in coordination with other agencies, to support activities which benefit the PHN sector in general. Such activities include the Bank's support to the Human Reproduction Research Program at the World Health Organization; its co-sponsorship of the Safe Motherhood Conference in 1987 and continued support to the Initiative; its involvement in the Task Force for Child Survival, and its efforts to build technical capacity in NGOs.

SUPPORT FOR NGOs

A substantial minority of PHN projects, about 21 percent, has provided finance for activities carried out by NGOs. Although the amount of assistance provided has usually been small, in Bangladesh over $4 million has been allocated to finance FP/MCH activities undertaken by NGOs. In India, the Fifth Population Project allocates over $5 million to encourage private sector activities in FP/MCH. But another important activity in this area, sponsored by the PHN division of the Bank's Policy, Planning and Research Department, is the effort to strengthen the institutional capabilities of NGOs in order that they may be more effectively used as agents in the PHN sector. Their strengths are their grass-roots understanding and experience of the people and communities in which they are based. Their weaknesses are that they are often small in size, heavily dependent on a few committed individuals, and without the resources to build the administrative structures required to attract and manage large amounts of funding. Since 1985 the Bank has supported the International Planned Parenthood Federation (IPPF) in efforts to strengthen the management capabilities of family planning associations in Africa, and in FY88 this assistance amounted to $300,000. Another grant went to the African Medical and Research Foundation (AMREF) to help it develop its technical capacity and attract donor funding. Other grants are being made to NGOs to encourage their participation in specific initiatives in the PHN field. One of the most important of these is the recent Safe Motherhood Initiative.

THE SAFE MOTHERHOOD INITIATIVE

The Bank played an instrumental role in launching this initiative through the Safe Motherhood Conference held in Nairobi in February 1987. An important driving factor was the realization that despite the effort going into MCH activities, maternal mortality was taking a high toll on women's lives in developing countries, and that little, if any, improvement had been made over the past twenty years, in contrast to the relative success in reducing infant and child mortality. Activities under this initiative comprise operational research, advocacy and lending. Lending for safe motherhood activities in Bank PHN projects is now estimated to be about 30% of project resources. Advocacy is pursued mainly through regional and national safe motherhood workshops supported not only by the Bank but other donors, and organized by Family Care International, a U.S-based NGO. The meetings provide an opportunity for participants from governments and NGOs to examine the levels and causes of maternal mortality and morbidity in their own countries and to begin developing national strategies and action plans to deal with the identified problems. The demand for and success of these workshops has exceeded initial expectations. Over 80 countries have either participated already, or have expressed interest in doing so. Seven regional workshops have already taken place – including one for 22 Francophone African countries in Niger, 1989; one for 13 Arab countries in Jordan, 1988; and one for 4

Portuguese–speaking nations in Brazil, in 1988 – countries in which traditionally it has been difficult to discuss such subjects as family planning and abortion. Support for operational research takes place through funding for the WHO-executed Safe Motherhood Operational Research Fund, to which, at the Nairobi Conference, Bank President Conable pledged $1 million over a 3 year period.

Task Force for Child Survival

This interagency group composed of WHO, UNICEF, UNDP, Rockefeller Foundation and the Bank has been very successful in accelerating child survival efforts, especially in the area of immunization. Immunization coverage of children under two now stands at over 50% in developing countries, up from about 25% when the Task Force was formed in 1984. Mr. Conable and the Senior Population Adviser to the Bank, Dr. Fred Sai, attended the "Bellagio III" meeting of the Task Force held in Talloires, France, in March 1988, and voiced strong support for the work of the Task Force.

The Special Program for Research, Development and Research Training in Human Reproduction (HRP).

This WHO program, originally established in 1972, was reconstituted in 1988, and the World Bank became a co-sponsor, together with UNDP, UNFPA and WHO. The Bank decided to support the program because of concern at the decline in international funding for contraceptive research and development in the 1980s, and the need for finding safer, more effective and more acceptable methods of contraception for use in developing countries. Much of HRP's research and development is conducted by centers established in developing countries, and one-quarter of its budget is devoted to this institutional development effort. The original focus of HRP was on the development and utilization of methods of fertility regulation, but lately the strategy has widened to include other reproductive health issues, including maternal health. The Bank currently contributes $2 million a year to the Program, which represents about 10% of its total funding.

CONCLUSION

This overview of the Bank's work in PHN indicates that its activities are strongly influenced by its role in development in general, and by its institutional character as a development bank. The Bank has access to the highest policy makers in its member countries and is, therefore, in a unique position to influence policy. It is involved in all sectors concerning national development, and better placed than more specialized agencies to encourage development planning that takes into account the needs of the social sectors. In addition, the Bank can complement assistance to family planning and MCH with activities in fields known to increase the demand for such services. Indeed, the Bank strongly believes that in some circumstances its support of education and women in development projects do as much for MCH as direct support. Its experience and expertise enable it to undertake a wide range of activities including projects, policy analysis and formulation, and research. It is impossible to provide dollar figures for the Bank's expenditure for any specified effort in MCH or FP since many PHN investments serve multiple purposes. PHN sector activities are unusually complex in comparison with other development projects. They involve organized efforts to change individual behavior, and a reaching out to the people they wish to help. The Bank has provided a great deal of assistance to countries in building up their health and family planning systems, particularly with respect to construction, equipment, training and management at the central government level. It is now moving toward greater efforts to improve service delivery at the periphery. Family planning and maternal and child health are priority concerns within the Bank's PHN activities, supported not only by country operations, but by efforts to mobilize and coordinate international programs leading to better health for the world's women and children.

REFERENCES

1. World Bank. The McNamara Years at The World Bank – Major Policy Addresses of Robert S. McNamara 1968-81. Baltimore, Johns Hopkins University Press, 1981, p. 12.

2. Clausen, A.W. Population Growth and Economic and Social Development: Addresses. Washington DC: The World Bank, 1984.

3. Conable, B.B.The Safe Motherhood Initiative: Addresses and Proposals for Action, Nairobi, Kenya, February 10, 1987. Washington D.C: The World Bank, 1987.

4. Conable, B.B. Address to the Board of Governors, Berlin, September 27, 1988. Washington DC: The World Bank, 1988, p. 6.

5. Simmons, G., and R. Maru.The World Bank's Population Lending and Sector Review, PPR Working Paper 94, Washington DC: The World Bank, 1988, p. 73.

6. Sai, F.T., and L.A. Chester. The Role of The World Bank in Shaping Third World Population Policy, Ch 11 in Roberts G. (ed). Population Policy: The U.S. and the Third World, New York: Praeger.

7. Barnum, H. Interaction of Infant Mortality and Fertility and the Effectiveness of Health and Family Planning Programs, PPR Working Paper 65. Washington DC: The World Bank, 1988.

8. Heaver, R. Reaching People at the Periphery: Can the World Bank's Population, Health and Nutrition Operations Do Better? PPR Working Paper 81, Washington DC: The World Bank, 1988.

Appendix Table
Features of PHN Projects, FY 81-87

Project	FY	Basic Health Services	Health Facilities De. Level 1	2	3	Family Planning Service	Para-Medical Training	Strengthening Management	Tropical Disease Control	Strengthening Pharmaceuticals	Nutrition	Cost Recovery	IEC	Location Urban	Rural
Tunisia II HP	81	X	X	X		X	X	X	X		X		X	X	X
Brazil I H	82	X	X	X			X	X					X		X
Kenya II P	82	X	X	X		X	X	X		X	X	X	X	X	X
Pakistan II P	83	X		X		X	X	X			X	X	X	X	
Yar I H	83						X	X		X	X	X	X		X
Oeru I PHC	83	X	X			X	X	X	X		X	X	X	X	X
Senegal I Rural H	83	X	X			X	X	X		X	X		X		X
Indonesia prov. H	83	X	X	X			X	X	X	X		X			X
Malawi I H	83	X	X			X	X	X		X		X	X	X	X
Pory I H	83	X	X			X	X	X					X		X
Comoros I HP	84	X	X			X	X	X		X	X	X	X	X	X
Mali I H	84	X	X	X		X	X	X		X	X		X	X	X
Brazil II	84	X	X	X		X	X	X			X		X		X
China I Rural H	84	X	X			X	X	X							X
India III P	84	X	X		X	X	X	X			X	X	X	X	X
Botswana I Fam. H	84	X	X			X	X	X		X	X		X		X
Nigeria I Sokoto H	85	X	X			X	X	X			X		X		X
Lesoiho I HO	85	X	X			X	X	X			X		X		X
Jordan I H	85	X	X	X		X	X	X			X		X	X	X
Indones II H Mpwr	85						X	X							
Morocco I H	85	X	X	X		X	X	X		X	X	X	X		X
Indonesia IV P	85	X	X			X	X	X	X		X	X	X	X	X
Burkina Faso H	85	X	X	X		X	X	X	X	X	X	X	X	X	X
India IV P	86	X	X	X		X	X	X			X	X	X	X	X
Colombia HS Integr	86	X	X			X	X	X			X	X			X
Ivory Coast H Demo	86	X	X			X	X	X			X			X	X
Indonesia N & Comm H	86	X	X			X	X	X			X	X	X		X
Bangladesh P & Fam H	86	X	X	X		X	X	X	X	X	X	X	X	X	X
Chana H & Ed	86	X	X			X	X	X			X	X	X	X	X
Niger H	86	X	X			X	X	X	X	X	X	X	X		X
Rwanda Family H	86	X	X	X		X	X	X			X		X		X
Sierra Leone HP	86	X	X	X		X	X	X		X	X	X	X		X
Brazil NE Basic H	86	X	X	X		X	X	X		X		X			X
China II	86	X	X	X		X	X	X		X		X			X
Zimbabwe Family H	87	X	X	X		X	X	X		X	X	X	X	X	X
Gambia I PH	87	X	X	X		X	X	X		X	X	X	X	X	X
Malawi II HP	87	X	X	X		X	X	X					X	X	X
Jamaica P/H	87	X	X	X		X	X	X			X	X	X		X
Oman M	87	X	X			X	X	X		X	X	X	X		X
Guinea Bissau PHN	87	X	X			X	X	X		X	X	X	X		X

47

THE POPULATION ASSISTANCE PROGRAM OF THE U.S. AGENCY FOR INTERNATIONAL DEVELOPMENT

DUFF G. GILLESPIE, PH.D., AND JUDITH R. SELTZER, PH.D.

PROGRAM OBJECTIVES

The population program of the Agency for International Development (USAID) began in 1965. USAID's population assistance is part of a much larger U.S.-foreign assistance effort to the Third World. Alongside programs in agriculture, education, health, human resources, and energy, the population program is about four to five percent of the total development assistance. While this percentage is small, USAID nevertheless has been, and still is, the single largest donor for population. Almost $3.4 billion has been provided since 1965. About half of this amount has been given since 1980.

The program has three objectives which encompass concerns for human rights, human welfare, and economic development. The three objectives of the population program are to:

1. enhance the freedom of individuals in developing countries to choose voluntarily the number and spacing of their children;
2. improve the health and survival of mothers and children by promoting adequate birthspacing; by encouraging childbearing during the safest years for women; and, by reducing abortions; and
3. encourage population growth consistent with the growth of economic resources and productivity.[1,2]

The underlying principles of U.S. population assistance are voluntarism and informed choice. Population assistance is not conditional; rather the assistance is provided to those developing countries that request it. In 1988, the program provided assistance for population activities in about 90 countries.

The population program supports activities in two broad areas: family planning service delivery (about 75 percent of total funding) and research designed to improve family planning technology. Service delivery areas supported by USAID include:

- policy dialogue in developing countries that can legitimize and promote family planning programs in both the public and private sectors;
- support of voluntary family planning programs, including a range of strategies for service delivery (e.g., clinic-based, subsidized commercial marketing, and community-based distribution);
- training of program personnel in reproductive health and fertility management;
- assistance in population and contraceptive information, education, and communication; and
- provision of contraceptive supplies (including oral contraceptives, IUDs, condoms).

A.I.D.'s research effort includes:

- biomedical research on safer, less expensive and more acceptable and effective methods of contraception;
- operations research to improve the management and operation of service delivery programs; and
- social science and demographic research to increase knowledge of the social (including health) and economic consequences of population change and to improve information on population dynamics and contraceptive use trends.[3]

ORGANIZATION OF ASSISTANCE

USAID is a mission-oriented agency with overseas Missions or representation in 69 countries and 13 regional development offices. Population assistance is provided through USAID Missions (under bilateral or country-to-country projects) monitored by the overseas USAID Mission staff; through regional projects monitored by the three Regional Bureaus (Africa, Asia/Near East, and Latin American/Caribbean); and by the Bureau for Science and Technology's Office of Population through centrally-funded projects.

The allocation of resources under the Agency's population account is:

- Bilateral programs, accounting for about 40 percent of population assistance, are carried out by USAID Missions in 32 countries.

- Office of Population accounts for 47 percent of the assistance. The assistance is provided through grant agreements and contracts (47 in 1988) with U.S. government and private agencies. The projects are developed by the Office of Population and carried out by these various organizations and are designed to complement USAID Mission programs. The projects support activities that are not readily included in the USAID bilateral programs. In countries that do not receive bilateral assistance, these projects are the primary, and in some cases, the only source of population support. In 1988, the Office of Population funded over 1,400 projects in about 90 countries.
- Regional population assistance programs account for about 11 percent of assistance.
- The remaining two percent supports special Agency initiatives in the population field.

FUNDING TRENDS

Congress appropriates funds for population assistance under the Population Planning Section of the Foreign Assistance Act. Funding has totalled nearly $3.4 billion over the last twenty-three years; $1.9 billion has been obligated since 1981. In 1988, the population budget amounted to $232 million. A reduction in population funds since 1985 largely reflects budgetary constraints throughout the Federal government. (See Table 1, next page, for a summary of USAID funding for 1965-1988).

PROGRAM INNOVATIONS

USAID's population assistance can be described in terms of a number of innovative program endeavors which have benefited the population programs in developing countries. Seven in particular are reviewed briefly.[4]

1. Fertility and contraceptive prevalence surveys have been essential for documenting the need for family planning and the effectiveness of service delivery efforts. Between 1974 and 1988, surveys have been conducted in 69 developing countries. This is clearly the largest social science effort ever undertaken.

2. Improved contraceptive methods have greatly enhanced the safety, effectiveness and acceptability of methods in developing countries. Several methods which have been greatly improved are female sterilization, copper IUDs, and low-dose oral contracep-

tives. In addition, a subdermal contraceptive implant (Norplant®) is being evaluated in clinical trials.

3. An operations research program has supported pilot and experimental projects and has been critical in demonstrating that family planning services are wanted and that they can be delivered efficiently in a variety of settings. This research has found that services can be effectively provided through a variety of delivery modalities including clinics, community-based and household distribution, and pharmacies.

Table 1
Summary of A.I.D. Population Assistance
1965-1988 (in $000,000)

	1965-1975	1976-1985	1986	1987	1988	Total
Office of Population	259.7	942.3	133.5	115.0	111.0	1561.5
Regional Programs						
Africa	35.0	74.7	26.1	33.8	36.9[b]	206.5
Asia	172.8	469.8	46.8	52.7	58.9[c]	860.6
Near East	21.2	38.4	0.0	0.0	0.0	0.0
Latin Amer/ Carib	92.2	108.0	30.2	24.6	22.1	277.1
UNFPA Support	97.0	315.9	0.0	0.0	0.0	412.9
All Other	41.7	12.3	0.9	4.4	4.6	63.9
Grand Total	719.6	1961.4	237.5	230.5[a]	233.5[d]	3382.5

Note: During 1985, the previously separate Asia and Near East regions of A.I.D. were combined into a single Asia/Near East (ANE) region. Prior to 1986, the funding levels reflect the previous division of program responsibilities.

[a] Excludes reprogrammed prior year deobligations.
[b] Development Fund for Africa
[c] Includes $8 million for Afghanistan
[d] Includes funds from Population Account and Development Fund for Africa

Source: U.S. Agency for International Development, Users Guide to the Office of Population, 1989.

4. Community-based distribution programs are a particularly effective means of outreach and have increased use of contraceptive prevalence at less cost than clinic-based delivery would have been. For example, outside Khartoum in the Sudan, contraceptive prevalence rose from 10.6 percent in 1980 to 33.5 percent by 1987 when village midwives provided family planning. In Muslim areas of southern Thailand, contraceptive prevalence increased from 12 to 39 percent after one year in which field workers were employed to sell pills and condoms.

5. A concerted effort to engage the private sector in developing countries has shown that the private sector (both for-profit and PVO) can be an effective channel for expanding access to family planning. While the non-profit private sector has pioneered the delivery of services in many countries, the for-profit sector is playing a growing role in countries as diverse as Egypt, Peru and Zimbabwe through commercial marketing of contraceptives and employee-based health insurance programs.

6. The Contraceptive Social Marketing project is one example of a successful private for-profit initiative. This project uses marketing and advertising techniques to increase the availability of services through commercial channels. In Mexico, a social marketing project was started with a government-subsidized chain of 17,000 grocery stores to make low-cost condoms available to low income groups. Sales in the first year of this project yielded $100,000 in revenue which is being used to purchase additional advertising.

7. A population communications project capitalizes on the commercial private sector to reach millions of couples with strong family planning messages for a fraction of the cost of the actual mass media time used. One example is an experimental rock video and hit song with a family planning message for young adults, performed by rock stars, Titiana and Johnny in Mexico. This experiment was successfully replicated in Nigeria and the Philippines by other rock stars.

PROGRAM IMPACT

Substantial declines in fertility have occurred in several regions of the world. Between the early 1960s and the early 1980s, fertility decreased by over

50 percent in East Asia (principally China) and by 25-30 percent in South Asia and Latin America. For the African continent, fertility declined by less than five percent. Most of this change occurred in North Africa since fertility in many African countries remained the same or increased somewhat.[5] Vigorous family planning programs in combination with social and economic development efforts have been credited with bringing about dramatic declines in fertility.[6] A number of countries which have experienced dramatic reductions in their birth rates have also benefited from substantial USAID population assistance. (See Table 2, next page). Two such countries are Thailand and Indonesia. Survey data show that in Thailand, average completed family size dropped from about 6.3 children to 2.3 between 1965 and 1987. In Indonesia, the average completed family size declined from 5.6 to 3.4 children over the same period.[7,8,9]

FUTURE NEEDS

Estimates of the future demand for family planning indicate that formidable challenges lie ahead.[10] Not only is the level of contraceptive prevalence likely to increase, but the number of potential users will increase dramatically simply due to growing populations. The cost and effort to provide services to the increasing number of potential users over the next twenty years will be enormous. The annual estimate for the year 2010 is between $9 and $10 billion. This estimate is three to four times the amount of resources currently being invested in family planning.

Given that donor funding for population has leveled off or even declined in terms of constant dollars, where will the additional resources come from to meet needs?

Greater emphasis is being placed on stimulating investments by developing-country governments and the private sector. USAID is concentrating much of its funding on activities which are highly leveraged, that is, which have a multiplier effect.

Among such efforts are encouraging policy reforms and increasing the availability of more effective and inexpensive contraceptives. Finally USAID population assistance is improving the efficiency of programs, for example, by training their program managers to improve their management skills and logistics management.

Table 2
Twenty Most Populous Developing Countries:
Changes in Crude Birth Rates, 1965-1988

Country	1988 Population (Million)	Crude Birth Rate 1965	Crude Birth Rate 1988	Percent Change
1. China	1.087	33	21	-34.4
2. India	817	43	33	-23.3
3. Indonesia	177	45	27	-40.0
4. Brazil	144	40	28	-30.0
5. Nigeria	112	51	46	-9.8
6. Bangladesh	110	50	43	-14.0
7. Pakistan	108	47	43	-8.5
8 Mexico	84	44	30	-31.8
9 Vietnam	65	42	34	-19.0
10. Philippines	63	42	35	-16.7
11. Thailand	55	43	29	-32.6
12. Egypt	53	42	38	-9.5
13. Turkey	53	40	31	-22.5
14. Iran	52	46	45	- 2.2
15. Ethiopia	48	50	46	- 8.0
16. S. Korea	43	36	19	-47.2
17. Burma	41	41	34	-17.1
18. Zaire	33	48	45	- 6.3
19 Colombia	31	42	28	-33.3
20 Morocco	25	50	36	-28.0
Total Developing Country Listed	3,201	40	31	-22.5
Total Developing Countries	3.931	40	32	-20.0
Total World	5.128	35	28	-20.0

*/ Countries receiving significant amount of A.I.D. population assistance during 1965 - 1988 are underlined.

Source: Population Reference Bureau, 1988

REFERENCES

1. U.S. Agency for International Development: Bureau for Program and Policy Coordination. A.I.D. Policy Paper: Population Assistance. Washington DC: USAID, Sept 1982.

2. Gillespie, D.G. International Population: The Continuing Challenge. Paper presented at the 29th Air Force Academy Assembly. March 1987.

3. U.S. Agency for International Development. User's Guide to the Office of Population. Washington DC: USAID, 1989.

4. Dumm, J.J. Twenty Years of A.I.D.'s Experience in Population. Paper presented at the Colloquium on International Population Assistance in the 1990s. April 1988.

5. Merrick, T.W. World Population in Transition. Pop Bull 41:2, April 1986.

6. Lapham, R.J., and W.P. Mauldin. Family planning program effort and birthrate decline in developing countries. Int Fam Planning Persp 10: 4, 1984, pp. 109-118.

7. Knodel, J., A. Chamratrithirong, and N. Devavalya. Thailand's Reproductive Revolution: Rapid Fertility Decline in a Third-World Setting. Madison WI: University of Wisconsin Press, 1987.

8. Chayovan, N., P. Kamnvansilpa, and J. Knodel. Thailand Demographic and Health Survey, Columbia, MD: Institute for Resource Development, Westinghouse, May 1983.

9. Central Bureau of Statistics, National Family Planning Coordinating Board, and Demographic and Health Surveys: National Indonesia Contraceptive Prevalence Survey 1987. Preliminary Report. Columbia, MD: Institute for Resources Development, Westinghouse, April 1988.

10. Gillespie, D.G., H.E. Cross, and J.G. Crowley, et al. Financing the Delivery of Contraceptives: The Challenge of the Next Twenty Years. Paper presented at the Conference on the Demographic and Programmatic Consequences of Contraceptive Innovations. National Academy of Sciences, Oct 1988.

11. Population Reference Bureau: 1988 World Population Data Sheet. Washington DC, 1988.

48

THE UNITED STATES AGENCY FOR INTERNATIONAL DEVELOPMENT'S CHILD SURVIVAL PROGRAM

PAMELA R. JOHNSON, PH.D., AND KENNETH J. BART, M.D., M.P.H.

INTRODUCTION

For millions of children in the developing world, good health remains an elusive goal. The major obstacles are readily apparent: diarrheal diseases; vaccine-preventable diseases such as measles, polio and neonatal tetanus; malaria and acute respiratory infections. Less obvious, but also significant as contributing to death, is malnutrition. Underlying these is the spectrum of social and economic factors that work against a child's well-being. Poverty, illiteracy and demographic factors such as the spacing and number of births also contribute to illness and death among developing world infants and children.[1] (Table 1, next page)

Long concerned with health in the developing world, since fiscal year 1985 the United States Agency for International Development (USAID) has accelerated its efforts to bring about declines in infant and child mortality in the developing countries it assists. Since that date, USAID has committed more than $600 million to child survival programs in more than 60 countries in a global effort carried out in cooperation with developing countries as well as the World Health Organization, United Nations Children's Fund (UNICEF), private voluntary organizations, educational and other institutions.

The child survival program is part of USAID's overall strategy for economic growth and development of its broader program of foreign assistance.[2] The Agency, first established in 1961 within the State Department, administers a foreign assistance program in 90 countries with an annual overall budget of $6 billion. Of this, approximately $300 million annually is directed to health assistance including child survival and AIDS activities. The foreign assistance program has multiple objectives, including humanitarian assistance for the poor and victims of natural disasters, and the fostering of economic growth and development and support for U.S. foreign policy objectives. USAID also shares responsibilities with the State Department and other federal agencies for such programs as Food Aid. USAID assistance usually takes the form of government-to-government agreements in which U.S. dollars are paired with host country resources in both cash and kind. Such bilateral programs are complemented by the activities of private voluntary organizations and by the efforts of other donors and organizations. To focus and coordinate efforts, staff in USAID field missions work with local counterparts to develop country-specific approaches within the framework of USAID's overall policies and strategies and reflecting the country's own needs and plans.

USAID'S HEALTH PROGRAM

The overall goal of USAID's health assistance program is to improve health status in assisted countries as reflected in increased life expectancy.[3] Most health problems in developing countries stem from infectious and para-

---

Table 1
The Burden of Mortality
A Comparison Between the Developed and Developing Worlds

	More Developed Countries	Less Developed Countries
Infant Mortality Rate	15/1,000	96/1,000
Child Mortality Rate	3/1,000	44/1,000
Maternal Deaths (per 100,000 live births)	30/100,000	550/100,000
GNP/Per Capita	$10,700	$780

Sources:
1. 1988 World Population Data Sheet of the Population Reference Bureau, Inc.
2. Mortality of Children Under Age 5: World Estimates and Projections, 1950-2025, United Nations, New York, 1988.
3. Population Reports, Series L, Number 7, Sept., 1988
4. Royston, Erica & Lopez, Alan D., "On the Assessment of Maternal Mortality", World Health Statistics Quarterly, 40 (1987)

sitic diseases, poor environmental conditions, lack of health care and knowledge, and malnutrition. Hundreds of millions of adults suffer from diseases unknown in temperate climates, but children are most likely to die from severe episodes of childhood diseases that today are virtually only known as minor illnesses or from diseases no longer considered public health problems in the developed world (Figure 1, next page). Fourteen million children under five die each year, most from potentially preventable causes. In addition, world-wide, more than half a million women die each year from causes associated with pregnancy and childbirth, a substantial proportion of which are also potentially preventable with known technologies.

Because of this, USAID's approach to increasing life expectancy and general health status in developing countries gives priority to the health problems of children and their mothers. The primary objectives of the Agency's health sector policy are to:

- reduce infant and early childhood mortality by increasing immunization coverage, reducing diarrheal disease mortality, improving nutrition in young children, and improving birth spacing and maternal health;
- reduce maternal mortality and morbidity;
- use child survival interventions as the basis for building a more comprehensive health care system which, over time, will ensure that gains made in improving child survival and health are sustained; and
- develop new technologies and improved delivery systems.

In keeping with the Agency's health policy, nearly 60 percent of all funds supporting health activities are used for child survival. In addition, the Agency's priorities in the sector are to prevent and control AIDS, improve health care financing, contribute to the greater availability of water supply and sanitation, develop improved technologies for priority health needs such as vaccines for malaria and other disease of childhood, improve maternal health care, and address uniquely tropical diseases, especially the resurgence of malaria and other vector-borne disease.

THE CHILD SURVIVAL PROGRAM

USAID's child survival strategy[4] is based on an understanding of the causes of death for infants and children in the developing world. More than half die from measles, neonatal tetanus, pertussis, and from causes associated with diarrheal disease. Others die from severe respiratory infections or malaria. Not usually cited as the primary cause of death, malnutrition is often an important contributing factor. As many as 60 percent of child deaths are due

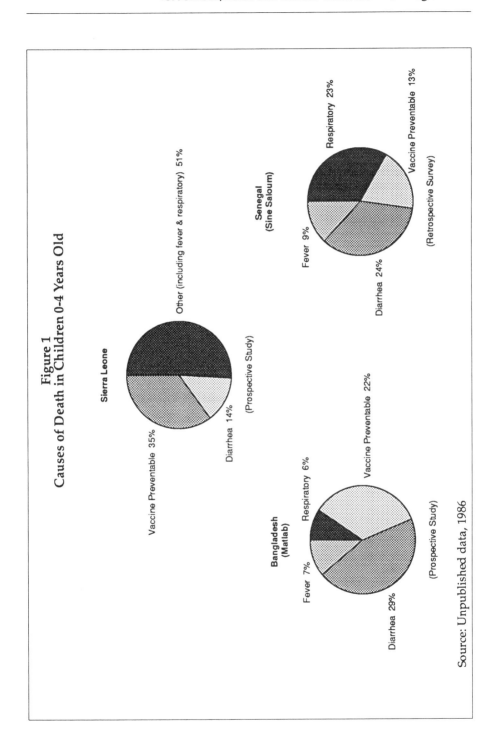

Figure 1
Causes of Death in Children 0-4 Years Old

Sierra Leone

Other (including fever & respiratory) 51%

Vaccine Preventable 35%

Diarrhea 14%

(Prospective Study)

**Senegal
(Sine Saloum)**

Respiratory 23%

Vaccine Preventable 13%

Fever 9%

Diarrhea 24%

(Retrospective Survey)

**Bangladesh
(Matlab)**

Respiratory 6%

Vaccine Preventable 22%

Fever 7%

Diarrhea 29%

(Prospective Study)

Source: Unpublished data, 1986

in part to the mortality of children made frail by malnutrition to respond adequately to the worst effects of illness. In many of those cases, the vicious circle – illness leading to poor nutrition resulting in additional illness – is the true cause of death.[5] In addition, behind a child's death there is often the unseen story that he or she was at increased risk from birth. Children who weigh less than 2500 grams at birth or who are born too soon after a sibling, for example, are more likely to die in their first year of life.[6] (Figure 2)

There is a range of views as how best to interrupt this tragic cycle of disease and malnutrition. It is argued that a broad range of problems should be addressed simultaneously to assure a lasting impact while others see single-purpose, focused programs as opportunity for rapid mortality reduction.

USAID's strategy recognizes merit in both points of view. At the core of the USAID strategy is the concentration of its resources on a few effective and affordable technologies directed at the leading causes of death, not only to bring about rapid and visible reductions in child mortality but also to serve as the foundation of the extension of the health services.

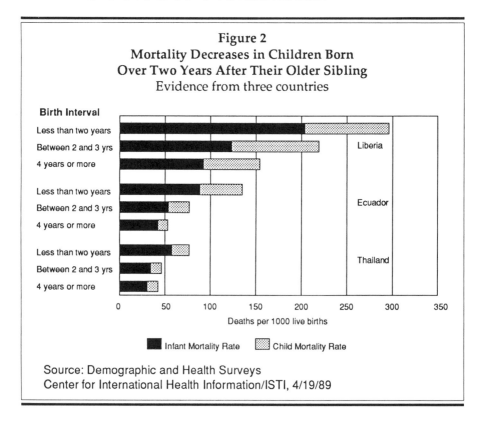

Figure 2
Mortality Decreases in Children Born
Over Two Years After Their Older Sibling
Evidence from three countries

Source: Demographic and Health Surveys
Center for International Health Information/ISTI, 4/19/89

The strategy calls for a principal focus on two technologies known to prevent the leading causes of death as the core of the child survival initiative: the management of acute dehydrating diarrheal disease, principally through oral rehydration therapy (ORT), and good feeding practices (breast feeding and/or feeding during diarrhea and post-diarrheal supplementation); and the prevention by immunization of six diseases of childhood. Building on the foundation of these interventions, USAID seeks to catalyze sustained improvements in the health and survival of children in the developing world and to help build strong, broad-based health systems that can deliver a range of essential services over time. The strategy also recognizes the importance of underlying causes of mortality and addresses reduction of high-risk births and improved nutrition practices.

USAID has chosen to give special emphasis to 22 countries which, together, account for two-thirds of the mortality in developing countries (excluding China). Figure 3 shows the distribution of fiscal year 1988 child survival resources among various child survival activities including diarrheal

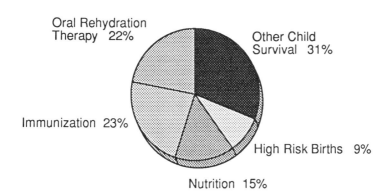

Figure 3
USAID Funding for Child Survival
Fiscal Year 1988

Total funding $169,868,000

Funding by Intervention

Oral Rehydration Therapy 22%

Other Child Survival 31%

Immunization 23%

High Risk Births 9%

Nutrition 15%

Source: USAID Health Information System CIHI, February 1989

disease management, immunization, the promotion of breast feeding, and promotion of spacing births to benefit the health of both mothers and children. (The Agency separately provides substantial support for family planning through its population program and also additional and separate resources for food and nutrition.) The remainder of child survival resources is directed at acute respiratory infections, malaria and other related activities.

On a country level, programs are developed in collaboration with and in support of host country programs. Thus, each country program is somewhat different. In Nepal, there is special attention to acute respiratory infections. In most African countries, malaria is given higher priority. In Latin America and the Caribbean, countries are building on a strong base to accelerate immunization efforts, especially those to eradicate polio, with a view to being the first region in the world to eliminate a major disease since smallpox.[8] And in Egypt, where oral rehydration therapy and immunization are broadly used, increasing attention is now being given to solidifying the financial basis to sustain high levels of performance in the future.

The involvement of the private sector is also an explicit goal of USAID's child survival strategy. USAID has fostered activities to stimulate the participation of the private sector – both voluntary and for-profit – to expand the availability of services and to generate additional revenues and energies. Private voluntary organizations (PVOs) from the United States and from developing countries themselves, have demonstrated remarkable resourcefulness in reaching some of the poorest and most remote populations with much needed services. Through a USAID-funded competitive grants program begun in 1985, 21 U.S. PVOs have received 67 grants to work in 20 countries. Bilateral programs have called upon U.S. PVOs, such as Save the Children in Haiti and CARE in India, and local groups, such as Eglise du Christ in Zaire. Overall, in fiscal year 1988, USAID provided $22 million to U.S. PVOs for child survival efforts as well as substantial additional funds for indigenous PVOs.

The priorities that have been established in USAID's child survival strategy reflect judgments as to both the most urgent problems as well as the most effective technologies for attacking those problems. Child survival programs will evolve, in part in response to the changing environment, in part because the technologies and approaches of the programs themselves will evolve. Success will also play a role in future priorities; as mortality is reduced from diarrheal and vaccine-preventable diseases, other causes of death will require attention. Investments in research and evaluation, while only a small part of USAID's overall program, will help design future programs in ways that benefit from the experience of the past and the technologies of the future.

IMPROVING TECHNOLOGY

Technology choice is one of the key factors affecting the sustainability of projects. A sound technology is one that works, and is affordable and accepted by the people for whom it is intended. The child survival technologies of the USAID program have been selected with these criteria in mind. Vaccination, if done properly, works and is far less expensive than the treatment of the diseases it prevents. ORT itself grew out of a recognition that the existing technology – intravenous therapy – was too costly and impractical to cope with the magnitude of diarrheal disease in the developing world.

But good technologies are put to hard tests in child survival programs. Vaccine temperatures must be measured accurately by illiterate mothers and used in adequate quantities. Scales used in growth monitoring programs must stand up to hard use. The cost of these technologies, even though measured in pennies, is still too high for some of the poorest countries of the world to afford in the volume that is needed.

Therefore, efforts to improve, adapt and lower the cost of basic technologies are part of USAID's overall program. For example, USAID is testing a temperature marker on measles vaccine vials. It is anticipated that such a tool will enable Ministries of Health to identify breaks in the cold chain, reduce vaccine wastage and give health workers at the periphery confidence that the vaccine they are injecting is potent.

USAID is working to develop and test new and improved vaccines. In the next decade, vaccines are expected to be available that will be easier to deliver, require fewer doses, cause fewer side effects and be more stable at higher temperatures. One example that is likely to affect programs in the near term is the use of new strains of measles vaccines. Because the current measles vaccine is not immunogenic in the presence of maternal antibodies, it cannot be used early enough in life to prevent many fatalities. Therefore, earlier immunization could reduce mortality among children six to nine months of age, a problem of major proportions in areas, especially in Africa, where measles is hyperendemic. USAID has supported research on alternative measles vaccines which may be administered as early as six months of age.[9]

Malaria is again growing as a problem of major health and economic dimensions in the developing world, especially in Africa. An estimated one million malaria deaths occur in Africa each year, and the most vulnerable are young, malnourished children and pregnant women. USAID in 1966 began the search for a malaria vaccine. Today USAID is supporting a network of institutions working on various aspects of vaccine development.

While vaccines remain one of the most effective preventive strategies, USAID-supported research is also developing and testing other approaches. Proper breast feeding is the rare intervention that has benefits across health, population and nutrition factors. Current research being supported by USAID is helping to define patterns that are optimal to achieve the fullest range of health, nutritional and contraceptive benefits. Studies of the impact of diarrheal diseases are expected to lead to treatment regimens that will both rehydrate and prevent nutritional depletion. Rice-based oral rehydration solutions are being investigated to provide much-needed calories during diarrhea episodes and also reduce stool output – a frequent complaint of mothers and a common reason for discontinuing ORT. Fortification of MSG with Vitamin A is being tested as an effective low-cost solution to vitamin A deficiency in countries where a single manufactured food is widely consumed by rich and poor alike. The role of vitamin A in reducing overall morbidity and mortality is being intensively investigated in several field studies supported by USAID.

OVERVIEW

Although progress has been slower in some countries, the increased availability of critical health services combined with improvement in socioeconomic conditions in the developing world is resulting in decline in infant and child mortality. Infant and child mortality will continue to decline if current trends are sustained. In the past few decades, the decline has been rapid in most of Asia, the Near East and Latin America and the Caribbean. In contrast, mortality has declined very slowly in most of Africa and parts of southeast Asia. However, even at the turn of the century, nearly half of all deaths in Africa are expected to be children under five years.[10] (Figure 4, next 3 pages)

USAID's child survival program is making an important contribution. With its emphasis on the major causes of infant and child death, and building to USAID's commitment on health in the developing world, the program has contributed to making a clear and measurable impact on the health and well-being of the world's children. The number of children dying remains unacceptably high. Nevertheless, in many countries, the prospects for survival for a child born today are clearly better than those born just five years ago.

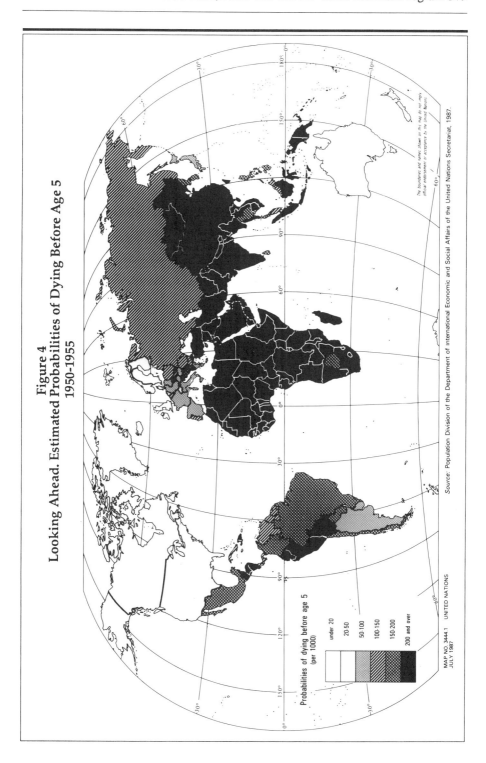

Figure 4
Looking Ahead. Estimated Probabilities of Dying Before Age 5
1950-1955

Probabilities of dying before age 5
(per 1000)

under 20
20-50
50-100
100-150
150-200
200 and over

Source: Population Division of the Department of International Economic and Social Affairs of the United Nations Secretariat, 1987.

MAP NO. 3444.1   UNITED NATIONS
JULY 1987

The boundaries and names shown on this map do not imply official endorsement or acceptance by the United Nations.

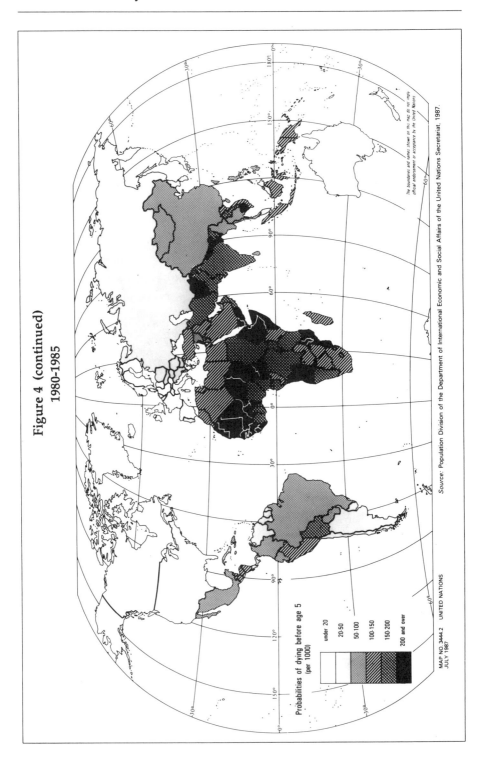

Figure 4 (continued)
1980–1985

Probabilities of dying before age 5
(per 1000)

under 20
20-50
50-100
100-150
150-200
200 and over

MAP NO. 3444.2   UNITED NATIONS
JULY 1987

Source: Population Division of the Department of International Economic and Social Affairs of the United Nations Secretariat, 1987.

The boundaries and names shown on this map do not imply official endorsement or acceptance by the United Nations.

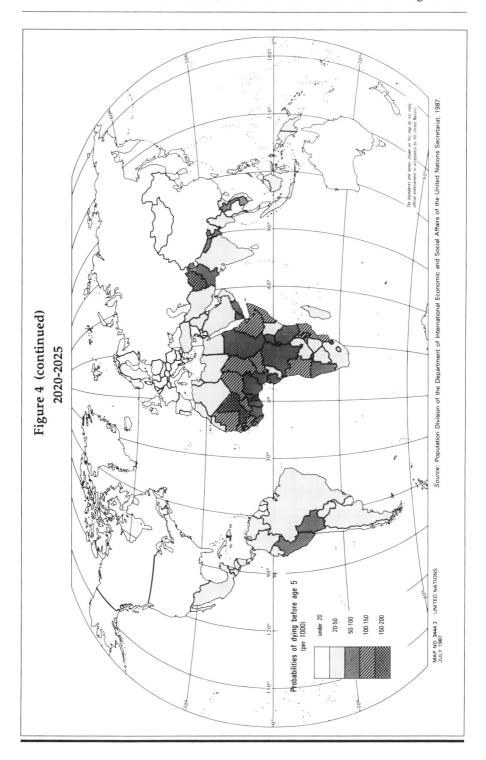

Figure 4 (continued)
2020-2025

Probabilities of dying before age 5
(per 1000)

under 20
20-50
50-100
100-150
150-200

MAP NO. 3444.3   UNITED NATIONS
JULY 1987

Source: Population Division of the Department of International Economic and Social Affairs of the United Nations Secretariat, 1987.

The boundaries and names shown on this map do not imply official endorsement or acceptance by the United Nations.

REFERENCES

1. The World Bank. World Development Report 1988. Washington DC: 1988.

2. U.S. Agency for International Development. Blueprint for Development. Washington DC, 1984.

3. U.S. Agency for International Development. AID Policy Paper: Health Assistance Revised. Washington DC, Dec 1987.

4. U.S. Agency for International Development. Child Survival Strategy. Washington DC, April 1986.

5. Scrimshaw, N.S. Interactions of malnutrition and infection: advances in understanding. In Protein-calorie Malnutrition. R.E. Olson (ed). New York: Academic Press, 1975.

6. Galway, K., B. Wolff, and R. Sturgis. Child survival: Risks and the road to health. Columbia, MD: Institute for Resource Development, Westinghouse. March 1987.

7. Walsh, J., and K.S. Warren. Strategies for Primary Health Care. Chicago: University of Chicago Press, 1986.

8. Hinman, A.R., W.H. Foege, and C.A. de Quadros, et al. The case for global eradication of poliomyelitis. Bull WHO, 65 (6): 835-840 (1987).

9. Markowitz, L.E., and R. Bernier. Immunization of young infants with Edmonston-Zagreb measles vaccine. Ped Inf Dis J 6:809-812, 1987.

10. United Nations. Mortality of children under age 5. Department of International Economic and Social Affairs. Population Studies no. 105. New York: UN, 1988.

Appendix

DEFINITIONS

Birgitta Bucht, Fil. KAND (M.A.)

1. **Live birth**   Live birth is the complete expulsion or extraction from its mother of a product of conception, irrespective of the duration of the pregnancy, which, after such separation, breathes or shows any other evidence of life, such as beating of the heart, pulsation of the umbilical cord, or definite movement of voluntary muscles, whether or not the umbilical cord has been cut or the placenta is attached; each product of such a birth is considered live-born.

2. **Crude birth rate**   Number of live births in a population during a specified period divided by the number of person-years lived by the population during the same period. It is frequently expressed as births per 1,000 population. The crude birth rate for a single year is usually calculated as the number of births during the year divided by the mid-year population.

3. **Age-specific birth rate**   Number of live births during a specified period to women of a specified age or age group, divided by the number of person-years lived during that period by women of that age or age group. When an age-specific fertility rate is calculated for a calendar year, the number of births to women of the specific age is usually divided by the mid-year population of women that age.

4. **Reproductive age**   The ages at which women are able to conceive. The reproductive age span is usually set to range between exact ages of 15 and 50 (that is, 15-49 in completed years).

5. **General fertility rate**   Ratio of the number of live births in a period to the number of person-years lived by women of reproductive age during the period. The general fertility rate for a year is usually calculated as the number of births divided by the number of women of reproductive age at mid-year.

585

6. **Crude death rate** Numbers of deaths in a population during a specified period divided by the number of person-years lived by the population during the same period. It is frequently expressed as deaths per 1,000 population. The crude death rate for a single year is usually calculated as the number of deaths during the year divided by the mid-year population.

7. **Infant** An infant is a child who has not yet reached its first birthday.

8. **Infant death** An infant death is the death of a live-born child who has not yet reached its first birthday.

9. **Infant mortality rate** The infant mortality rate is a measure of the risk of dying between birth and exact age one, i.e., the probability of dying between birth and exact age one ($_1q_0$ in life table notation). It is expressed in terms of number of deaths of children under age one per 1,000 live births.

10. **Neonatal** The term neonatal refers to a period of four weeks or 28 days after birth.

11. **Neonatal death** A neonatal death is the death of a live-born child who is less than 28 days old.

12. **Neonatal mortality rate** The ratio of neonatal deaths during a given period to the number of live births during the same period.

13. **Post-neonatal** The term post-neonatal refers to a period between 28 days and one year after birth.

14. **Post-neonatal death** A post-neonatal death is the death of a child who is between 28 days and one year old.

15. **Post-neonatal mortality rate** The ratio of post-neonatal deaths in a given period to the number of live births during the same period.

16. **Fetal death** Fetal death is death prior to the complete expulsion or extraction from its mother of a product of conception, irrespective of the duration of pregnancy; the death is indicated by the fact that after such separation the fetus does not breathe or show any other evidence of life, such as beating of the heart, pulsation of the umbilical cord, or definite movement of voluntary muscles.

17. **Perinatal** The term perinatal refers to a period between the 28th week of pregnancy and the end of the first week after birth.

18. **Perinatal mortality rate** Perinatal deaths include late fetal deaths (fetal deaths of 28 or more weeks of gestation) and deaths of infants less than

one week old. The perinatal mortality rate is the ratio of perinatal deaths in a given period to live births during the same period.

19. **Low birth weight** A live-born infant with a birth weight of less than 2,500 grams (5 1/2 lbs) is said to have low birth weight.

20. **Maternal death** A maternal death is defined as the death of a woman while pregnant or within 42 days of delivery or termination of pregnancy, irrespective of the duration or the site of the pregnancy, from any cause related to or aggravated by the pregnancy or its management but not from accidental or incidental causes.

21. **Maternal mortality rate** Number of maternal deaths in a given period divided by the number of live births during the same period. The maternal mortality rate is usually expressed per 100,000 live births.

22. **Child mortality rate** Number of deaths occurring in a given period to children between ages 1 and 5, divided by the number of person-years lived during the same period by children between ages 1 and 5. When a child mortality rate is calculated for a calendar year, the number of deaths of children between age 1 and 5 is divided by the mid-year population of children the same age.

23. **Under-five mortality** Under-five mortality is a measure of the risk of dying between birth and exact age 5, i.e., the probability of dying between birth and exact age 5 ($_5q_0$ in life table notation). It is expressed as deaths of children under age 5 per 1,000 live births.

REFERENCES

1. World Health Organization, Manual of the International Statistical Classification of Diseases, Injuries, and Causes of Death, Ninth Rev, 1975. Adopted by the Twenty-ninth World Health Assembly. Volume 1. Geneva: WHO,1977, pp. 763-764.

2. Van de Walle, E. (ed). Multilingual Demographic Dictionary. International Union for the Scientific Study of Population. Liege: Ordina Editions, 1982, pp. 59-60.

3. United Nations. Manual X: Indirect Techniques for Demographic Estimation. United Nations publication, Sales no. E.83.XII.2, 1983, p. 302.

AUTHORS' INDEX

SUBJECT INDEX

A

Abortion: 215, 512
  adolescent, induced, 457, 497
  spontaneous, 179, 184
  unsafe/illegal, 170, 199, 221, 457
Abuse: alcohol, 459, 476
  sexual, 459
  substance, 313
Accidents: and injuries, 428-439, 456, 461
  common (table), 431
  morbidity, 435
  mortality, 312, 435
  prevention, 436-439, 444
  traffic, 431, 434
Acquired immunodeficiency syndrome
    (AIDS): and drug abuse, 460
  diagnosing, 73
  in adolescents, 458
  in mother and child, 68-78, 373
  Pattern I, II, III countries, 69
  pediatric diagnosis, 74
Acute respiratory infections (ARI):
    86, 123, 285, 306, 349-360, 372
  ARI control program, 354
  as cause of child death, 366
  classification, 349, 356, 357
  prevention, 359
  rates, 349
  therapy, 354
Adolescence, 253
  defined, 453, 454, 470, 491
  health and nutrition status of girls
    during, 257
Adolescent: behavior and health, 456, 491
  contraceptive use, 494, 498
  fertility, 470-474
  health, 265, 453-468
    principles of intervention for, 467
  health needs, 421, 454
  health problems, 454
  health promotion, 463
  mortality, 301, 312
  obstetric risk, 496
  pregnancy, 255, 495
  sexual behavior, 457, 491-493
  sexual maturation in, 470, 491

Age-specific birth rate, defined, 585
Agency for International Development
    (US). See USAID.
AIDS. See Acquired immunodeficiency
    syndrome.
Alcohol use in adolescents, 459, 476
  See also Intrauterine growth
    retardation.
Alma-Ata conference (WHO), 80, 97, 103,
    115, 239, 532
  recommendations, xviii
Anemia, iron deficiency. See Nutritional
    deficiency.
Antenatal care. See Prenatal care.
ARI. See Acute respiratory infections.
Arm circumference: as surrogate for
    birthweight, 121
  to diagnose malnutrition, 124

B

Bacterial ARIs (table), 351
Bamako initiative, 369, 537
Birth control methods. See
    Contraceptive(s).
Birth spacing. See Child spacing.
Births, world distribution of (figure), 29
Bites, animal, 433
Breastfeeding, 12, 257, 321-324, 369, 397
  and child health, 522
  and fertility, 323, 513
  and HIV infection, 76
  duration of, 6, 322
  early, 122
  to reduce ARI morbidity, 360
  to reduce mortality, 7, 123, 286, 330,
    360, 366
  See also Weaning.
Bronchiolitis (ARI), 351, 352
Burn injuries, 431

C

Campylobacteriosis, 329-330
Child care, as social benefit, 50
Child Care Standard Act (NYC), Model,
    408

Y